MEDICAL CONSEQUENCES OF NUCLEAR WARFARE

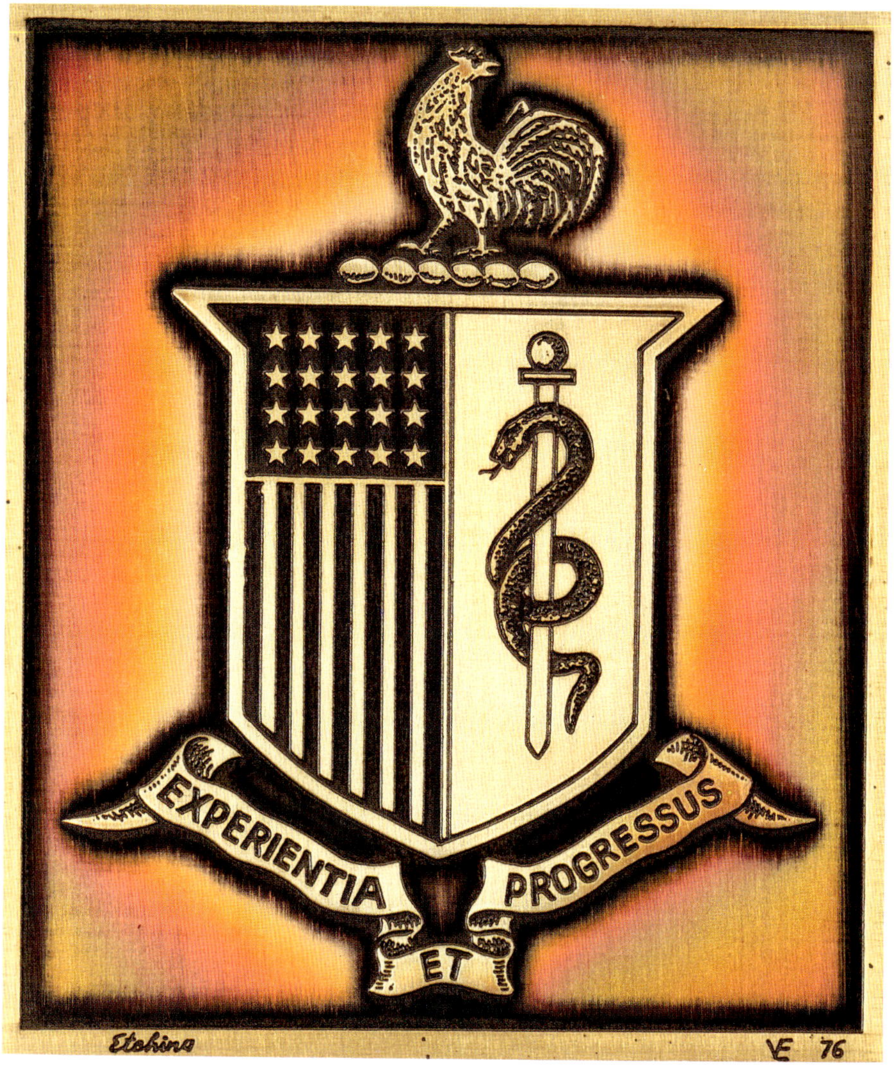

The Coat of Arms
1818
Medical Department of the Army

A 1976 etching by Vassil Ekimov of an original color print that appeared in *The Military Surgeon*, Vol. XLI, No. 2, 1917

The first line of medical defense in wartime is the combat medic. Although in ancient times medics carried the *caduceus* into battle to signify the neutral, humanitarian nature of their tasks, they have never been immune to the perils of war. They have made the highest sacrifices to save the lives of others, and their dedication to the wounded soldier is the foundation of military medical care.

Textbook of Military Medicine

SERIES ON COMBAT CASUALTY CARE

Published by the

Office of the Surgeon General
Department of the Army, United States of America

Senior Editor

Colonel Russ Zajtchuk, MC, U.S. Army
Deputy Commander,
Walter Reed Army Medical Center
Former Deputy Director, Directorate of Professional Services,
Office of the Surgeon General
Professor of Surgery, Uniformed Services University of the Health Sciences

Managing Editor

Donald P. Jenkins, Ph.D.
Office of the Surgeon General
Associate Professor of Surgery, Georgetown University
Visiting Associate Professor of Anatomy,
Uniformed Services University of the Health Sciences

Associate Editor

Colonel Ronald F. Bellamy, MC, U.S. Army
Thoracic Surgery Service, Walter Reed Army Medical Center
Associate Professor of Military Medicine and Surgery,
Uniformed Services University of the Health Sciences

Production Editor

Virginia M. Ingram
TMM Publications, Office of the Surgeon General
and the American Registry of Pathology

The TMM Series

Part I. *Warfare, Weaponry, and the Casualty*

Volume

1 BATTLEFIELD ENVIRONMENT

2 MEDICAL CONSEQUENCES OF NUCLEAR WARFARE

3 MEDICAL CONSEQUENCES OF BIOLOGICAL WARFARE

4 MEDICAL CONSEQUENCES OF CHEMICAL WARFARE

5 CONVENTIONAL WARFARE: BALLISTIC, BLAST, AND BURN INJURIES

6 COMBAT STRESS

Part II. *Principles of Medical Command and Support*

Volume

1 MEDICAL COMMAND AND SUPPORT IN AIRLAND BATTLE

2 MEDICINE IN LOW-INTENSITY CONFLICT

Part III. *Military Preventive Medicine and the Environment*

Volume

1 DEPLOYMENT AND MOBILIZATION

2 OCCUPATIONAL HEALTH: THE SOLDIER IN THE INDUSTRIAL BASE

3 PERSONAL AND PHYSICAL READINESS OF THE SOLDIER

4 THE NATURAL ENVIRONMENT: ALTITUDE, COLD, AND HEAT

Part IV. *Surgical Combat Casualty Care*

Volume

1 THE CASUALTY

2 MEDICAL IMAGING

3 ANESTHESIA AND CRITICAL CARE

4 HEAD AND NECK SURGERY

5 OPHTHALMIC SURGERY AND NEUROSURGERY

6 CARDIOTHORACIC SURGERY

7 ABDOMINAL AND UROGENITAL SURGERY

8 ORTHOPEDIC SURGERY

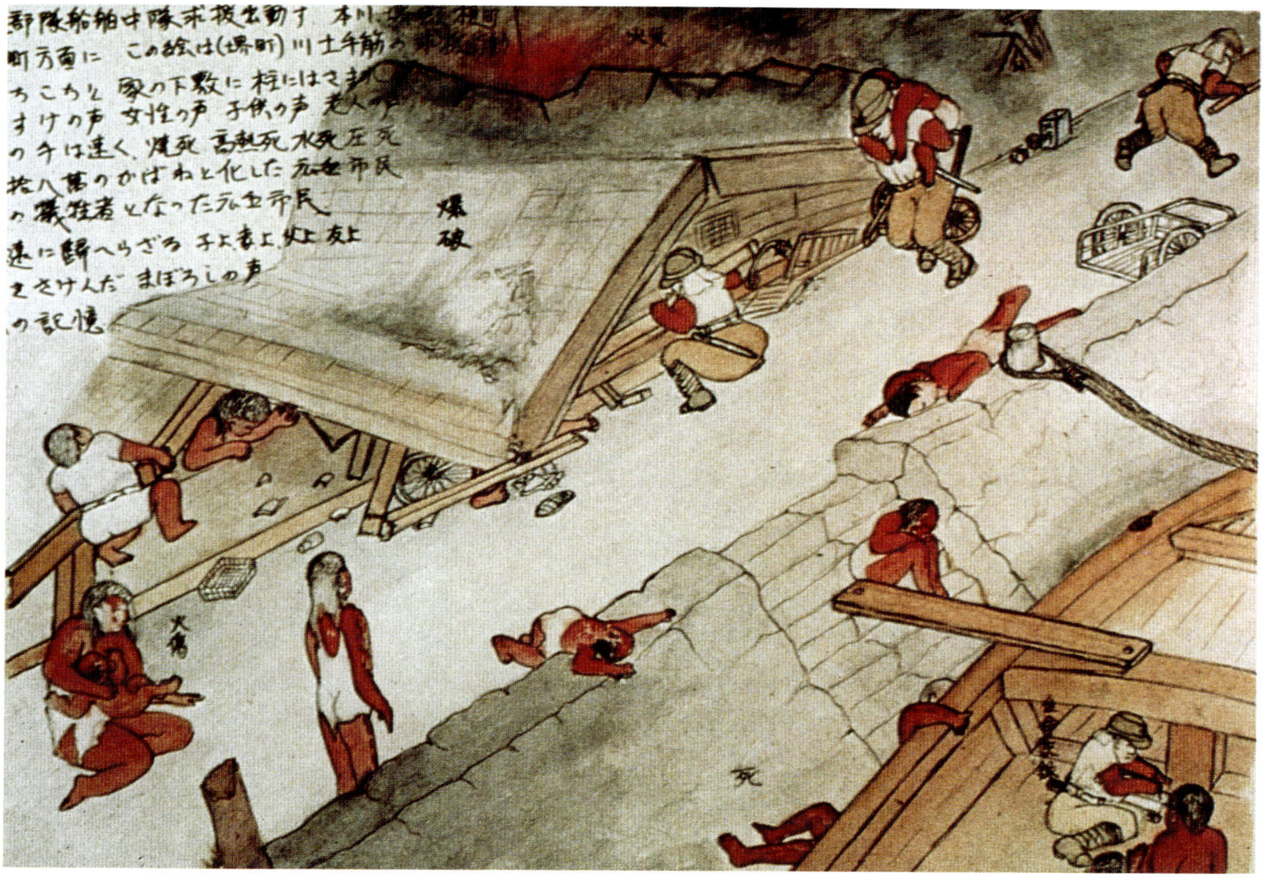

The artist, Ken Nakagawa, witnessed rescue operations performed by Japanese naval personnel along a riverbank in Hiroshima at 0840 on 6 August 1945. Approximately 280,000 deaths occurred as a consequence of this first atomic bombing. The reactions of other survivors are explored in Chapter 8.

MEDICAL CONSEQUENCES OF NUCLEAR WARFARE

Specialty Editors

RICHARD I. WALKER
T. JAN CERVENY

Contributing Authors

LEONARD A. ALT
VICTOR BOGO
ROBERT F. DONS
NUSHIN K. FARZANEH
C. DOUGLAS FORCINO
LEO I. GIAMBARRESI
LARRY W. LUCKETT
THOMAS J. MacVITTIE
G. ANDREW MICKLEY
BRUCE E. VESPER
THOMAS L. WALDEN, Jr.
BRUCE R. WEST
ROBERT W. YOUNG

Armed Forces Radiobiology Research Institute
Bethesda, Maryland

Defense Nuclear Agency
Alexandria, Virginia

Published by TMM Publications, Office of the Surgeon General,
5111 Leesburg Pike, Falls Church, Virginia 22041-3258

Colleen Mathews Quick, Publications Specialist

Library of Congress Cataloging in Publication Data

Medical Consequences of Nuclear Warfare

Includes index.
1. Radiation-Physiological effect. 2. Nuclear weapons-Physiological effect. (eds.) Zajtchuk, R.; Jenkins, D. P.; Bellamy, R. F.; Ingram, V. M.
I. Walker, Richard I. II. Cerveny, T. Jan

PRINTED IN THE UNITED STATES OF AMERICA

96 95 94 93 92 91 90 89 5 4 3 2 1

Contents

Foreword

The dramatic technological, social, and economic progress of the twentieth century has yet to prevent the use of armed conflict to resolve political differences among nations. As those of us in military medicine prepare to support our forces into the next century, we must continually be ready for the many challenges presented by modern warfare.

The Army Medical Department has embarked on an ambitious readiness initiative. This new doctrine focuses on far-foward surgical care, increased intensive-care capabilities, a policy of returning soldiers to duty as far foward as possible, improved ground and air evacuation capabilities, new medical logistics systems that incorporate blood-distribution networks, and improved management of combat stress. Our goals are to maintain our momentum as we conserve fighting strength and to support our soldiers and their families both in peacetime and in time of war.

The military health-care system is the largest comprehensive health-care organization in the United States. Because the vast majority of our patients are not active duty military personnel, it may seem that our day-to-day activities are far removed from what we would be required to do during time of war. The ability to deploy a highly trained medical corps to any area of the world, however, is our highest priority. To be effective, we must not only maintain the highest standards of technical competence, but must also be prepared to use our skills creatively and courageously in situations that may be primitive, dangerous, or unknown. Major General James H. Rumbaugh, the late commander of Walter Reed Army Medical Center (who aptly described his organization as "the largest live-fire range in the Army"), understood that everything we do in our daily practice hones our expertise. Our readiness initiative will provide a clearer combat context in which to apply that expertise. Lessons of medical survival have been learned in previous conflicts at great cost. We cannot afford to forget them.

It is my hope that you will find the *Textbook of Military Medicine* series a useful addition to your readiness training programs, and that it will stimulate you to think about and plan for what will be required of each of us should the need arise to make a transition from peace to war.

Lieutenant General Frank F. Ledford, Jr.
The Surgeon General
U.S. Army

April 1989
Washington, D.C.

Preface

Medical Consequences of Nuclear Warfare is the second volume of Part I, *Warfare, Weaponry, and the Casualty*. It addresses the increasingly important medical challenges of the consequences and management of radiation injuries.

The presence of vast nuclear arsenals has had a paradoxical effect on our collective human consciousness: because we are unavoidably aware of the potential destruction stored in those warheads, we are less likely to use them in a global thermonuclear war. However, maintaining this deterrent carries its own high price. The likelihood of accidental detonations, small-yield nuclear attacks in regional conflicts, and radiation injuries in reactors and weapons plants increases as familiarity with this powerful force spreads. Arms limitations agreements among superpowers are important, but third-world nations now too have access to the materials and technology necessary to enter the nuclear arena. The volatility of world politics may be moving beyond the ability of any policy- or lawmaking group to control. Given the devastating medical consequences that would follow a nuclear detonation or accident, the training of the medical corps in treating radiation syndromes will be a crucial factor in the effective management of casualties.

The rapidly expanding science of medical radiobiology has greatly affected the prospective readiness of the military medical corps to deal with these injuries. The Armed Forces Radiobiology Research Institute has been a leader in the establishment of the base of scientific and clinical knowledge from which the current concepts of medical management have evolved. In addition to research, the institute is involved in continuing medical education and in our nation's emergency response system. It is in a unique position to understand the importance of converting vast amounts of laboratory data into practical, efficient medical techniques and treatments. The authors have written their chapters from a combined academic and military perspective in order to specifically help the military physician.

Captain Richard I. Walker, MC, U.S. Navy, and Major T. Jan Cerveny, MC, U.S. Air Force, provided the expertise in the organization of this textbook. The first chapter is an overview of nuclear events and their consequences. The following chapters examine the effects of radiation exposure on humans and the ways they will affect triage, diagnosis, and treatment protocols as well as military logistics. A discussion of the latest prospects for radioprotection concludes the text.

It is possible that no amount of knowledge or training will help any medical unit to deal with the mass casualties that a large-scale radiation incident or accident would incur. However, data from accidental and therapeutic radiation exposures, together with ongoing clinical research results, are all useful in determining the treatment of individual victims of smaller incidents who are in a position to be saved.

The *Textbook of Military Medicine* series is a reality because of the vision and support of the late Major General James H. Rumbaugh; Lieutenant General Frank F. Ledford, Jr., the Surgeon General of the Army; Lieutenant General (ret.) Quinn H. Becker, our former Surgeon General; and Major General Robert H. Buker, Deputy Surgeon General of the Army.

The editors gratefully acknowledge the assistance in the preparation of this volume of Junith Van Deusen, Modeste E. Greenville, Sonia Jones, and Carolyn B. Wooden of the Publications Division of the Armed Forces Radiobiology Research Institute.

Colonel Russ Zajtchuk
U.S. Army

April 1989

Chapter 1

NUCLEAR EVENTS AND THEIR CONSEQUENCES

LEONARD A. ALT, M.S.,* C. DOUGLAS FORCINO, Ph.D.,** and RICHARD I. WALKER, Ph.D.***

*Major, United States Army; Program Manager, Radiation Sources Department, Armed Forces Radiobiology Research Institute, Bethesda, Maryland 20814-5145
**Lieutenant, United States Navy; Department of Military Medicine, Uniformed Services University of the Health Sciences, Bethesda, Maryland 20814-4799
***Captain, United States Navy; Director, Enteric Diseases Program, Naval Medical Research Institute, Bethesda, Maryland 20814-5055 and Armed Forces Radiobiology Research Institute, Bethesda, Maryland 20814-5145

INTRODUCTION

Radiation damage to human cells was first recognized just 4 months after the reported discovery of X rays by Wilhelm Conrad Roentgen. In 1896, Dr. J. Daniels found that the irradiation of his colleague's skull resulted in loss of hair. Since then, many other biomedical effects of radiation have been described.

The understanding of atomic physics increased rapidly in the early twentieth century and culminated in the Manhattan Project, which harnessed the power of the atom in a bomb. Thus began the nuclear era in international relations and warfare, bringing new challenges to the military physician.

Today, more and more countries are developing nuclear weapons, with those in the United States and the Soviet Union achieving the greatest capabilities. One modern American or Soviet submarine carries nuclear weapons that can release energy equivalent to 500 bombs of the size used at Hiroshima in 1945. This vast power is greater than the energy released from all weapons in all previous wars combined. Of course, the extensive use of these nuclear weapons in a confrontation would nullify an effective medical response. Rational minds must continue to recognize this potentially devastating nuclear power and maintain a general peace, as they have for over 40 years.

The deterrent effect of nuclear weapons does not mean that military physicians can ignore the possibility of their use. The most likely situations requiring a medical response are the use of weapons against a deployed naval force, a remote city, or a remote facility; a third-world conflict; a terrorist act; or an accident involving a nuclear weapon.

Military medical preparedness can focus beyond nuclear weapon events. Today, nuclear material is used in medicine, industry, and power generation, bringing increased risk of occupational and accidental exposures. New radiation hazards in space will have to be overcome if successful peacetime and military uses of that frontier are to be realized. Military physicians trained to respond to weapons-related injuries can bring expertise to these situations.

NUCLEAR AND PHYSICAL PROCESSES IN WEAPONS

Weapons-related injuries can be best understood after examining the destructive forces—*blast, thermal*, and *radiation*—that produce them. In comparison with a conventional explosive weapon, a nuclear weapon's effectiveness is due to its unequalled capacity to liberate a tremendous quantity of energy in a very small space in an extremely short time. This section presents a simple description of the physical processes taking place within the first few thousandths of a second after a nuclear weapon detonation.

Nuclear Energy

Energy may be broadly classified as potential or kinetic. Potential energy is energy of configuration or position, or the capacity to perform work. For example, the relatively unstable chemical bonds among the atoms that comprise trinitrotoluene (TNT) possess chemical potential energy. Potential energy can, under suitable conditions, be transformed into kinetic energy, which is energy of motion. When a conventional explosive such as TNT is detonated, the relatively unstable chemical bonds are converted into bonds that are more stable, producing kinetic energy in the form of blast and thermal energies. This process of transforming a chemical system's bonds from lesser to greater stability is exothermic (there is a net production of energy). Likewise, a nuclear detonation derives its energy from transformations of the powerful nuclear bonds that hold the neutrons and protons together within the nucleus. The conversion of relatively less stable nuclear bonds into bonds with greater stability leads not only to the liberation of vast quantities of kinetic energy in blast and thermal forms, but also to the generation of ionizing radiations.

To discover where these energies come from, consider the nucleus of the helium atom, which is composed of two neutrons and two protons bound

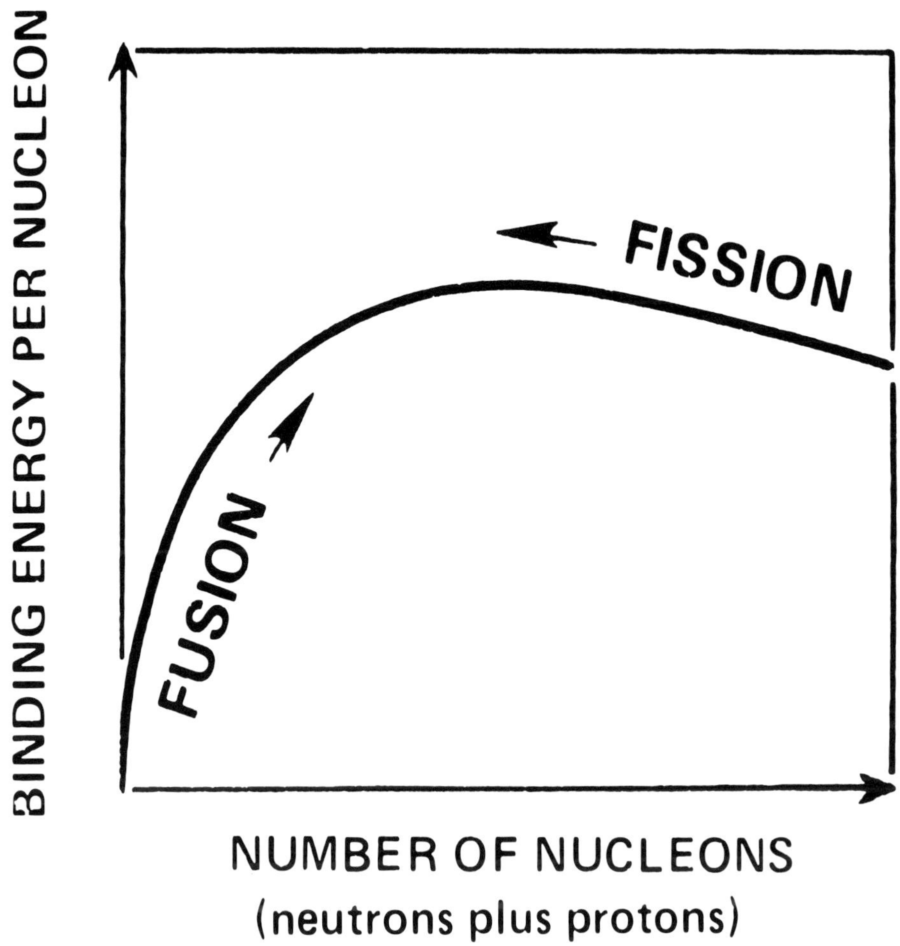

Fig. 1-1. Curve of binding energy per nucleon

tightly together by the *strong* (or specifically nuclear) *force*. If we compare the bound neutrons and protons to those in the unbound state, we find that the total mass of the separate neutrons and protons is greater than their mass when they bind together to form the helium nucleus. The mass that has been lost in the process of forming the nuclear bonds is called the *mass defect*. Einstein's famous equation, $E = mc^2$ (energy equals mass multiplied by the speed of light squared), quantifies the conversion of this missing mass into the binding energy that holds together the helium nucleus. This is the potential energy stored in the bonds of the strong force. A small amount of mass, when multiplied by the speed of light squared (an extremely large number), has a large amount of binding energy. If the total binding energy for each element is calculated and divided by its total number of nucleons (that is, neutrons plus protons; for helium, two neutrons plus two protons equals four nucleons), a measure is obtained of how tightly the average nucleon is bound for that particular atom. A plot of this "average binding energy per nucleon" for each element gives the curve in Figure 1-1.

It is significant that this curve has a broad maximum. This means that there is a range of elements for which the neutrons and protons are most tightly bound and, thus, have the most stable nuclear bonds. If nuclei having less stable nuclear bonds can be converted into nuclei having more stable bonds, the system will pass from a state of lesser to greater stability, and energy will be released. This is the energy source of nuclear weapons. The process can occur in two ways: *fission* or *fusion*. Fission is the process of breaking less stable larger elements (such as uranium and plutonium) into two of the more stable midrange elements. Fusion is the process of combining lighter nuclei (such as those of deuterium and tritium, which are isotopes of hydrogen) into heavier elements lying farther up the curve of binding energy per nucleon.

Energy Release in Nuclear Weapons

A fission nuclear device is practical for only three elements: uranium-233, uranium-235, and plutonium-239. In order to construct an efficient weapon, instability is induced in one of these nuclei by striking it with a neutron. The unstable nuclear bonds are broken, the nucleus splits apart, and relatively more stable nuclear bonds are reformed by each of the two midrange fission fragments. This is accompanied by the release of a large quantity of energy and the prompt emission of gamma rays and neutrons (*initial nuclear radiation*). It is important to note that approximately 82% of the fission energy is released as kinetic energy of the two large fission fragments. These fragments, being massive and highly charged particles, interact readily with matter. They transfer their energy quickly to the surrounding weapon materials, which rapidly become heated. The fission fragments consist of over 300 different isotopes of thirty-eight separate chemical elements. Most of the fragments are highly unstable radioactively and will later contribute to the radiologically and chemically complex fallout field.

One fission event alone does not make a weapon, which requires a self-perpetuating, exponentially escalating chain reaction of fissions. This is achieved by the suitable physical arrangement of certain nuclear materials. Also, since the weapon must not reach the proper, or *critical*, configuration until the desired time of detonation, some way must be found to make the transition on demand from a safe, or *subcritical*, condition to the critical state. In a functioning fission device, this is done by altering the mass, shape, or density of the nuclear materials.

The two basic classes of fission weapons are the *gun-assembled device* and the *implosion device*. The gun-assembled weapon is a mechanically simple design that uses a "gun tube" arrangement to blow together two small masses of uranium-235 to form a supercritical mass. The 15-kiloton-yield weapon used at Hiroshima was a gun-assembled device (1 kiloton, or kt, equals the energy released by detonation of 1,000 tons of TNT, and 1 megaton, or MT, equals 1,000,000 tons of TNT). The implosion weapon uses an extremely complex system of precisely formed, conventional chemical-explosive lenses to crush a mass of plutonium-239 to supercritical density. The first tested nuclear weapon (the Trinity device) and the 21-kt-yield weapon used at Nagasaki were implosion devices. From the viewpoint of a weapon's accessibility, it is fortunate that the much more easily constructed gun-assembled weapon cannot effectively use the more readily producible plutonium-239. Instead, it must be fueled with uranium-235, which is more difficult to obtain.

The limit on a fission weapon's yield, from an engineering viewpoint, is several hundred kilotons. Therefore, the multi-megaton weapons in the American and Soviet inventories are fusion weapons, deriving much of their power from the combination of light isotopes of hydrogen (deuterium and tritium) into heavier nuclei lying farther up the curve of binding energy per nucleon. Due to the presence of powerful forces of electrostatic repulsion, initiation of the fusion of deuterium and tritium requires extremely high temperatures, about 50,000,000°C. The only practical way to achieve those temperatures in a weapon on earth is to detonate a fission device inside the fusion materials. The deuterium and tritium then fuse and release energy, partly in the form of highly energetic and penetrating fusion neutrons, which have energies about ten times the typical energies of fission-generated neutrons. The fusion weapon then uses these high-energy fusion neutrons to cause secondary fissions. Thus, a fusion weapon actually generates power from both fission and fusion processes, usually in roughly equal proportions.

An *enhanced radiation weapon*, or neutron bomb, might be produced by altering the design of a standard small-yield fusion weapon to permit the high-energy fusion neutrons to better escape the device. This modification increases the initial production of neutron radiation, reduces the proportion of the weapon's energy expressed in blast and thermal effects, and reduces the amount of residual fallout radiation. Thus, a given total yield produces more biologically damaging neutron radiation, less destruction of matériel from blast and thermal effects, and less residual radiation fallout.

Production of Blast and Thermal Effects

The blast and thermal effects of detonation produce by far the greatest number of immediate hu-

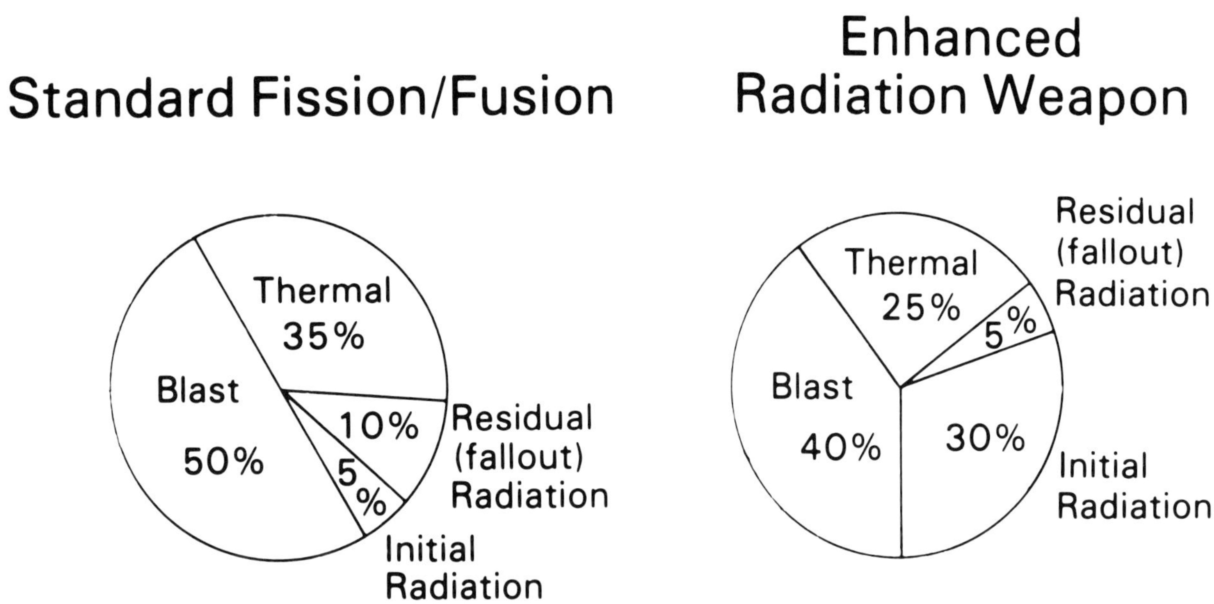

Fig. 1-2. Energy partition of a nuclear weapon

man casualties in nuclear warfare. The nuclear reactions within the weapon have died out after the first one-millionth of a second, and the fission and fusion events have produced a vast quantity of energy, which has been rapidly and locally transferred to the bomb materials in the form of heat. The weapon's materials (bomb casing, electronics, chemical explosive residues, and 80% of the original nuclear fuels, which even in a relatively efficient device remain unreacted) now exist as a highly energetic plasma of positive ions and free electrons at high temperature and high pressure. Through a process of electron-ion interaction known as *bremsstrahlung*, the plasma becomes an intense source of X rays. These X rays leave the vicinity of the bomb materials at the speed of light, heat the first several meters of air surrounding the weapon, and generate a fireball with an initial temperature of 1,000,000°C. The intensely hot fireball reradiates thermal energy in the form of electromagnetic radiation at infrared, visible, and ultraviolet frequencies.

At about the same time, the weapon's materials have started to expand supersonically outward, dramatically compressing and heating the surrounding air. This phenomenon, called *case shock*, is the source of the destructive blast wave and further thermal radiations. A unique interaction between the X-ray-heated air and the case-shock-heated air is responsible for the nuclear weapon's characteristic double pulse of thermal output. Added to these blast and thermal effects is the initial nuclear radiation (primarily neutrons and gamma rays) which is produced promptly by the fission and fusion processes, and the *residual radiation* (primarily gamma rays and high-energy electrons) which are produced later by decay of the radioactive fission fragments composing the fallout field. Figure 1-2 depicts the typical energy partition for a standard fission or fusion device and the energy partition expected from a typical enhanced-radiation weapon (neutron bomb).

The range of the blast, thermal, and radiation effects produced by the detonation of a nuclear weapon depends on many factors, perhaps the most significant of which, for the battlefield soldier, is total weapon yield. Figure 1-3 shows the range over which the various effects are lethal, as a function of yield. It is noteworthy that initial radiation is the dominant threat for only very small tactical devices, and thermal effects are dominant for large-yield strategic weapons.

BLAST, THERMAL, AND RADIATION EFFECTS

The destructive blast, thermal, and radiation effects of a fission or fusion weapon all stem from the device's capacity to transform the very strong nuclear bonds of uranium, plutonium, deuterium, and tritium from a relatively unstable state to a more stable one. The quantitative difference between the effects of a nuclear weapon and the effects of a conventional explosive is the result of the dramatically greater strength of the nuclear bonds. A qualitative difference arises from the production of *(a)* initial nuclear radiations from the fission and fusion processes themselves and *(b)* delayed radioactivity from decay of the unstable fission fragment byproducts.

Blast Effects

During the detonation of a standard fission or fusion nuclear device, the rapidly expanding plasma gives rise to a shock or blast that is responsible for dissipating about 50% of the total energy of the weapon. This represents a tremendous amount of energy, even in small, tactical-sized weapons of a few kilotons. As the blast wave travels outward from the site of the explosion, it is composed of static and dynamic components that are capable of producing medical injuries and structural damage. The static component of the blast wave is a wall of compressed air that exerts a crushing effect on objects in its path. The dynamic component is the movement of air caused by and proportional to the difference between the static overpressure and the ambient pressure. In this discussion, the static and dynamic components will be called the *blast wave* and *blast wind*, respectively.

In discussing the structural damage to buildings after a nuclear detonation, it is difficult to separate the effects of the static component from those of the dynamic component. For example, the 5-psi (pounds per square inch) blast wave and 160-mph blast winds associated with the blast wave's passage would destroy a two-story brick house.

However, the medical problems resulting from exposure to the shock wave can be divided into those that result from the static component and those that result from the dynamic component. Injuries resulting from the blast waves will be caused by exposure to high pressures with very short rise times, and will consist primarily of internal injuries. For example, the threshold level for rupture of the eardrum is about 5 psi. Although this injury is very painful, it would not limit the accomplishment of a critical military mission. The 160-mph winds that accompany the passage of a 5-psi blast wave would be sufficiently strong to cause displacement and possible injuries. At the other end of the spectrum, a pressure level of 15 psi will produce serious intrathoracic injuries, including alveolar and pulmonary vascular rupture, interstitial hemorrhage, edema, and air emboli. If the air emboli make their way into the arterial circulation, cerebral and myocardial infarctions may ensue. The initial outward signs of such pulmonary damage are frothy bleeding through the nostrils, dyspnea, and coughing. Victims may be in shock without any visible wounds. In addition, serious abdominal injuries, including hepatic and splenic rupture, may result from a rapid and violent compression of the abdomen.

The blast winds that accompany the blast wave can also produce injuries. Debris carried by the wind may cause missile injuries ranging from lacerations and contusions to fractures and blunt trauma, depending on the projectile's size, shape, and mass. Wind velocity of 100 mph will displace a person, resulting in lacerations, contusions, and fractures from tumbling across the terrain or from being thrown against stationary structures. Winds capable of causing displacement injuries or missile injuries would be produced by a blast wave with an overpressure of less than 5 psi. At this pressure level, the blast winds are more significant in producing injury than is the static component of the blast wave. At high pressure levels, both the static and dynamic components are capable of producing serious injuries.

Although the LD_{50} (lethal dose, or fatal injury, for 50% of cases) from tumbling occurs at about 50 mph, the LD_{50} from impact occurs at about 20–25 mph. The LD_{50} from blast is estimated to occur at 6 psi, due primarily to the force of blast winds. For a small tactical weapon or terrorist device with a yield of 0.5 kt, the range for this level of overpressure would extend to slightly less than 0.5 km. For larger tactical or strategic weapons with yields of 50 and 500 kt, the range for LD_{50} at 6 psi would expand to just under 2 km and just under 4 km, respectively.

Protection from the effects of the blast wave is difficult to achieve because it is an engulfing phenomenon. The best protection can be found in a blast-resistant shelter. However, protection from the effects of the blast winds can be achieved in any location offering shielding from the wind. If adequate shelter is not found, the best defense against blast effects is to lie face down on the ground with feet pointed toward ground zero. This reduces the body's surface area that is exposed to wind-borne debris and offers less resistance to the force of the blast wind.

Thermal Effects

Following the detonation of a standard fission or fusion device, approximately 35% of the weapon's energy is dissipated as thermal energy. The general types of injuries resulting from this energy are burns, including *flash burns* and *flame burns*, and certain eye injuries, including *flash blindness* and *retinal burns*.

The thermal output after a nuclear detonation occurs in two distinct pulses, as a result of the interaction of the shock wave with the leading edge of the fireball. The first pulse contains only about 1% of the total thermal energy output and is composed primarily of energy in the ultraviolet range. Because the first pulse is of very short duration and the ultraviolet energy is rapidly absorbed by the atmosphere, it does not contribute significantly to producing casualties. The second pulse is composed primarily of energy in the infrared and visible portions of the electromagnetic spectrum, contains about 99% of the thermal energy liberated by the nuclear detonation, and is responsible for subsequent burns and vision problems.

Burn Injury. The two types of burn injury, flash burn and flame burn, are caused by different events and have different prognoses. Flash burn results from the skin's exposure to a large quantity of thermal energy in a very brief time. This often leaves the affected area of the skin with a charred appearance. However, since the heat pulse occurs rapidly and the thermal conductivity of the skin is low, the burn is often superficial, killing only the outer dermal layers and leaving the germinal layer essentially undamaged. In contrast, flame burn results from contact with a conventional fire, such as clothing or the remains of a building ignited by the fireball's thermal pulse. In most cases, the healing of a flame burn is abnormal because the germinal layer has been damaged.

Since the heat pulse travels at the speed of light, protection from burns is not possible unless warning is given in time to find cover. The electromagnetic energy of the thermal pulse travels in a straight line, so any barrier placed in its path will offer some protection. Even clothing will provide some protection from the deposition of thermal energy onto the skin. Since light colors tend to reflect rather than absorb thermal energy, light-colored clothing will offer more protection than dark-colored clothing.

Figure 1-3 shows the range of LD_{50} for burn injury from weapons of different yields. Notice that for weapons of very low yield, the range for burn injury LD_{50} is about equal to the range for the LD_{50} from blast and radiation. As the weapon yield increases, the range for burn injury increases much more rapidly than the range for blast injury or radiation injury. This means that burns will always be present after the detonation of a nuclear device, and for weapons with a yield above 10 kt, burns will be the predominant injury. Because of the large number of burn casualties and the time- and labor-intensive treatment that they require, burn injury is the most difficult problem to be faced by the military medical community in a nuclear conflict.

Eye Injury. Thermal energy may also cause eye injury. The two types of eye injury that would occur would not burden a medical facility. Flash blindness is a temporary condition that results from a depletion of photopigment from the retinal receptors. This happens when a person indirectly observes the brilliant flash of intense light energy from a fireball. The duration of flash blindness can be as short as several seconds during the day, followed by a darkened afterimage for several minutes. At night, flash blindness can last three times longer, with a loss of dark adaptation for up to 30 minutes. This could seriously compromise military operations.

Another eye injury is retinal burn, which results from looking directly at the fireball and focusing its image on the retina. This intense light energy is strong enough to kill the retinal receptors and create a permanent blind spot. It is surprising that retinal burn is no more detrimental to mission accomplishment than is flash blindness.

To protect against injury, the eyes can be closed and shielded after the individual receives warning of a detonation. Using one of the lead-lanthanum-zirconium-titanium goggles that have been developed may provide further protection.

Effects of Initial and Residual Radiations

A detonating fission or fusion weapon produces

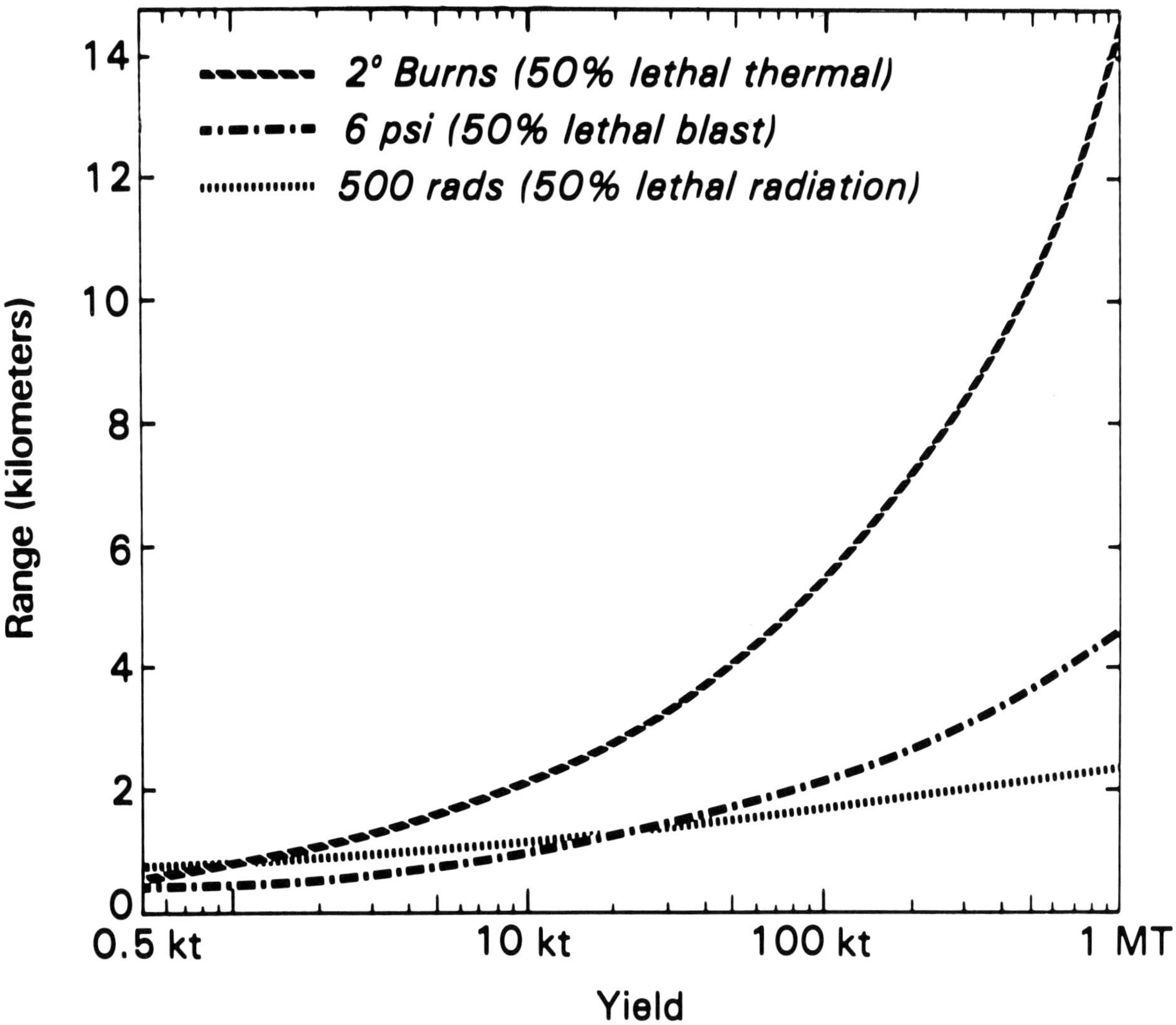

Fig. 1-3. Range of effects of a nuclear weapon

a variety of nuclear radiations. Initial radiation occurs at the time of the nuclear reactions, and residual radiation occurs long after the immediate blast and thermal effects have ended. The nuclear radiations include neutrons, gamma rays, alpha particles, and beta particles, which are biologically damaging and may significantly affect human health and performance. Initial radiation consists of neutrons and gamma rays produced within the first minute after detonation. Mechanisms for producing initial radiation are *(a)* the generation of neutrons and gamma rays directly from the fission and fusion processes, *(b)* the production of gamma rays through inelastic scatter reactions with elements in the atmosphere surrounding the weapon, and *(c)* the isomeric-decay and neutron-capture gamma rays. Residual radiation primarily includes gamma rays, beta particles, and alpha particles generated beyond the first minute after detonation. Most of these radiations are produced by the decay of the fission fragments generated by weapon fission processes, but some are activated bomb components and surface materials made radioactive by exposure to the intense neutron flux generated by fission and fusion events.

The broad classes of initial radiation and residual radiation come from an analysis of a 20-kt ground burst. The hot fireball produced by this weapon, laden with highly radioactive fission fragments, rises upward through the atmosphere so quickly that, after about 60 seconds, it reaches a height from which the initial radiations no longer strike the ground. A person on the ground would therefore be safe from the initial radiations after 1 minute. As the yield of the weapon is increased, the fireball rises more quickly, but the 60-second point remains approximately the same. The main hazard from initial radiation is acute external whole-body irradiation by neutrons and gamma rays. Figure 1-3 shows that it is only for very small tactical weapons that the initial radiation is potentially fatal at distances where the blast and thermal effects are survivable. Therefore, significant initial radiation hazards are restricted to the first minute after detonation and to several hundred meters surrounding a small-yield tactical weapon. Conversely, residual fallout covers a wide geographic area and remains a significant biological hazard long after detonation.

Fallout. Our consideration of the origin of radioactive debris begins with a review of the basic nuclear and physical processes that occur as the device detonates. As the fissile material splits, the massive and highly charged fragments carry away 82% of the fission energy, and release it as heat within the bomb components. This transforms the components into an extremely hot plasma. Bremsstrahlung interactions between the electrons and positive ions within this plasma generate an intense source of low-energy X rays, which leave the plasma and interact with the first several meters of air surrounding the weapon. The X rays heat this air to an extremely high temperature and initiate the development of the fireball that is characteristic of nuclear explosions. The rapid outward expansion of weapon material dramatically compresses and heats the air around the weapon (case shock), further contributing to the generation of the fireball. This hot bubble of gas, containing highly radioactive fission fragments and activated weapon material, is the origin of the fallout radiation.

Sources of fallout include *(a)* highly unstable fragments produced by the fissioning of plutonium or uranium, *(b)* roughly 80% of the nuclear fuels that remain unreacted after the weapon has blown itself apart (uranium or plutonium for all weapons, as well as tritium for fusion devices), and *(c)* activation products (weapon components and ground elements made radioactive by exposure to the weapon's intense neutron flux). Another contributor to fallout is *salting*, the inclusion of materials in a weapon that will activate when exposed to the initial neutron flux, thus increasing the amount of residual radioactive isotopes. Because of operational limitations in using a salted weapon, it is expected that this technique will be rarely used. Since the fission fragments produced by the fissioning of uranium or plutonium account for most of the activity in the fallout field, the fusion process is relatively "clean" regarding the production of residual radiation.

Early fallout is radioactive material deposited within the first day after detonation. This fallout is the most significant for the military because it is highly radioactive, geographically concentrated, and local. It tends to consist of larger particles (approximately 0.01–1.0 cm in diameter) usually deposited within a few hundred miles of ground zero. Because the material has had little time to decay, it is radiologically very active. The biological hazards from early fallout are external whole-body gamma-ray irradiation from gamma emitters deposited on the ground; external beta-particle irradiation from beta emitters deposited on the skin; and internal beta-particle irradiation from beta-emitting isotopes that are ingested, injected, or inhaled.

Delayed fallout generally consists of the smaller particles deposited after the first 24 hours. This material is less significant as an immediate hazard to the military because it has a longer time to decay and it is deposited over a wider area. Under certain circumstances, delayed fallout may be distributed worldwide, presenting a long-term health hazard, primarily through internalized exposure.

The ultimate deposition of nuclear fallout on the ground is influenced by the physical interactions of the rising fireball with the atmosphere. For a ground or near-surface burst, the interaction of the fireball with ground debris also affects the fallout deposition. As the hot gas bubble quickly rises through the atmosphere, it creates and is followed by a strong vacuum directly from below. This generates winds that rush radially inward toward ground zero and upward toward the ascending fireball. For a near-surface burst, these winds can pick up large quantities of dirt and debris from the ground and inject them into the fireball (a process called *stem formation*). This material, along with any other ground material directly vaporized by a surface burst, then provides condensation centers within the fireball. The gaseous fission fragments condense more quickly on these relatively larger debris particles than they would have otherwise, greatly increasing early local fallout. This fallout is deposited quickly in a concentrated area relatively near ground zero. Thus, a ground or near-surface detonation is the most significant fallout hazard to the military. The activation of surface materials through irradiation of ground elements by the direct neutron flux of a near-surface burst may also increase the local fallout hazard to troops traveling through that area soon after detonation.

In the case of a pure airburst detonation with no secondary ground materials injected into the fireball, the cloud rises and cools, and the fission fragment vapors begin to cool and condense at certain temperatures (characteristic of their particular elements). Therefore, because the time for airburst fission-product condensation is delayed and because fission products do not condense on large particles of ground debris, the proportion of fallout activity expressed as early local fallout is greatly reduced.

Characteristics of Fallout and the Prediction of Hazards. The factors that determine the extent of anticipated fallout hazard are:

- The total fission yield (fission fragments are the largest contributor to fallout activity)
- The ratio of energy produced in a fusion weapon, by fission process versus fusion process (the higher the fission fraction, the more fission products and consequently the greater the radiological hazard)
- The specific design of the weapon (for example, an enhanced radiation weapon will produce proportionately less fallout than an equivalent-yield standard nuclear weapon)
- The altitude of burst (a ground or near-surface detonation produces the greatest early local hazard)
- The composition of surface elements near ground zero in a near-surface burst (accounting for the neutron flux-induced activation potential of surface materials)
- The meteorological conditions (winds and precipitation introduce by far the greatest uncertainties in predicting where and when the fallout will be deposited)
- The time after detonation (the more time allowed for radiological decay, the less the activity of the fallout field)

In terms of absolute quantity of energy from fallout, approximately 10% of the quoted energy yield of a typical fission weapon will be decay radiation; for fusion weapons, it will be approximately 5%.

The elemental distribution of fission fragments is almost independent of whether the fissile material is plutonium or uranium. In each case, approximately 38 different chemical elements are produced, consisting of about 300 separate radionuclides. Thus, the chemical and radiological characteristics of the fallout field are extremely complex and, in practice, are amenable only to empirical analysis. The fission fragments are highly unstable and decay primarily by emitting gamma rays and beta particles. Activated weapon materials and ground elements, as well as unspent tritium from a fusion weapon, will decay by the same means. The unspent uranium and plutonium from fission processes decay by emitting alpha particles, which are a hazard primarily if they are inhaled. The immediate detection of fallout radiation is not possible with the physical senses, so appropriate instruments must be used. However, the heavy early, local fallout material is usually visible as a dust-like deposit that may look like a film on shiny surfaces. These visible particles are the most hazardous component of fallout.

MEDICAL CONSEQUENCES OF NUCLEAR WEAPONS

Military planners are concerned with the effect of nuclear weapons on the human component of operational systems. It is futile to harden machinery to large amounts of radiation if the human operator is incapacitated by relatively small doses. Radiobiology research can help reduce the logistical drain on medical resources caused by large numbers of severely injured casualties. Targeting and contingency planning depend on knowing radiation effects on military personnel.

The Chernobyl Accident

Unlike controlled radiotherapy, radiation associated with weapon detonations or accidents can result in uncontrolled and usually unpredictable exposures, which make radioprotective measures difficult. As seen in the 1986 accident in Chernobyl, USSR, *dosimetry* (measurement of radiation dose) is also difficult. Physical dosimeters, if available, may

TABLE 1-1

PERCENT DISTRIBUTION OF INJURIES SUSTAINED IN A NUCLEAR WAR

Type of Injury	Percent Distribution
Single Injuries (30%–40%)	
Irradiation*	15–20
Burns	15–20
Wounds	≤ 5
Combined Injuries (65%–70%)	
Burns + Irradiation	40
Burns + Wounds + Irradiation	20
Wounds + Irradiation	5
Wounds + Burns	5

*Including fallout

be lost during a nuclear event or may record cumulative doses with no information on dose rate. Furthermore, dosimeters provide point data rather than whole-body data. Biological dosimetry is also imperfect, and the time-consuming tests of lymphocyte depletion and cytogenetic damage (such as those used for Chernobyl victims) give different results. Dosimetry with uncontrolled exposures is complicated by two other factors with which military physicians may have to cope.

One is the uneven distribution of exposures on a victim due to shielding. Thus, pockets of critical cells that are necessary to regenerate affected tissues may survive, even if some parts of the body receive very high doses of radiation. Bone-marrow transplants were generally unsuccessful in Chernobyl victims, partially because of the survival of some host stem cells in the bone marrow; as surviving marrow was regenerated, it rejected the transplanted marrow cells.

Another complication of dosimetry in accidents or warfare is that other injuries, such as burns or mechanical trauma, can be superimposed on radiation injuries. The prognosis for these combined injuries is much graver than for radiation injuries alone, so combined injuries must be carefully considered during *triage* (sorting of casualties). It is estimated that 65%–70% of weapon-related injuries will be combined injuries, with burns and radiation being the most common combination (Table 1-1).

Burns and radiation effects were the most common injuries seen in seriously injured victims of the Chernobyl disaster. Thousands of medical and paramedical personnel were available for the relatively small number of patients at Chernobyl, but this will not be the case in military situations. If a nuclear weapon is detonated, physicians will have to adapt to mass-casualty management techniques, which require simplified and standardized care.

Today, scientists are exploiting the tremendous advances in biotechnology—the new knowledge and techniques in gene regulation, immunology, neurobiology, and related sciences—and will soon develop significant protection for the human body from the consequences of radiation exposure and associated injuries.

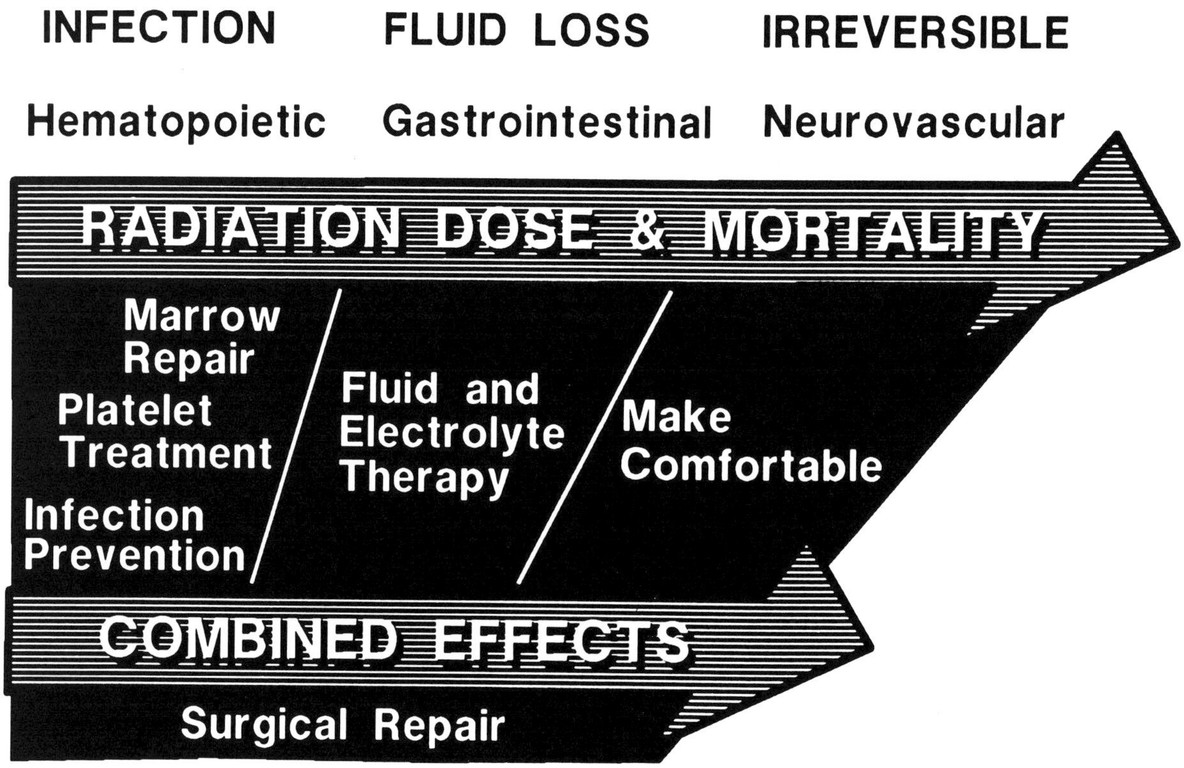

Fig. 1-4. Major acute radiation subsyndromes after injury to bone marrow, intestine, or neurovascular system

Nature of Radiation Injuries

Almost every major organ system can be affected by radiation exposure, and management in a nuclear accident or warfare will require the coordinated efforts of physicians, allied health professionals, and health-physics personnel.

A nuclear device detonated over a major city will cause tremendous numbers of casualties. The day after the detonation, 45,000 dead and 90,000 injured were counted in Hiroshima. Modern weapons would result in a much larger number of casualties. As the number of persons killed immediately due to blast and thermal injuries increases, so does the number of individuals at some distance from the epicenter who have serious but potentially survivable injuries. Therefore, an understanding of these injuries is extremely important to preserve human life and ensure the success of military operations.

Damage to the human body by ionizing radiation is caused by the deposition of energy. This is true for both electromagnetic radiation (such as X rays and gamma rays) and particulate radiation (such as beta particles, which are high-speed electrons, or neutrons). This energy deposition results in reactive chemical products, including free radicals (such as the hydroxide radical). These free radicals can further combine with body chemicals, primarily water, to form reactive species (such as hydrogen peroxide). These elements then combine with cellular components to cause damage. The primary targets of damage within the cell are deoxyribonucleic acid (which can be attacked not only by reactive chemical products but also by direct effects of the radiation itself), cellular and nuclear membranes, and enzymes.

The amount of damage sustained is a function of the radiation's quality, dose, and dose rate, and of the individual cell's sensitivity. The higher the dose, or the greater the deposition of radiation energy, the greater the damage expected. *Quality* refers to particular types of radiation (such as gamma radiation or neutron radiation) and their relative

TABLE 1-2

MEDICAL CONSEQUENCES OF NUCLEAR WEAPONS

Performance Decrement	Acute Effects	Delayed Effects
ETI* / Hypotension	Infection	Cancer
Motor	Bleeding	Life shortening
Cognitive	Dehydration	
Emesis/Diarrhea	Delayed wound healing	

*Early Transient Incapacitation

abilities to damage humans. Neutrons seem to be more effective in producing organism death, and gamma rays appear to be more effective in inducing performance decrement. In general, the more quickly a dose of radiation is delivered to the body, the more severe the consequences. The most sensitive cells are those that tend to divide rapidly, such as the bone-marrow cells and the cells lining the crypts of the gastrointestinal tract. Less sensitivity is exhibited by cells that divide more slowly or not at all, such as cells in the central nervous system (CNS).

The irradiation of cells has both acute and delayed effects (Table 1-2). Acute effects involve cell death, cell injury, and the release of disruptive mediators within the cell, which can lead to performance decrements. Other acute effects are infection and uncontrolled bleeding due to destruction of the bone marrow, dehydration and electrolyte imbalance due to denudation of the epithelial lining of the intestine, and slow healing of wounds. Delayed effects include cancer and nonspecific life shortening. Eventually, either the organism dies, or regeneration and recovery occur.

Military attention is focused primarily on acute effects because they are of the most immediate concern to the tactical military commander. Performance decrement occurs within minutes or hours after relatively low exposures to radiation. It includes a phenomenon called *early transient incapacitation* (ETI), a temporary inability to perform physically or cognitively demanding tasks. This inability can be accompanied by hypotension, emesis, or diarrhea. A pilot or a soldier in a nuclear/biological/chemical protective suit could be critically affected by a symptom like emesis. Performance decrement may be due to lesions other than those associated with the lethal consequences of radiation injury to cells. This hypothesis might be significant in the development of practical radioprotectants.

Acute Radiation Syndrome and Associated Subsyndromes

With increasing doses of radiation, changes take place in body tissues or organs, some of which are life threatening. The symptoms that appear soon after radiation exposure are called the *acute radiation syndrome* (ARS). This large category may be broken down into the *hematopoietic*, *gastrointestinal*, and *neurovascular subsyndromes* (Figure 1-4).

The hematopoietic subsyndrome is seen within two weeks after biologically significant radiation doses of 1.0–2.5 grays (Gy). This damage to the body's blood-forming organs, specifically to the bone marrow, can lead to suppressed production of white blood cells and platelets, which in turn leads to increased susceptibility to infection and uncontrolled bleeding. Treatment consists of administering platelets and preventing infection during the time required for bone-marrow repair. Much research is directed toward finding means to enhance the repair or replacement of this tissue.

The gastrointestinal subsyndrome appears within a week or two after exposure to higher doses, which are sometimes survivable. After this exposure, crypt cells in the epithelial lining of the intestine are destroyed. This leads to excessive fluid

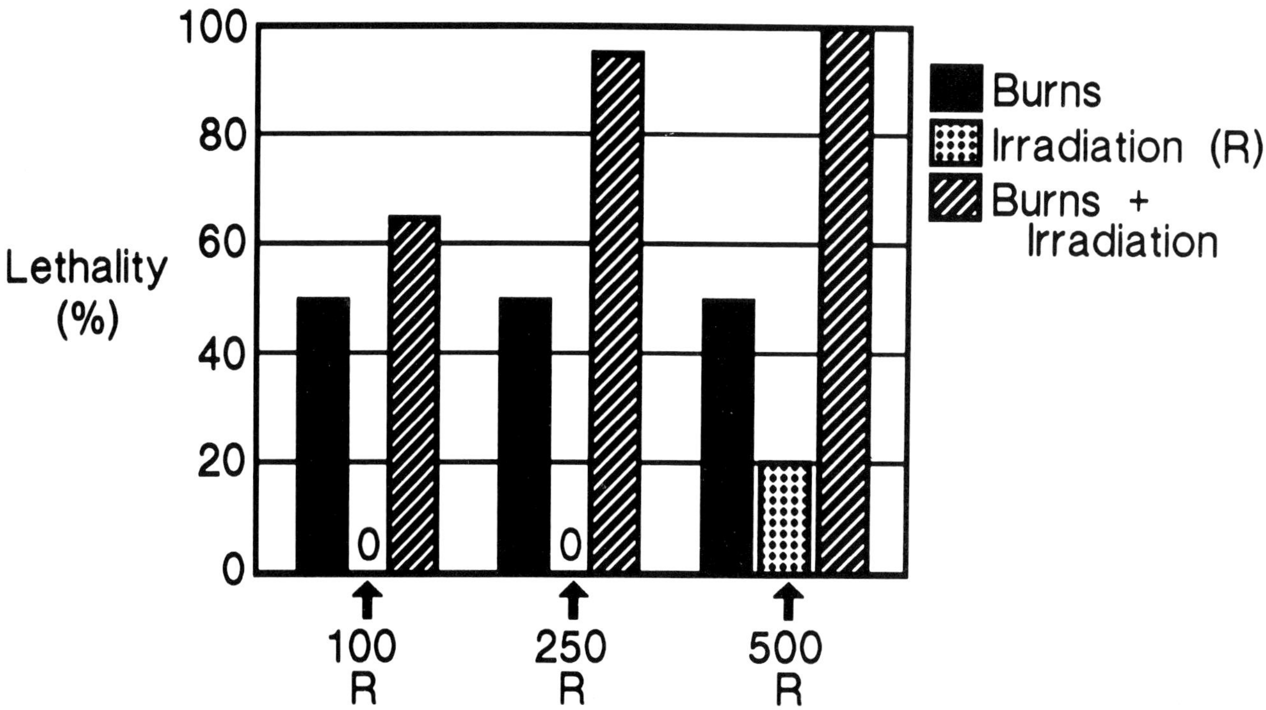

Fig. 1-5. Combined effects of simultaneous burns and whole-body irradiation on rats

loss and imbalance of electrolytes within the body, which may result in loss of the intestinal wall. Treatment focuses on preventing fluid loss and on balancing electrolytes during the time required for gastrointestinal repair.

The neurovascular subsyndrome appears within a few days after much higher doses of radiation, and consists of irreversible damage to the CNS. There is no treatment, other than making the patient as comfortable as possible.

Combined Injury

ARS and its medical effects are significantly complicated when radiation injury is combined with conventional blast trauma or thermal burn injuries. The following data show that the insult to the body from combined radiation and conventional injuries is much more severe than it would be from a single injury.

In Figure 1-5, the percent of mortality in rats that received an LD_{50} burn is compared to the percent of mortality when this insult was combined with sublethal to minimally lethal doses of radiation. Rats receiving 1.0 or 2.5 Gy of radiation alone had no mortality, while those receiving 5.0 Gy alone had about 20% mortality. Animals that received an LD_{50} burn and 1.0 Gy of radiation (which by itself was not lethal) had increased mortality up to 70%. Animals that received 2.5 Gy of radiation in combination with an LD_{50} burn had mortality approaching 95%. Those that received an LD_{50} burn and an LD_{20} irradiation with 5.0 Gy showed 100% mortality. Thus, radiation combines synergistically with either burn or blast injuries to increase lethality.[1]

REFERENCE

1. Alpen, E. L., and Sheline, G. E. 1954. The combined effects of thermal burns and whole-body X-radiation on survival time and mortality. *Ann. Surg.* 140: 113-118.

Chapter 2

ACUTE RADIATION SYNDROME IN HUMANS

T. JAN CERVENY, Ph.D.,* THOMAS J. MacVITTIE, Ph.D.,** and ROBERT W. YOUNG, Ph.D.***

INTRODUCTION

PATHOPHYSIOLOGICAL SUBSYNDROMES

- Hematopoietic Subsyndrome
- Gastrointestinal Subsyndrome
- Neurovascular Subsyndrome

DETERMINANTS OF RADIATION EFFECTS ON HUMANS

- Lethality Curve
- Modification of Dose-Response Curve
- Influence of Radiation Quality and Exposure Geometry on LD_{50}
- Influence of Trauma on LD_{50}
- Effect of Clinical-Support Therapy on LD_{50} Dose-Effect Curve
- Exposure Geometry: Heterogeneous Partial-Body and Nonuniform Exposure
- Considerations on Establishing the Human LD_{50}
  - *Radiotherapy*
  - *Radiation Accidents*

PRESENT VIEW OF RADIATION EFFECTS ON HUMANS

*Major, United States Air Force; Program Manager, Bioenvironmental Hazards, Air Force Office of Scientific Research, Bolling Air Force Base, Washington, D.C. 20332-6448
**Chairman, Experimental Hematology, Armed Forces Radiobiology Research Institute, Bethesda, Maryland 20814-5145
***Human Response Program Manager, Radiation Policy Division, Defense Nuclear Agency, 6801 Telegraph Road, Alexandria, Virginia 22310-3398

INTRODUCTION

The importance of human sensitivity to ionizing radiation was recognized even before the detonation of the first nuclear weapon. However, the exact relationship of dose to human mortality is still not precisely known because clear human data are lacking, and analyses of human mortality have been based primarily on data from radiation accidents, radiation therapy patients, and atomic-bomb victims. These studies have been faulted because of the small numbers of subjects, imprecise dosimetry, or patients' pre-existing health problems and treatments. Therefore, many studies with laboratory animals have been undertaken in an effort to define the relationship between radiation exposures and effects. Several comprehensive analyses of human data and animal data have been conducted in an effort to derive a dose-response for humans.

Information on humans and animals has made it possible to describe the symptomatology associated with the acute radiation syndrome (ARS). In humans, ARS is defined as the symptoms manifested after exposure to ionizing radiation, and is often called radiation sickness. From a physiological standpoint, ARS is a combination of subsyndromes. They appear in stages and are directly related to the level of radiation received (Figure 2-1). These subsyndromes begin to occur within hours after exposure and may last for several weeks.

PATHOPHYSIOLOGICAL SUBSYNDROMES

Radiation damage results from the sensitivity of cells to radiation, and those that replicate most rapidly are the most sensitive to radiation exposure. In descending order of sensitivity, these cell types are spermatogonia; lymphocytes; erythroblasts; other hematopoietic cells; cells of the small intestine, stomach, colon, epithelium, skin, CNS, muscle, and bone; and the protein collagen. Mature cells that are more highly differentiated appear to be the least affected by radiation. This difference in cell sensitivity is the basis for the distinction among the three subsyndromes of ARS.

In order of their occurrence with increasing doses of radiation, ARS is divided into hematopoetic, gastrointestinal, and neurovascular subsyndromes.

Each subsyndrome can be further divided into four stages: *prodromal, latent, manifest illness*, and *recovery*. Prodromal symptoms begin a few hours to 4 days after exposure. The severity, time of onset, and duration of symptoms relate directly to the exposure dose received. The latent period is a brief reprieve from symptoms, when the patient may appear to have recovered. This reprieve may last up to 4 weeks, depending on the dose, and then is likely to be followed by 2–3 weeks of manifest illness. The manifest illness stage is the most difficult to manage from a therapeutic standpoint, for this is the maximum state of immunoincompetence that the patient will suffer. If the patient survives the manifest illness stage, recovery is almost assured. Therefore, treatment during the first 6 weeks to 2 months after exposure is crucial to ensure recovery from a rapidly received, high dose (less than 5 Gy) of ionizing radiation.

Hematopoietic Subsyndrome

The target cells of the hematopoietic tissue are the stem cells. Their anatomical location in the bone marrow distributes them throughout the body. Dorsal exposure would maximize damage to the hematopoietic system, because the greatest percentage of active bone marrow lies in the spine and dorsal regions of the ribs and pelvis. Vertical exposure would be the least damaging per equivalent dose, due to absorption and consequent nonuniform dose distribution, thus sparing the dorsal marrow. A dose-dependent suppression of bone marrow may lead to marrow atrophy and pancytopenia. Prompt radiation doses of about 1–8 Gy cause significant damage to the bone marrow. Doses of approximately 3 Gy may result in death to 50% of exposed persons.[1] The biological response of bone-marrow stem and progenitor cells to radiation exposure is exponential in nature. For ex-

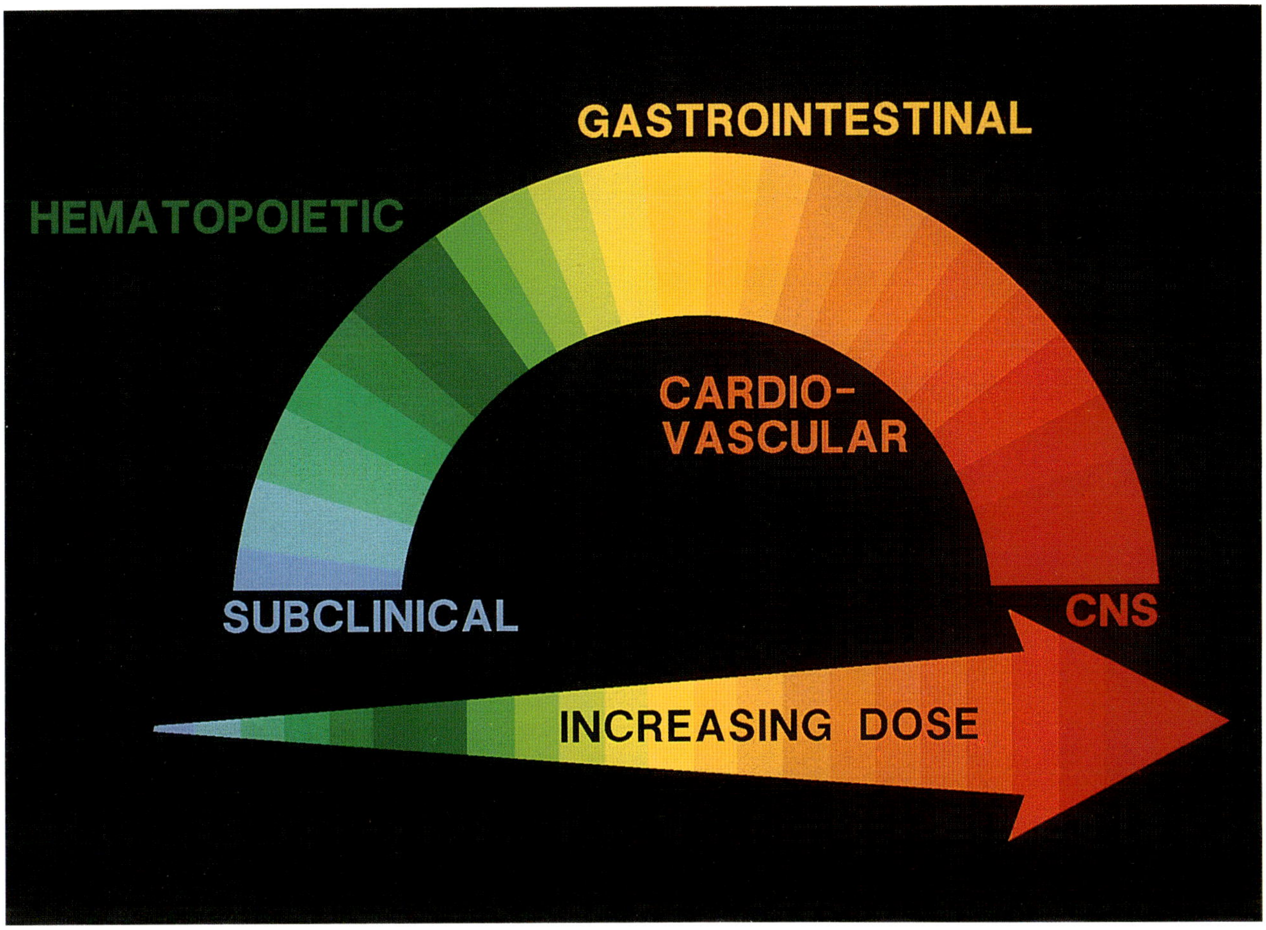

Fig. 2-1. Increasing severity of radiation effects with increasing dose. (Label for each radiation effect is color-coded to dose range [on arc] producing that effect.)

ample, halving the dose received does not increase the survival of stem cells from 1% to 50%, but to only 10%. Therefore, shielding remains the best protection of bone marrow.

Prodromal symptoms may include nausea, vomiting, anorexia, and diarrhea. If severe diarrhea occurs during the first 2 days, the radiation dose may have been lethal. The hematopoietic prodrome may last up to 3 days. This is followed by about 3 weeks of latency, during which the patient will suffer from significant fatigue and weakness. The clinical symptoms of manifest illness appear 21–30 days after exposure, and may last up to 2 weeks. Severe hemorrhage from platelet loss and infection associated with pancytopenia from bone-marrow suppression are the lethal factors in the hematopoietic subsyndrome. Platelet counts of fewer than 20,000/mm^3 (hemocytometer counting chamber), decreased erythrocyte counts, and severely suppressed white cell counts (fewer than 1,000) may be seen. Clinical hematological studies (complete blood count with platelets) may follow a course similar to that shown in Figure 2-2. There is a progressive decrease in peripheral cellular elements with increasing radiation dose. Specifically, a 50% decrease of absolute lymphocytes within the first 24 hours, followed by a second drop within 48 hours, is pathognomonic of potentially lethal injury from penetrating ionizing radiation.

The nuclear accident in Chernobyl provided information indicating that the total hematological profile must be used in predicting the radiation dose.[2] As shown in Figure 2-2, the systemic granulocyte count will increase at varying times after exposure, and may result from increased chemotaxis due to cell damage after irradiation. This transient increase may provide a false low interpretation of dose, and therefore should not be used as the sole indicator of dose received. However, a lowered granulocyte count may indicate the beginning of an immunocompromised state, which will likely be followed by the onset of fever and possi-

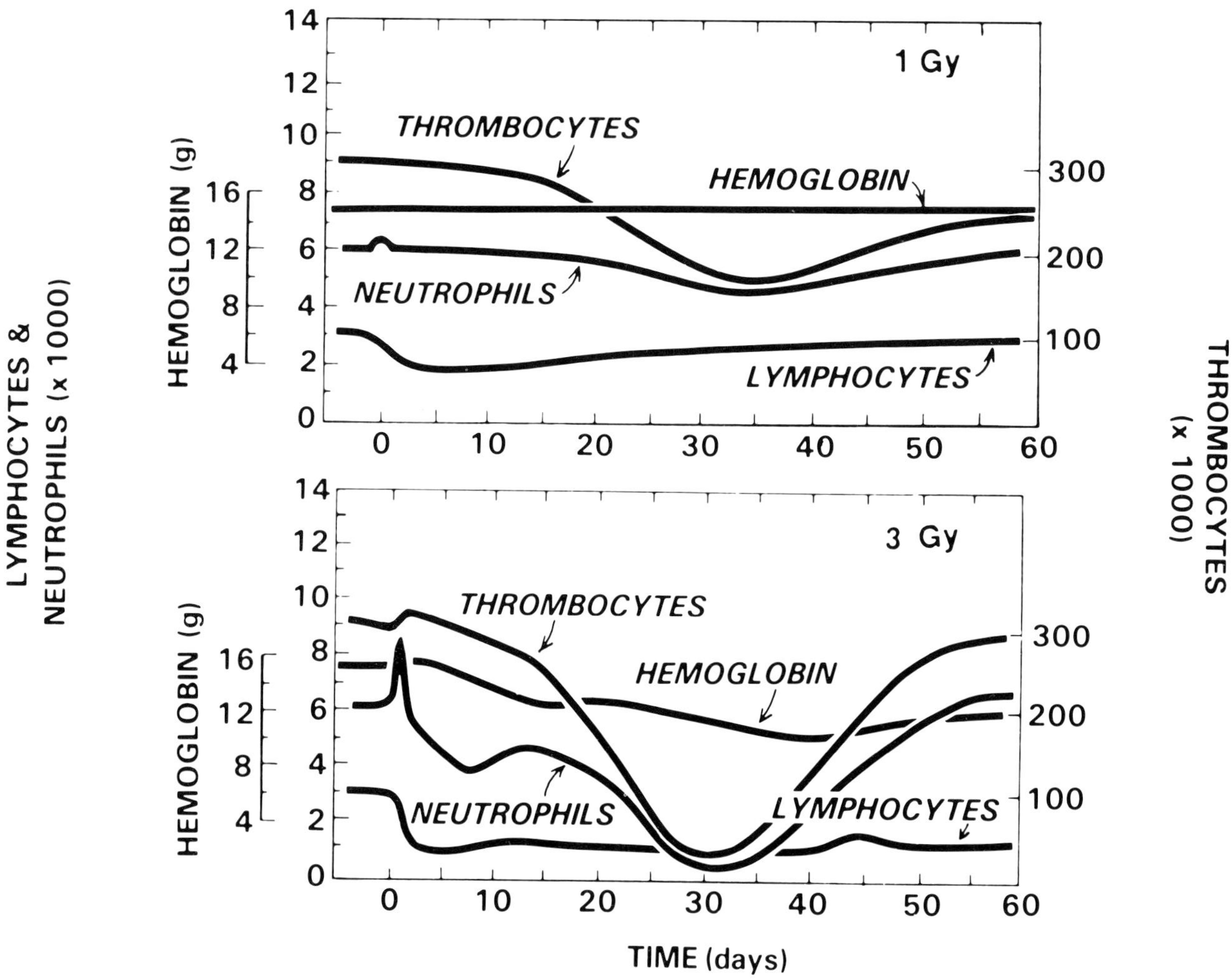

Fig. 2-2. Hematological response to whole-body exposure. Comparison of 1-Gy and 3-Gy gamma-radiation effects on hematopoietic system.

bly severe infection.

Overall, the systemic effects that can occur from the hematopoietic subsyndrome include immunodysfunction, increased infectious complications, hemorrhage, anemia, and impaired wound healing. Impaired wound healing may be due in part to endothelial damage, which significantly depresses the revascularization of injured tissue.[3]

Gastrointestinal Subsyndrome

The gastrointestinal subsyndrome overlaps the hematopoietic subsyndrome, but its consequences are more immediate. At radiation doses above 12 Gy, this subsyndrome supersedes the hematopoietic subsyndrome in lethality. Its prodromal stage includes severe nausea, vomiting, watery diarrhea, and cramps occurring within hours after irradiation, followed by a much shorter asymptomatic latent period of 5–7 days. Then the manifest illness begins, with vomiting and severe diarrhea accompanied by fever. At higher doses, bloody diarrhea, shock, and death may ensue.

The intestinal mucosa suffers severe pathological damage following radiation exposure. The turnover time of 3–5 days for intestinal mucosal epithelial cells explains the shortened latent period. Since severely damaged crypt stem cells do not divide, the aging mucosal lining is shed and not replaced. This results in loss of absorption and provides a portal for intestinal flora to enter the systemic circulation. Figure 2-3 depicts vascular coalescence, which also significantly decreases intestinal absorption abilities. Severe mucosal hemorrhage has been seen in experimental animal models (Figures 2-4 and 2-5). The overall intestinal pathology includes

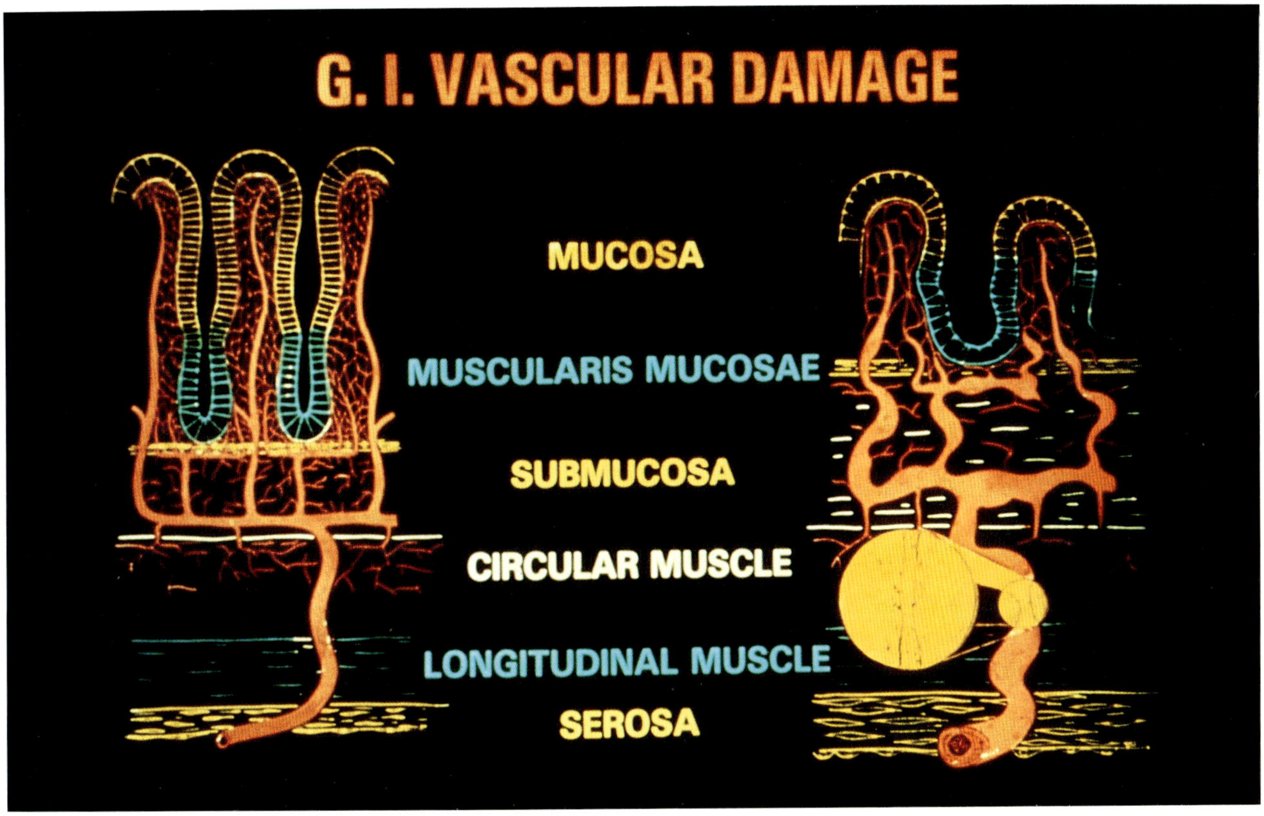

Fig. 2-3. Normal intestinal tissue (left) and irradiated intestinal tissue (right). Dramatic changes are manifested by loss of mucosal lining, damage to crypt cells, and coalescence of capillary networks into large cisternae. (Label for each layer of tissue is color-coded to its portion of each illustration.)

disturbance of absorption and secretion, glycocalyx disruption, mucosal ulceration, alteration of enteric flora, depletion of gut lymphoid tissue, and motility disturbances.[4]

Systemic effects of this subsyndrome may include malnutrition resulting from malabsorption; vomiting and abdominal distension from paralytic ileus; dehydration, acute renal failure, and cardiovascular collapse from shifts in fluids and electrolytes; anemia from gastrointestinal bleeding; and sepsis from damaged intestinal lining.

Neurovascular Subsyndrome

This subsyndrome is difficult to define. The lethal dose is over 30 Gy, but there is little information on these doses for human exposure, and the causes of death are confusing.[1,3,5] Cardiovascular shock accompanies such high doses, resulting in a massive loss of serum and electrolytes through leakage into extravascular tissues. The ensuing circulatory problems of edema, increased intracranial pressure, and cerebral anoxia can bring death within 2 days.

The stages of the neurovascular subsyndrome are extremely compressed. The prodromal period may include a burning sensation that occurs within minutes, nausea and vomiting that occur within 1 hour, and confusion, prostration, and loss of balance. During the latent period, apparent improvement for a few hours is likely to be followed by severe manifest illness. Within 5–6 hours, the overt clinical picture proceeds with the return of severe watery diarrhea, respiratory distress, and gross CNS signs. After receiving doses in this range, two victims of separate uranium or plutonium recovery accidents survived fewer than 48 hours, even though they received optimal life support in excellent care facilities.

The pathology of this subsyndrome may be due to massive damage of the microcirculation. This has been postulated as a causative mechanism in the damage of some organs. Preliminary experimental evidence indicates that the cause of initial hypotension may be an early, overwhelming surge of histamine released from degranulated mast cells.[5,6] In fact, animal models did not suffer this hypotension when pretreated with histamine (H_1)

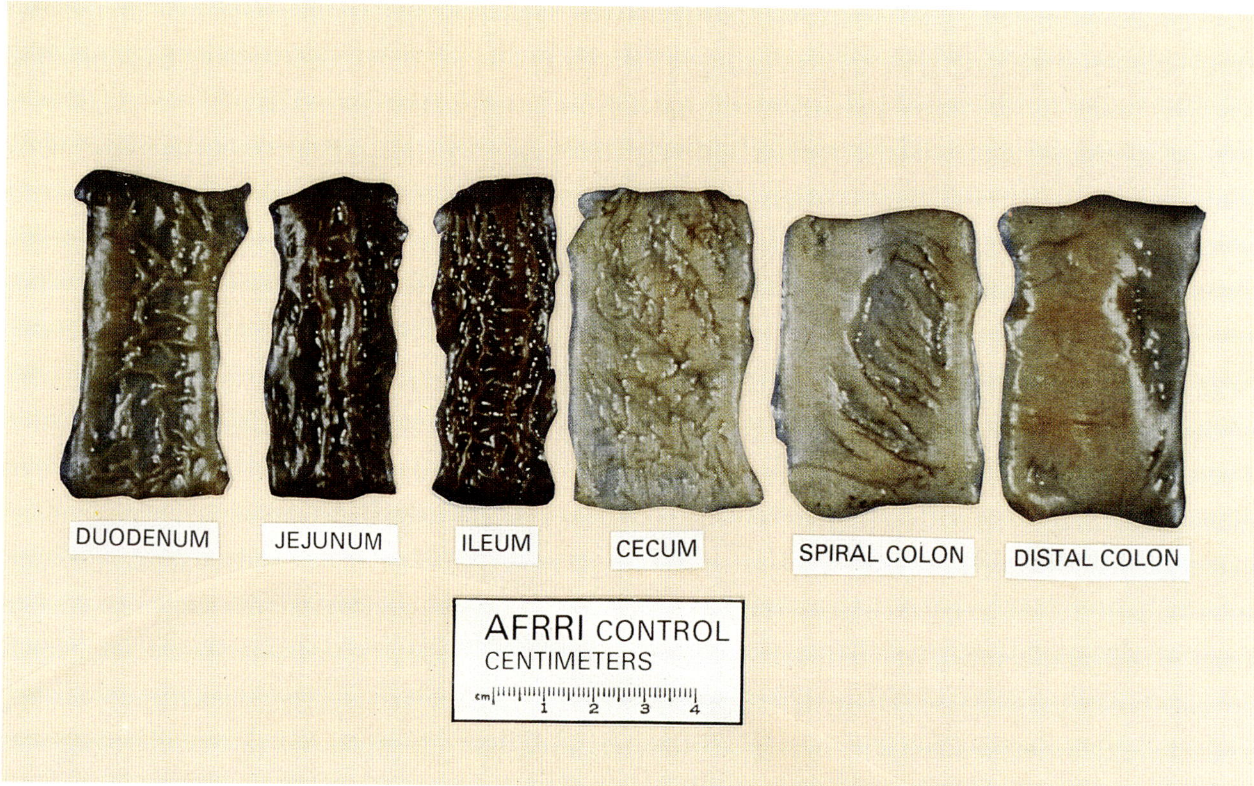

Fig. 2-4. Porcine intestinal segments from normal animals. Normal tissue appears pink to gray.

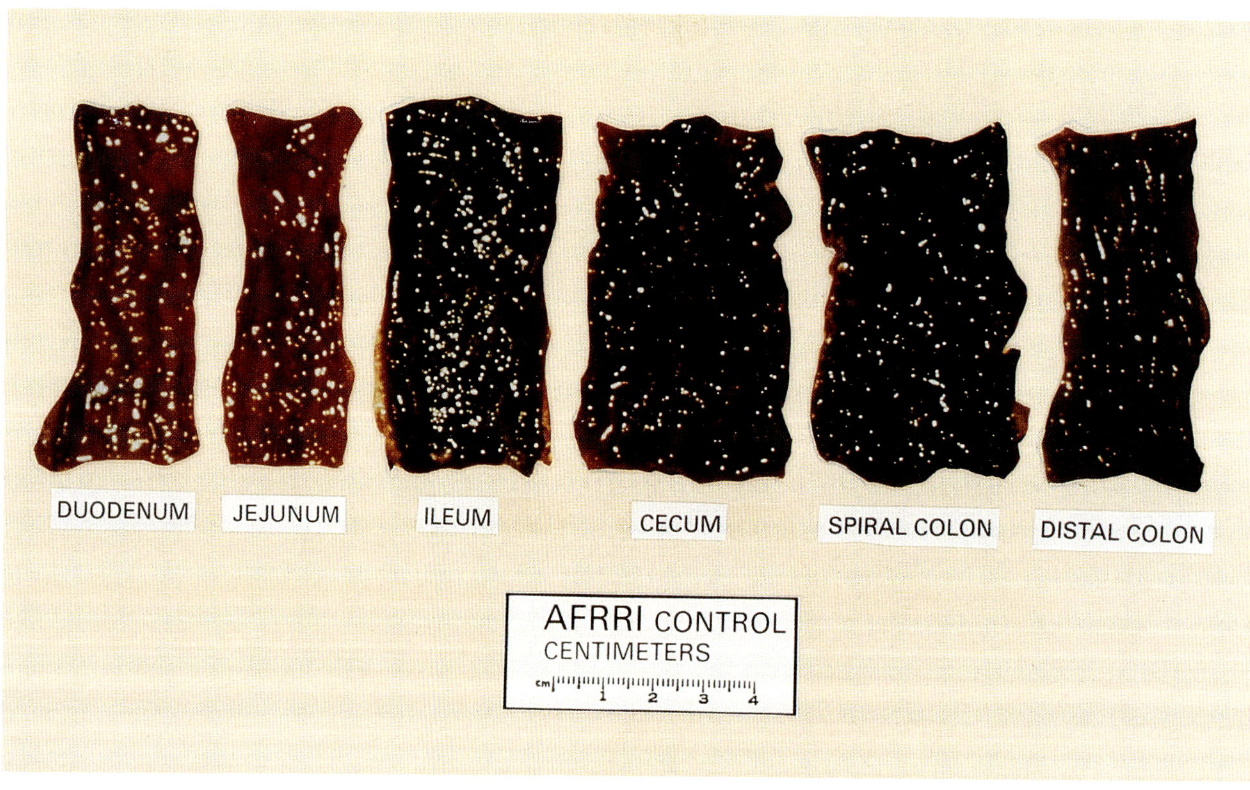

Fig. 2-5. Porcine intestinal segments from 4-Gy-irradiated animals. Irradiated tissues from all segments show signs of severe hemorrhage and ulceration.

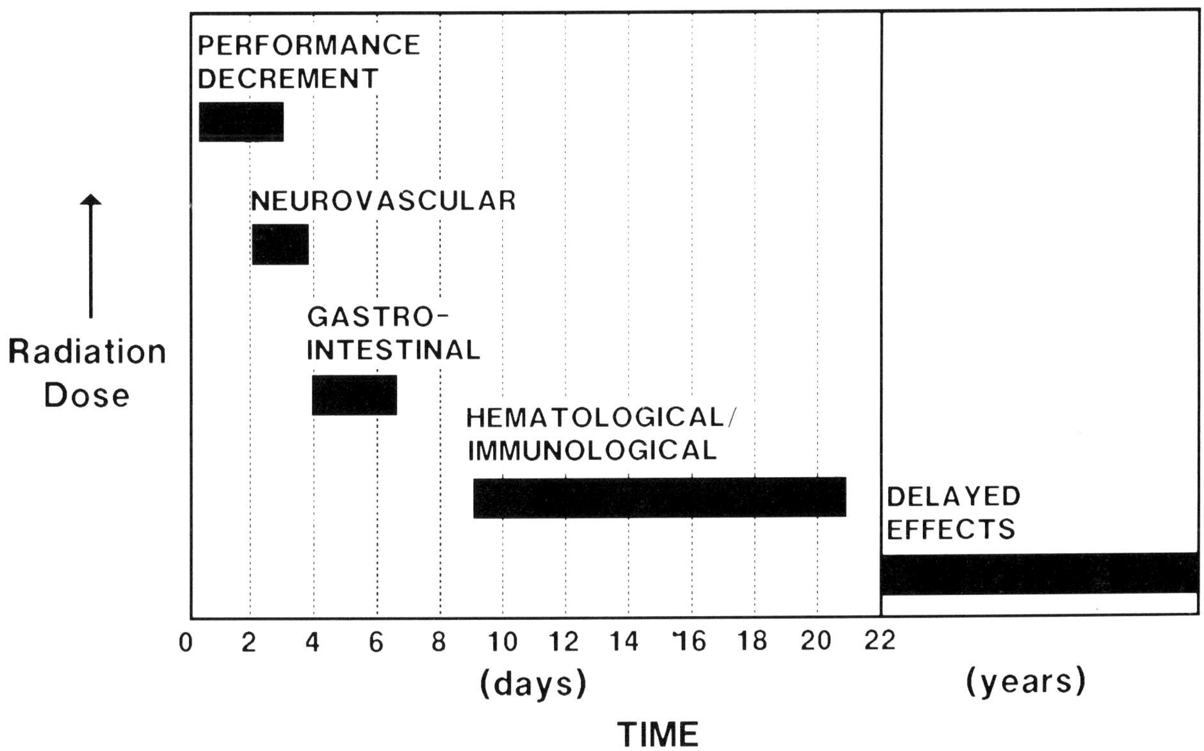

Fig. 2-6. Occurrence of radiation effects in relation to dose and time. As radiation dose increases, time to manifestation of effect decreases.

blockers.[7,8]

The radiation threshold for this dual subsyndrome is not as well defined as it is for the others. Experimental evidence indicates that 50 Gy will elicit the neurovascular subsyndrome. Whether the dose is 50 or 100 Gy is inconsequential; either is a supralethal dose resulting in severe performance decrement. Figure 2-6 shows the occurrence of radiation effects in relation to dose and time. Table 2-1 charts the pathophysiological events.

DETERMINANTS OF RADIATION EFFECTS ON HUMANS

Energy deposition, known as *linear energy transfer* (LET), can be correlated to the severity of damage to the tissue. Gamma and X rays, which are primarily responsible for ARS, pass through tissue almost unimpeded by the skin or protective clothing. Thick shielding (such as lead, concrete, or dirt) is required to protect a person from these radiations. These rays are called *low LET* because they do not leave a great deal of their energy behind. Exposure to gamma emitters (such as cobalt-60) results in an accumulation of the dose within the first few centimeters of tissue, followed by a gradual decline of the dose level to 50% at the radiation's exit from the body. In contrast, *high-LET* neutron exposure results in significant absorption of energy within the first few centimeters, with diminution of dose at increasing tissue depth. In these cases, unilateral radiation results in more uniform exposure with gamma than with neutron radiation. Bilateral or multilateral exposure increases the uniformity of dose in all cases.

Alpha and most beta particles have low energy levels and cannot pass through skin (high-energy beta excepted) or clothing. Therefore, internalization (ingestion, inhalation, or absorption through a wound) and systemic contamination with alpha or

TABLE 2-1

PATHOPHYSIOLOGICAL EVENTS OF ACUTE RADIATION SYNDROME

	Pathophysiological Events		
Dose Range (Gy)	Prodromal Effects	Manifest-Illness Effects	Survival
0.5–1.0	Mild	Slight decrease in blood cell count	Almost certain
1.0–2.0	Mild to Moderate	Early symptoms of bone-marrow damage	Probable (>90%)
2.0–3.5	Moderate	Moderate to severe bone-marrow damage	Possible**
3.5–5.5	Severe	Severe bone-marrow damage; slight intestinal damage	Death within 3.5–6.0 weeks†
5.5–7.5	Severe	Bone-marrow pancytopenia and moderate intestinal damage	Death within 2–3 weeks
7.5–10.0	Severe	Combined gastrointestinal and bone-marrow damage; hypotension	Death within 1.0–2.5 weeks
10.0–20.0	Severe gastrointestinal damage; upper half of range: ETI;* gastrointestinal death		Death within 5–12 days
20.0–30.0	Gastrointestinal and cardiovascular damage		Death within 2–5 days

*Early Transient Incapacitation

**Top third of range: $LD_{50/60}$
Middle third: $LD_{10/60}$
Bottom third: $LD_{5/60}$

†Top half: $LD_{99/60}$
Bottom half: $LD_{90/60}$

Source: Data from reference 1.

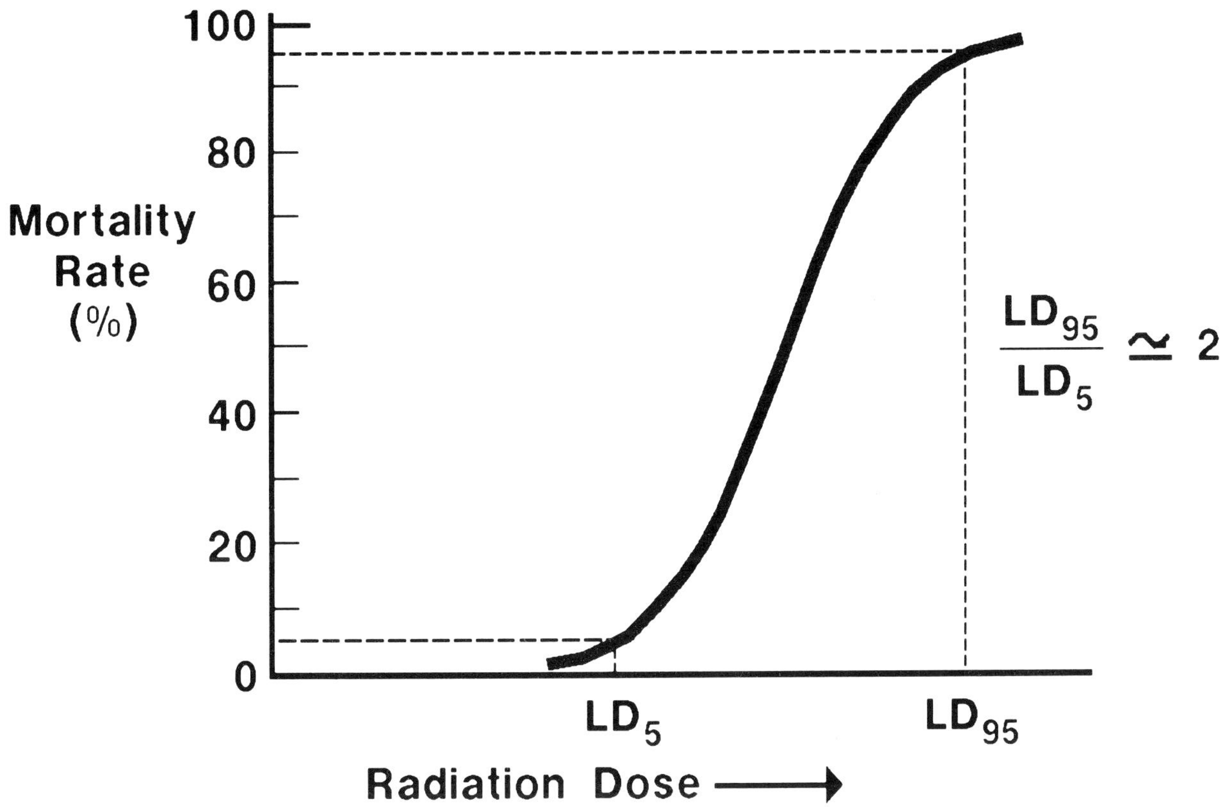

Fig. 2-7. Standard dose-response curve

beta radionuclides must occur for these radioactive particles to cause problems. Once internalized, they are a significant threat, because almost all of their energy is deposited in a short path through tissue or even in a single cell.

Lethality Curve

The slope of a lethality curve is weighted heavily by data at each extreme of its distribution. In the majority of experimental cases, the ratio of the data points is less than 2, independent of species (Figure 2-7). The more inbred and homogenous the population, the steeper the slope. This fact underscores the importance of reliable dosimetry, not only in the experimental situation but also in accurately determining the human exposure doses after a nuclear accident. In a recent examination, this correlation of a steep dose-effect relationship (slope) was evaluated using available data from canine studies.[9] Purebred and inbred populations did not appear to be either more sensitive or more resistant than mongrels. Given the genetic heterogeneity of humans, this ratio has been useful in extrapolating from animal data to the human dose-response curve, and in defining a lethal dose of radiation that will kill 50% of the healthy, untreated, exposed personnel (the LD_{50}) within 30 to 60 days after exposure. In spite of the heterogeneity surrounding LD_{50} values, it "seems possible to conclude that the doses giving between 90%–95% mortality in most animal experiments are about twice those giving 5%–10% mortality."[10] In a recent review of animal data, a uniform dose normalized to the LD_{50} (D/LD_{50}) revealed that no deaths occurred when D/LD_{50} was less than 0.54.[11] When D/LD_{50} was greater than 1.3, mortality was 100%. Total survival in a population can apparently be changed to total mortality by increasing the dose by a factor of 2.4. Relationships between dose and lethality, drawn from a large number of animal studies, emphasize two important points on extrapolation to the human radiation response: *(a)* reliable dosimetry is extremely valuable, and *(b)* either therapy or trauma can significantly shift the dose-response relationship. An error in dosimetry of 0.5–1.0 Gy can result in large shifts along the dose-response curve, and effective therapy can increase the LD_{50} by approximately 1.0

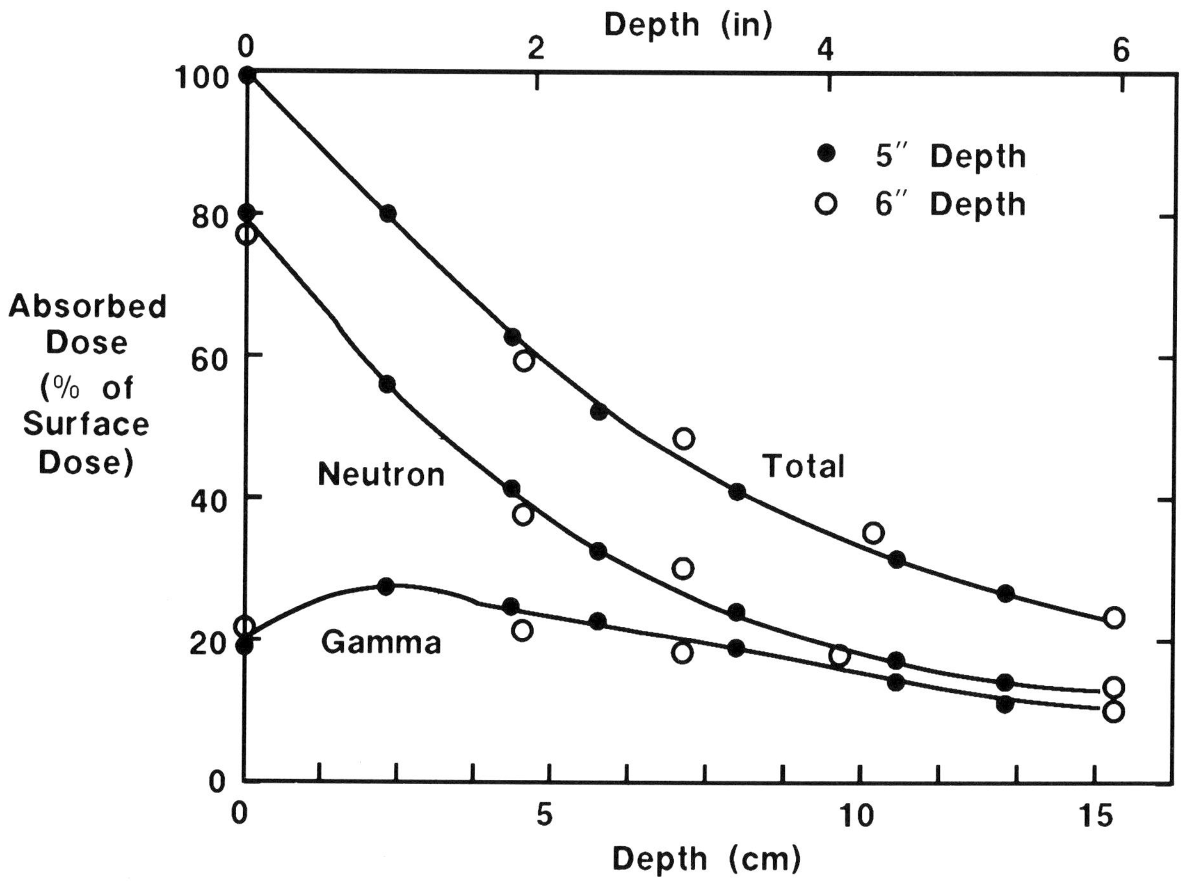

Fig. 2-8. Depth-dose relationship in phantoms. Effect of tissue depth on absorbed radiation dose from unilateral mixed-fission gamma and 1-MeV neutron radiations. Low-LET, high-energy gamma radiation produces a more uniform exposure than does fission neutron radiation.

Gy. The degree of trauma depends on the duration and intensity of the radiation exposure, and it can shift along the mortality curve.

Modification of Dose-Response Curve

Radiation lethality may be a consequence of changes in the cellular kinetics of renewal systems critical for survival.[12,13] If this is correct, then modification of the dose-response relationship is achievable by replacement of the mature functional cells or their essential factors, or by actual substitutions in the damaged cell-renewal system.

Factors that compromise or damage the hematopoietic system or the immune system will also negatively affect the dose-response curve. Severe trauma, poor nutritional status, and stress are in this category. Other factors that significantly modify the dose-effect curve are radiation quality, exposure geometry (such as partial-body exposure or nonuniform exposure), and dose rate.

Influence of Radiation Quality and Exposure Geometry on LD_{50}

Distribution of radiation dose (energy deposition) throughout the target tissue varies significantly with the energy and quality of radiation and with the geometry of the exposure. Figure 2-8 illustrates the effects of tissue depth on absorbed radiation dose from unilateral cobalt-60 and 1 MeV (million electron-volts) of mixed neutron-gamma radiations. To reconstruct the effects of an accidental exposure involving neutrons, we must consider the tissue depth of a large-animal model (such as the canine) and that of humans, relative to the absorption characteristics of these two different radiation types (gamma and neutron, 1 MeV).

Equivalent doses of different types of radiation, or of the same type at different energy levels, do not produce equivalent biological effects. However, the *relative biological effectiveness* (RBE) of two types of radiation can be compared. A significant number of studies establishes the LD_{50} for hematopoietic death in canines at approximately 2.60 Gy for 1,000 kVp (plate voltage in kiloelectron-volts) of cobalt-60 radiation, or 2,000 kVp of X radiation. For lower-energy X radiation (50–250 kVp), an average dose of 2.28 Gy would yield this LD_{50}.[14-21] These values suggest an RBE of approximately 0.87 for radiation higher than the standard 250 kVp of X-ray energy. Canine exposure to mixed-fission neutron-gamma radiation yields an LD_{50} value of 1.48 Gy (compared to a derived value of 2.60 Gy for cobalt-60).[15] This results in an RBE of approximately 1.7. Using a neutron spectrum of similar energy, an LD_{50} of 2.03 Gy (compared to 2.80 Gy for 1 MVp of X radiation) was determined to have an RBE value of 1.38.[22] An RBE value of approximately 2.0 has been reported for rhesus monkeys exposed to fission neutrons of 1 MeV energy (the LD_{50} value was 2.60 Gy) and for X radiation of 300 kVp energy (the LD_{50} value was 5.25 Gy).[23] A significant RBE has been observed in the rhesus (LD_{50}) using gamma-neutron exposure, compared to the RBE for 250 kVp of X radiation.[24,25] Several studies used mice to establish RBE values for fission and high-energy neutrons pertaining to X radiation and cobalt-60 radiation.[25-28]

A radiation dose delivered to hematopoeitic stem cells in bone marrow is the most damaging to the organism. Therefore, unilateral exposure with either gamma or neutron radiation will result in nonuniform dose distribution, whereas bilateral or rotational whole-body neutron exposure will have a greater RBE. Unilateral exposure usually occurs in accidents or warfare. Exposure to any type of unilateral radiation can result in lower doses to stem-cell populations that are distant from the source, with a consequent rise in the LD_{50}value (Table 2-2).

Influence of Trauma on LD_{50}

The combination of radiation exposure and trauma produces a set of circumstances not encountered by most military and civilian physicians. In combined injury, two (or more) injuries that are sublethal or minimally lethal when occurring alone will act synergistically, resulting in much greater mortality than the simple sum of both injuries would have produced. The mechanisms responsible for combined-injury sequelae are unknown, but they can significantly increase the consequences of radiation exposure across the entire dose-response curve. It must be emphasized that the survival of a patient following exposure in the hematopoietic dose range requires *(a)* a minimum critical number of surviving stem cells to regenerate a competent host defense system, *(b)* the functional competence of surviving cells composing the specific and nonspecific immune system, or *(c)* effective replacement or substitution therapy during the critical postexposure cytopenic phase. Trauma alone, depending on its intensity, may effectively depress host resistance to infection.[29-35] When imposed on a radiation-injured system, it can be lethal. In most instances, trauma symptoms will either mask or exacerbate the first reliable signs of radiation injury. This will cloud the situation if one is relying on biological dosimetry and prodromal symptoms for estimation of dose. In addition, the choice of treatment in these cases should include consideration of not only the patient's initial status but also the condition that will exist 7–21 days later when the radiation effects are seen.

Relatively few animal models of combined injury are available for determining effective therapy. The few reported studies demonstrate the synergistic effect of combined injuries. Sheep were exposed to 4 Gy of mixed neutron-gamma radiation and then 1 hour later subjected to an abrupt overpressure; this resulted in increased mortality from 25% for irradiated-only animals to 50% for the combined-injury animals.[36] A rat model showed a synergistic effect when a 250-kVp X-ray dose (LD_{50}) was followed in 7 days by a low-lethal (5%) level of air blast.[37] Mortality increased from approximately 46% for the irradiated-only animals to 76% for the combined-injury animals, and was related to radiation-induced thrombocytopenia, which compromised normal coagulation and maintenance of the capillary endothelium.

An open skin wound (combined injury) markedly increases the chances of infection. The immediate closure of wounds has been recommended.[38] Mortality in mice from exposure to 5.1 Gy of gamma radiation alone rose from 25% to 90% when combined with open dorsal skin wounds occurring 2 days after exposure. If wounds were immedi-

TABLE 2-2

MODIFICATION OF LETHAL DOSE ACCORDING TO LATERALITY OF EXPOSURE*

Factor		Dog	Sheep	Pig
Body Mass (kg)		7–13	32–57	62 (average)
Radiation		X rays (1 MeV)	X rays (1 MeV)	X rays (2 MeV)
LD_{50} Mean ± SE		(Roentgen at midplane of exposure volume in absence of animal)		
	Unilateral Exposure (UE)	386 ± 10	303 ± 13	434 ± 13
	Bilateral Exposure (BE)	321 ± 9	252 ± 17	362 ± 13
	Difference (UE - BE)	65	51	72
	Ratio (UE /BE)	1.20	1.20	1.20

*A unilateral exposure from any radiation type may result in the sparing of distant stem-cell populations, thereby raising the LD_{50}.

ately closed, mortality decreased to 18%. Closing of the skin wound obviously affected the mechanism of pathogenesis.

In combined injuries, burns produce the most significant synergistic increases in mortality. The dog, pig, rat, and guinea pig have been studied as animal models.[34,39-43] Table 2-3 summarizes this synergistic effect on the lethality of combined radiation and trauma. As little as 0.25 Gy, combined with a burn of 20% body surface area, increased mortality in dogs from 12% to 20%.[43]

In the early 1980s, investigators performed the most comprehensive analysis to date of the effect of combined injury (thermal and skin wound) on lethality and on the suppression of host resistance to subsequent bacterial challenge.[44,45] In addition, they used cobalt-60 gamma versus mixed-fission neutron-gamma radiations in various ratios of LD_{50} on mice that had either thermal injuries or skin wounds. The addition of fission-energy neutrons to gamma radiation significantly lowered the LD_{50} in radiation-only experiments to give RBE values as high as 2.5. The addition of trauma to radiation exposures also significantly reduced the LD_{50}. The effect of combined injury on lethality was dominated by radiation. The RBE did not change with the addition of trauma.

Injuries to the abdomen may present significant problems to the irradiated subject. Blast overpressure, blunt trauma, and penetrating trauma are all significant causes of abdominal injury. The impact of laparotomy or splenectomy in mice that had received whole-body radiation has been evaluated.[38] Exposure to 5.1 Gy alone caused mortality of 27%, whereas laparotomy or splenectomy alone caused an approximate 5% mortality. Splenectomy at 2, 4, or 8 days after irradiation increased the mortality to 60%, 75%, and 85%, respectively. Laparotomy combined with radiation caused maximum mortality when surgery was performed on day 8. The role of the spleen in nonspecific resistance to bacterial infection has recently been demonstrated.[46]

The impact of combined injuries on the radiation dose-effect curve depends on the intensity and the

TABLE 2-3

COMBINED EFFECTS OF WHOLE-BODY RADIATION AND BURNS ON VARIOUS ANIMAL MODELS*

Subjects	Percent Lethality
Dog	
20% burns	12
100 R exposure	0
20% burns + 100 R	73
Pig	
10%–15% burns	0
400 R exposure	20
10%–15% burns + 400 R	90
Rat	
31%–35% burns	50
250 R exposure	0
500 R exposure	20
15%–31% burns + 100 R	65
31%–35% burns + 250 R	95
31%–35% burns + 500 R	100
Guinea Pig	
1.5% burns	9
250 R exposure	11
1.5% burns + 250 R	38

*Significant increases in mortality occur when radiation is superimposed on concomitant conventional trauma.

time of injury relative to radiation exposure.[47,48] The biological consequences of these combined injuries will significantly affect the patient's abilities to survive and recover, and will markedly increase the casualty burden on medical personnel. Those patients in Hiroshima and Nagasaki who suffered conventional trauma along with radiation exposure developed significant complications 2–3 weeks later, corresponding to the time of hematopoietic depression. Until the 1986 reactor disaster in Chernobyl, the victims of Hiroshima and Nagasaki provided the only documentation on human radiation injuries and associated trauma. Hospitalized Chernobyl victims also experienced medical complications associated with bone-marrow damage and immunosuppression.

Effect of Clinical-Support Therapy on LD_{50} Dose-Effect Curve

Modification of survival throughout the LD_{50} dose range is achievable using a simple regimen of clinical support to replace or substitute the depleted functional cells after stem-cell destruction. In the cases of large-animal models (monkey, canine, and swine) and the human, therapy is directed at replacing the functions of the granulocytes and platelets. Experimental work performed more than 20 years ago showed the efficacy of supportive care centered on systemic antibiotics and transfusions of fresh platelets. Several canine studies indicated that antibiotics, singly or in combination, were successful in reducing mortality in the LD_{50} range.[18,49-51] Combination antibiotics, in conjunction with fresh whole-blood transfusions and parenteral fluids, have been effective in controlling dehydration and thereby reducing mortality. Reports that hemorrhage is easier to control than infection may be traced to the fact that several types of opportunistic pathogens are capable of overwhelming a compromised host.[18]

In an attempt to determine the lowest dose at which spontaneous regeneration would not occur, the dose range was extended in a later animal study from 4.0 to 5.5 Gy, well into 100% lethality (LD_{100}). The dose of 4.2 Gy resulted in an LD_{100}. Survival was significantly increased with good clinical support. This support consisted of *(a)* several antibiotics (penicillin G, dihydrostreptomycin, and tetracycline) administered at the onset of fever (8–13 days after exposure) and continued until fever subsided for 3–4 days and white cell count was greater than $1,000/mm^3$; *(b)* the infusion of fresh platelet-rich plasma from 50 ml of blood, given when blood platelet levels were below $5,000/mm^3$ (10–12 days after exposure); and *(c)* fluid therapy (isotonic saline or 5% dextrose) given during the period of anorexia. Soft food was usually given during this period to entice the animals to eat. The success with these regimens supports the hypothesis that infection and hemorrhage are the main contributors to lethal consequences of radiation exposure in the hematopoietic subsyndrome range. Controlling infection during the critical granulocytopenic and thrombocytopenic phase is the limiting factor in successful treatment.[49,51]

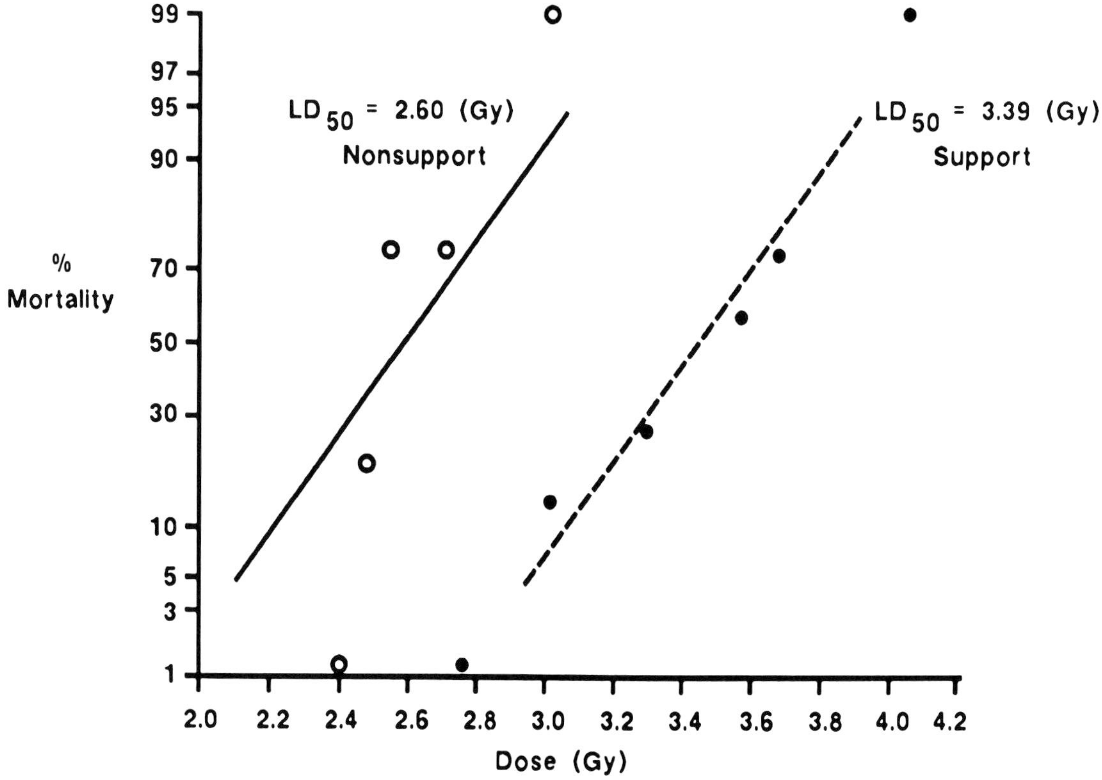

Fig. 2-9. Effect of clinical support therapy on LD_{50}. Parenteral fluids, platelets, and antibiotics to control infection during critical nadirs in granulocyte and platelet counts provide the basis for successful treatment.

These studies have been extended over a dose range that is capable of determining the shift in LD_{50} that is due to treatment. Figure 2-9 shows the shift in the canine LD_{50} from 2.60 Gy to approximately 3.39 Gy measured as midline tissue dose. This results in a dose reduction factor of 1.3. The treatment regimen was essentially the same as above, with the addition of the newer antibiotics, gentamicin and claforan (cephotaxime-SO_4).[15] These collective data indicate that modest clinical care consisting of the infusion of fluids, antibiotics, and fresh platelets is capable of shifting the LD_{50} by a factor of 1.5. A more intensive regimen of support, including use of a sterile barrier and selective decontamination of intestinal bacteria, should allow an even greater shift in the LD_{50}. It must be emphasized that the practical application of these concepts requires that the damage to the stem-cell system be reversible; that is, the surviving fraction of hematopoietic stem cells must be capable of spontaneous regeneration.

Exposure Geometry: Heterogeneous Partial-Body and Nonuniform Exposure

Partial-body exposure can result in death through irradiation of specific target organs, such as the brain, lungs, and gastrointestinal structures. However, significant variations in the hematopoietic subsyndrome and related lethality can be seen when portions of the active marrow are either shielded physically from exposure or receive a smaller radiation dose due to nonuniform dose distribution through the body tissue. The earliest report of a shielding effect on the hematopoietic system was in 1963.[52] Exteriorized spleens of mice were shielded, which increased the LD_{50} from 550 to 975 R (roentgens). It was concluded that the shielded spleen contained competent and mobilizable hematopoietic stem cells that were capable of totally repopulating the depleted marrow space and significantly modifying the hematopoietic subsyndrome's dose-effect relationship. Many later experiments supported this finding by shielding either the hind limbs or tails of mice. A further comparison in mice has been made of the therapeutic efficacy of this autorepopulation versus the efficacy of autologous and/or syngeneic bone-marrow transplantation.[26] In this study, one leg was shielded from lethal total-body exposure, allowing stem cells of the shielded leg to reseed the irradiated marrow space. Another set of mice received a similar exposure with the shielded leg later amputated. The marrow contents were harvested by a grinding technique and then autotransplanted. (The grinding allowed greater efficiency in the stem-cell harvest.) Results indicated that autorepopulation of the marrow was more efficient than marrow transplant.

A series of experiments using canines further illustrated the protective effects of partial-body shielding.[53,54] Large-animal models can not only illustrate the relationships between tissue depth and dose, but can also approximate the nonuniform effects of exposure for more reliable extrapolation to the human radiation response. Shielding the lower body indicated an approximately sevenfold increase in LD_{50}.[54] One report emphasized that considerable hematopoietic tissue may be spared by nonuniform exposures to cobalt-60 gamma radiation.[55] Results indicated that the greater the dose gradient and the more nonuniform the exposure, the greater the survival of stem cells that are capable of repopulation.

These canine experiments illustrate the complexity of determining the dose received during an accidental exposure. Accidental whole-body irradiation will most likely not be strictly unilateral, due to backscatter and reflection of the radiation. It is also possible that some body regions may be shielded. These factors, as well as the anatomical position of the exposed subjects, can either increase or decrease the total dose received. Shielding and nonuniform dose distribution can therefore differ markedly in how much hematopoietic tissue they spare. The biological response of marrow stem and progenitor cells to radiation is exponential in nature.

Considerations on Establishing the Human LD_{50}

Similarly, it is difficult to calculate accurately the dose that a human has received after accidental radiation exposure. Radiation quality or type, dose rate, shielding, exposure geometry, and coincident trauma can significantly modify the relationship of dose and response.

Several comprehensive analyses of human and animal data have been conducted over the years in an effort to derive a dose-response curve for humans. Some reports serve as landmarks, but none has been completely successful. The quest for an LD_{50} for humans began in the late 1940s and continues today.[10,56,57] The most recent activity on this subject has shifted from the United States to the United Kingdom, where interest from the British Home Office produced comprehensive analyses.[10,58,59] The suggestion emerging from these analyses—that the LD_{50} might be as high as 6 Gy (body surface, free-in-air dose)—was controversial in light of the long-held view that the value was 4.5 Gy or less. The 6-Gy free-in-air dose corresponds to an approximately 4.5-Gy bone-marrow dose, and the 4.5-Gy free-in-air dose corresponds to a 3.6-Gy bone-marrow dose. The 1986 LD_{50} value of 1.54 Gy to the bone marrow added to the controversy and sparked new interest in resolving these discrepancies.[59]

Available data on uncomplicated radiation exposures to the human within the hematopoietic-subsyndrome range are relatively limited. The evidence to date (excluding the 1986 nuclear disaster in Chernobyl and the 1987 radiation isotope incident in Goiânia, Brazil) is from three sources: *(a)* twenty cases of radiotherapy with whole-body, bilateral exposure to gamma radiation; *(b)* two nuclear criticality accidents involving mixed neutron-gamma exposure of nine persons, one of whom died; and *(c)* the cases of thousands of persons exposed to the nuclear detonations over Hiroshima and Nagasaki in 1945. The following descriptions of the radiotherapy patients and nuclear criticality patients illustrate the type of information that, until recently, was used in determining the human LD_{50}.

Radiotherapy. Twenty adolescent patients (nineteen with Ewing's sarcoma and one misdiagnosed who actually had leukemia) were uniformly exposed to 3.0 Gy of whole-body cobalt-60 gamma radiation as a midline tissue dose at a dose rate of 0.2 Gy/minute.[60] All patients survived for at least 1 year. It appears that this experience would set the lower limit for the lethal dose at a dose greater than 3.0 Gy. However, several modifying factors must be considered. These patients were given excellent supportive clinical care during their hospital stay. They received fluids, electrolytes, and blood replacement (platelets for some) as necessary, and simple antibiotic treatment while under barrier nursing. It has been recently revealed that many of

TABLE 2-4

ANIMAL-MODEL PREDICTIONS OF LETHAL RADIATION DOSES TO HUMANS*

Lethal Dose	Dose Rate (Gy/minute)					
	0.01	0.02	0.05	0.10	0.20	0.50
LD_5	194	177	156	143	130	115
LD_{10}	210	192	171	157	144	128
LD_{50}	275	257	234	218	204	186
LD_{90}	341	321	297	279	263	243
LD_{95}	360	339	313	295	278	257

*The predictions from the model express the relationship between the dose rate and the LD_{50}.

these patients received local radiation to the sites of the tumors before, and in some cases after, the whole-body exposure. These prior exposures complicate the picture because of possible abscopal effects on distant hematopoietic tissue. It is difficult to determine the effect of hospital-based care and support, but the Chernobyl experience and animal data point to a significant decrease in lethal consequences.

Radiation Accidents. Of many radiation accidents reviewed (Chernobyl excluded), two involved shielding, dose uniformity, and acute exposure (estimated as 2–10 Gy) that were comparable to LD_{50} values in humans. Both accidents were criticality accidents that involved fission neutrons, low-energy photons, and high-energy gamma rays. Four of the seven male workers exposed in the 1958 Y-12 Oak Ridge, Tennessee, accident and five of the workers exposed in the 1958 Vinca, Yugoslavia, accident are considered to have received relevant radiation doses.

Reconstruction of the Y-12 accident dose indicates a total marrow dose range of 3.25–4.40 Gy for upper limits to 1.9–2.6 Gy for lower limits, assuming lateral or anterior-posterior exposure.[10] These workers most likely were exposed to two pulses separated by several seconds. The accident occurred during maintenance operations at a fuel-reprocessing plant. A uranyl nitrate solution was inadvertently allowed to collect, and a fission chain reaction began, followed by a second reaction and perhaps more. The first reaction probably gave the greatest part of the total dose to the workers. Seven persons received 1.0 Gy or more, and of them, four are considered to have received the higher homogeneous doses, which are more relevant.

Nausea and vomiting occurred in three workers within 2 hours after exposure, and one vomited on the second day. Diarrhea was not evident. Some complaints of soreness, fatigue, and weakness were registered. All showed hematological changes reflecting severe marrow damage. Hospital treatment was conservative, and the patients were discharged 39 days after exposure.

At Vinca, the exposure of five persons ranged from a lower limit of 1.8–2.3 Gy to an upper limit of 2.3–3.1 Gy,[10] occurring over several minutes when an unshielded research reactor temporarily ran out of control.[61,62] This led to the emission of a "softer" neutron spectrum than that which occurred in the accident at Y-12. Low-energy neutrons are not very penetrating, but do give rise to a measurable tissue gamma dose. Therefore, a calculation of marrow dose had to be estimated. Although the dose levels at both accidents were similar, the clinical responses of the victims differed significantly.

For the Vinca victims, severe nausea and vomiting occurred within the first hour. A larger dose to the superficial tissues was indicated by erythema, conjunctivitis, and loss of body hair. The most highly irradiated victim suffered severe diarrhea. Victims were nursed under sterile conditions, receiving fluids, electrolytes, blood-cell transfusions, and antibiotics. The hematological picture worsened through the 3 weeks after exposure, and five patients were injected with donor-matched bone-marrow cells at 4–5 weeks after exposure. The value of the marrow transplant is moot. It has been argued that the recipients were on their way to recovery and that the benefits of these transplants were temporary at best. One man, who received the highest dose of radiation, did not respond to treatment; he died of gastrointestinal complications on day 32.

PRESENT VIEW OF RADIATION EFFECTS ON HUMANS

Several new studies relate to the establishment of an LD_{50} for a low-LET radiation dose to the bone marrow of healthy young adults. These studies include several important observations that must be considered when estimating the radiation mortality response of humans. First, in selecting data groups for analysis, the influence of postirradiation clinical treatment must be taken into account. Carefully controlled experiments clearly indicate that treatment will elevate the estimate of the LD_{50} by as much as 30%.[63] The calculated LD_{50} of approximately 6 Gy for the Chernobyl patients treated for ARS also indicates a benefit from intensive clinical support. This observation is reinforced by the fact that many of these patients had complicating burns, which have been shown to lower the LD_{50} in the Nagasaki victims and in studies of laboratory animals. These observations suggest that the British value of 4.5 Gy overestimates the bone-marrow LD_{50} , since this value is derived entirely from persons who received supportive therapy.[60] The data from the Ewing's sarcoma patients in this study seem particularly compromised, because these patients received not only antibiotics and platelets but also barrier nursing and possibly tumor pretreatment with X rays before receiving the 3 Gy of total-body radiation.[60] If this pretreatment with X rays can be confirmed, we must assume that the sensitivity of the patients to subsequent radiation therapy was reduced. These several factors suggest that anchoring the low end of a dose-response curve with these data is not justified.

The second observation to emerge from these new studies is the dependence of LD_{50} on dose rate, particularly at rates of 0.6 Gy/hour or less, as seen in data from human experience and studies with laboratory animals.[11,64] This dependence is particularly important when attempting to use low-dose-rate studies as estimates of prompt LD_{50}. Table 2-4 shows a model for the relationship between dose rate and LD_{50}.[11]

The third observation is that the LD_{50} for the human cannot be modeled on a 70-kg animal. This is true even if the analysis is based on all animal studies to date, if the model is carefully controlled for body weight, and if the dose rate is below 0.5 Gy/minute. The LD_{50} may be more species-independent at prompt dose rates, where data from several large mammals, including humans, appear to converge.[65]

A fourth observation is that although the LD_{50} for the human may not be exactly like that of another 70-kg mammal, the slope derived from the animal model is much more credible than the unacceptably shallow slope observed in the Hiroshima and Nagasaki analyses. These differences in slope may be due to differences in *(a)* the accuracy of dose determination, *(b)* the homogeneity of the sample populations for humans and animals, or *(c)* the postirradiation treatment. With no acceptable slope that can be empirically derived directly from human data, the recommendation is to use the slope obtained from the Oak Ridge National Laboratory animal model (Figure 2-10). The LD_{90} and LD_{10} should be taken as the values for the limits of the dose-response curve because the extrapolations are totally unreliable beyond that range. The slope should be expressed as the ratio of the LD_{90} to the LD_{10}. This expression maintains linearity over the entire curve and has a value of 1.9, which is in good agreement with other such values.[64,65]

The final observation is the degree of agreement

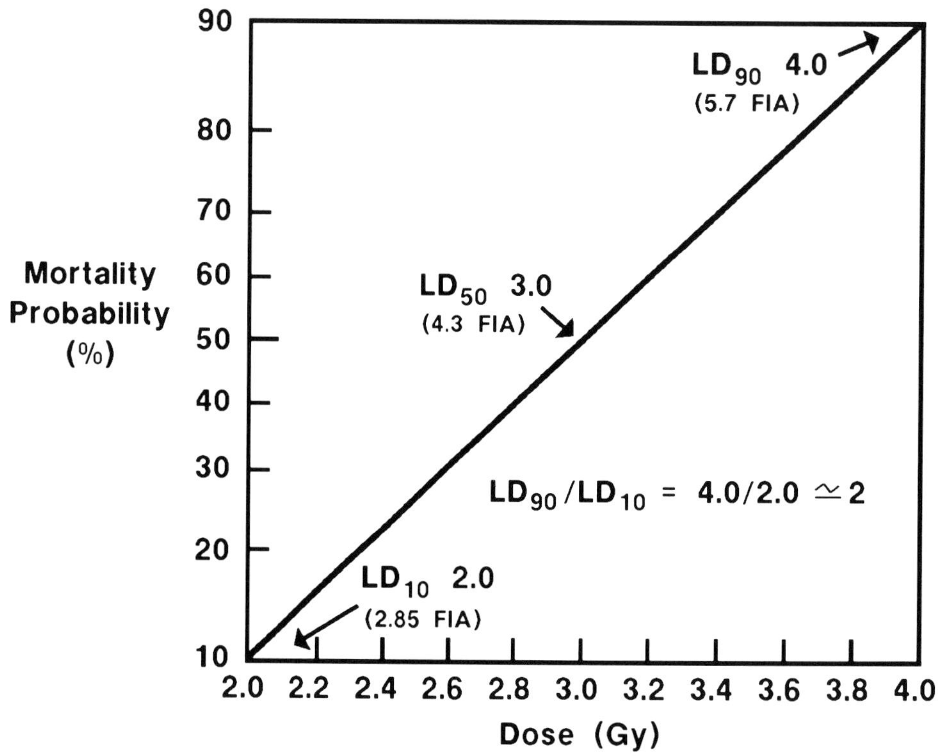

Fig. 2-10. Human mortality for high-dose-rate, low-LET radiation doses to bone marrow. Doses beyond LD_{90} or below LD_{10} cannot be reliably extrapolated. Slope, calculated from this animal model, is expressed as ratio of LD_{90} to LD_{10}.

that is emerging among the values for the LD_{50}, especially from the Hiroshima and Nagasaki data. Recently, a value of 1.54 Gy for the midlethal bone-marrow dose for Hiroshima was published.[59] This value was derived from survey data relating the mortality of persons in wooden houses to their distance from the hypocenter of the bomb. Using preliminary calculations of dose versus ground range, the Hiroshima LD_{50} was determined to be 1.54 Gy.[59] However, if one uses the latest calculations, the value becomes 2.3 Gy to the bone marrow. This value is in general agreement with the reported value of 2.24–2.50 Gy, based on doses and essentially the same model.[66] Both of these values were skewed by the inclusion of data from deaths due to burns and blast effects. If one increases these values by 17.5% (the difference in LD_{50} for radiation only, and radiation combined with blast injuries and burns), the values increase to 2.75–3.0 Gy. Another recent analysis of the data from Hiroshima estimates the LD_{50} to be 2.72 Gy by correlating white blood-cell counts to the percentage of mortality. Considering the diversity of these analyses and the approaches by which they were derived, their agreement is remarkable. Even more remarkable is the fact that these values agree with the human values obtained 20 years ago for patients, when adjusted for bone-marrow dose and prompt dose rates.

There is good agreement among the data (particularly the recent data from Hiroshima and Nagasaki) that the NATO human LD_{50} should not be raised for healthy untreated persons. Based on the range of values discussed, the recommended value for the LD_{50} is 3.0 Gy to bone marrow (4.3 Gy free in air).

REFERENCES

1. Young, R. W. 1987. Acute radiation syndrome. In *Military Radiobiology,* edited by J. J. Conklin and R. I. Walker, 165-190. Orlando, FL: Academic Press.

2. Annex 7. 1986. Medical-biological problems from the USSR State Committee on the Utilization of Atomic Energy. In *The Accident at the Chernobyl Nuclear Power Plant and Its Consequences.* Vienna: International Atomic Energy Agency Experts Meeting.

3. Bowers, G. J. The combined injury syndrome. In reference 1, 191-217.

4. Gunter-Smith, P. J. Effect of ionizing radiation on gastrointestinal physiology. In reference 1, 135-151.

5. Hawkins, R. N., and Cockerham, L. G. Postirradiation cardiovascular dysfunction. In reference 1, 153-163.

6. Cockerham, L. G.; Doyle, T. F.; Donlon, M. A.; and Helgeson, E. A. 1984. Canine postradiation histamine levels and subsequent response to Compound 48/80. *Aviat. Space Environ. Med.* 55(11): 1041-1045.

7. Cockerham, L. G.; Pautler, E. L.; Carraway, R. E.; Cochrane, D. E.; and Hampton, J. D. Effect of disodium cromoglycate (DSCG) and antihistamines on postirradiation cerebral blood flow and plasma levels of histamine and neurotensin. *Fundam. Appl. Toxicol.,* in press.

8. Cockerham, L. G.; Prell, G. D.; Cerveny, T. J.; O'Brien, M.; and Hampton, J. D. Effects of aminoguanidine on pre- and postirradiation regional cerebral blood flow and systemic blood pressure in the primate. In preparation.

9. Jones, T. D. 1981. Hematologic syndrome in man modelled from mammalian lethality. *Health Phys.* 41: 83-103.

10. Baverstock, K. F., and Ash, P. J. N. D. 1983. A review of radiation accidents involving whole body exposure and the relevance to the $LD_{50/60}$ for man. *Br. J. Radiol.* 56: 837.

11. Jones, T. D.; Morris, M. D.; Wells, S. M.; and Young, R. W. 1986. *Animal mortality resulting from uniform exposures to photon radiations: Calculated LD_{50}s and a compilation of animal data* [Publication 6338]. Oak Ridge, TN: Oak Ridge National Laboratory.

12. Bond, V. P.; Fleidner, T. M.; and Archambeau, J. V. 1965. *Mammalian radiation lethality.* New York: Academic Press.

13. Bond, V. P., and Sugahara, T. 1969. *Comparative cellular and species radiosensitivity.* Baltimore: Williams and Wilkins Co.

14. Ainsworth, E. J.; Leong, G. F.; and Alpen, E. L. 1984. Early radiation mortality and recovery in large animals and primates. In *Response of Different Species to Total Body Irradiation,* edited by J. J. Broerse, and T. J. MacVittie, 87-111. Dordrecht, The Netherlands: Martinus Nijhoff Publishers.

15. MacVittie, T. J.; Monroy, R. L.; Patchen, M. L.; and Darden, J. H. Acute lethality and radiosensitivity of the canine hematopoietic system to cobalt-60 gamma and mixed neutron-gamma irradiation. In reference 14, 113-129.

16. Krebs, J. S., and Jones, D. C. L. 1975. *Radiobiology of large animals* [Final report for contract DAHc20-70-C-0219, Defense Civil Preparedness Agency work unit 24310, SRI Project PYU-8150]. Washington, DC: Defense Technical Information Center.

17. Norris, W. P.; Fritz, T. E.; Rehfeld, C. E.; and Poole, C. M. 1968. The response of the beagle dog to cobalt-60 gamma radiation: Determination of the $LD_{50(30)}$ and description of associated changes. *Radiat. Res.* 35: 681.

18. Sorensen, D. K.; Bond, V. P.; Cronkite, E. P.; and Perman, V. 1960. An effective therapeutic regimen for the hematopoietic phase of the acute radiation syndrome in dogs. *Radiat. Res.* 13: 669.

19. Alpen, E. L.; Jones, D. M.; Hechter, H. H.; and Bond, V. P. 1958. The comparative biological response of dogs to 250 kVp X-rays and 100 kVp X-rays. *Radiology* 70: 541.

20. Shively, J. N.; Michaelson, S. M.; and Howland, J. W. 1958. The response of the dog to bilateral whole-body cobalt-60 irradiation. I. Lethal dose determination. *Radiat. Res.* 9: 445.

21. Vriesendorp, H. M., and van Bekkum, D. W. Susceptibility to total body irradiation. In reference 14, 43-57.

22. Ainsworth, E. J.; Leong, G. F.; Kendall, K.; and Alpen, E. L. 1965. Comparative lethality responses of neutron- and X-irradiated dogs: Influence of dose-rate and exposure aspect. *Radiat. Res.* 26: 32.

23. Broerse, J. J.; van Bekkum, D. W.; Hollander, C. V.; and Davids, J. A. G. 1978. Mortality of monkeys after exposure to fission neutrons and the effort of autologous bone marrow transplanation. *Int. J. Radiat. Biol.* 34: 253.

24. Wise, D., and Turbyfill, C. L. 1968. *The acute mortality response of monkeys (Macaca mulatta) to pulsed mixed gamma-neutron radiations.* [Scientific Report SR68-17]. Bethesda, MD: Armed Forces Radiobiology Research Institute.

25. Stanley, R. E.; Seigneur, L. J.; and Strike, T. A. 1966. *The acute mortality responses of monkeys (Macaca mulatta) to mixed gamma-neutron radiations and 250 KVP rays* [Special Report SP66-23]. Bethesda, MD: Armed Forces Radiobiology Research Institute.

26. Carsten, A. L. Acute lethality—the hematopoietic syndrome in different species. In reference 14, 59-86.

27. Ainsworth, E. J.; Long, G. F.; Kendall, K.; and Alpen, L. 1964. The effects of pulsed neutron or gamma irradiation in mice. *Radiat. Res.* 21: 75-85.

28. Davis, J. A. G. 1966. Relative biological effectiveness of fission neutrons for production of the bone marrow syndrome in mice. *Int. J. Radiat. Biol.* 10: 299.

29. Duque, R. E.; Phan, S. H.; Hudson, J. L.; Till, G. D.; and Ward, P. A. 1985. Functional defects in phagocytic cells following thermal injury. Application of flow cytometric analysis. *Am. J. Pathol.* 118: 116.

30. Shires, G. T., and Dineen, P. 1982. Sepsis following burns, trauma, and intra-abdominal infections. *Arch. Intern. Med.* 142: 2012-2022.

31. Munster, A. M. 1976. Post-traumatic immunosuppression is due to activation of suppressor T cells. *Lancet* 1: 1329-1330.

32. Saba, J. M., and Scovill, W. A. 1975. Effects of surgical trauma on host defense. *Ann. Surg.* 7: 71-81.

33. Alexander, J. W., and Wixson, D. 1970. Neutrophil dysfunction and sepsis following burn injury. *Surg. Gynecol. Obstet.* 130: 431-438.

34. Korlof, B. 1956. Infection in burns. *Acta. Chir. Scand.* [Suppl.] 209: 117-139.

35. Balch, H. H. 1955. The effect of severe battle injury and of post traumatic renal failure on resistance to infection. *Ann. Surg.* 142: 45-153.

36. Jones, R. K.; Chiffelle, T. L.; and Richmond, D. R. 1968. A study of effects of combined blast and radiation injury in sheep. In *Intermedes Proceedings 1968: Combined Injuries and Shock,* 57-66. Stockholm: Forsvarets Forskningsanstalt.

37. Richmond, D. R.; Jones, R. K.; and White, C. S. The effects of blast and ionizing radiation in rats. In reference 36, 67-74.

38. Messerschmidt, O. 1966. Untersuchungen uber Kombinationsschaden. Uber die Lebenserwartung von Mausen, die mit Ganzkorperbestrahlungen in Kombination mit offenen oder geschlossenen Hautverletzungen, Bauchoperationen oder Kompressionsschaden belastet wurden. *Strahlentherapie* 131: 298-311.

39. Valeriote, F. A., and Baker, D. G. 1964. The combined effects of thermal trauma and x-irradiation on early mortality. *Radiat. Res.* 22: 693-703.

40. Vogel, C. E. H. 1961. Burns and other trauma associated with radiation exposure. *Milit. Med.* 126: 688-692.

41. Alpen, E. L., and Sheline, G. E. 1954. The combined effects of thermal burns and whole body X-irradiation on survival time and mortality. *Ann. Surg.* 140: 113-118.

42. Baxter, H.; Drummond, J. A.; Stephens-Newsham, L. G.; and Randall, R. G. 1953. Reduction of mortality in swine from combined total body radiation and thermal burns by streptomycin. *Ann. Surg.* 137: 450-455.

43. Brooks, J. W.; Evans, E. I.; Ham, W. T.; and Reid, R. D. 1952. The influence of external body radiation on mortality from thermal burns. *Ann. Surg.* 136: 533-545.

44. Ledney, G. D.; Stewart, D. A.; and Exum, E. D. 1980. Proliferative responses of lymphomyelopoietic cells of mice after wound trauma. *J. Trauma* 20: 141-147.

45. Ledney, G. D.; Stewart, D. A.; Exum, E. D.; and Sheehy, P. A. 1981. Skin wound-enhanced survival and myelocytopoieses in mice after whole-body irradiation. *Acta Radiol.* [Oncol.] 20: 29-38.

46. Singer, D. 1976. Postsplenectomy sepsis. *Perspect. Pediatr. Pathol.* 1: 285-311.

47. Schildt, B., and Thoren, L. 1968. Experimental and clinical aspects of combined injuries. In *Combined Injuries and Shock*, edited by B. Schildt and L. Thoren, 3-15. Stockholm: Forsvarets Forskningsanstalt.

48. Schraibor, M. I., and Korchanov, L. S. Relevance of radiation injury in the combined injury syndrome. In reference 36, 17-20.

49. Perman, V.; Sorensen, D. K.; Usenik, E. A.; Bond, V. P.; and Cronkite, E. P. 1962. Hematopoietic regeneration in control and recovered heavily irradiated dogs following severe hemorrhage. *Blood* 19: 738-742.

50. Perman, V.; Cronkite, E. P.; Bond, V. P.; and Sorensen, D. K. 1962. The regenerative ability of hematopoietic tissue following lethal x-irradiation in dogs. *Blood* 19: 724-737.

51. Jackson, D. P.; Sorenson, D. K.; Cronkite, E. P.; Bond, V. P.; and Fliedner, T. M. 1959. Effectiveness of transfusions of fresh and lyophilized platelets in controlling bleeding due to thrombocytopenia. *J. Clin. Invest.* 38: 1689-1697.

52. Jacobson, L. O.; Marks, E. K.; and Gaston, E. O. 1963. Observations on the effect of spleen-shielding and the injection of cell suspensions on survival following irradiation. *Proc. Soc. Exp. Biol. Med.* 119: 122.

53. Maille, H. D.; Krasavage, W.; and Mermagen, H. 1966. On the partial-body irradiation of the dog. *Health Phys.* 12: 883.

54. Hansen, C. L.; Michaelson, S. M.; and Howland, S. W. 1961. Lethality of upper body exposure in beagles. *Public Health Rep.* 76: 242.

55. Gozenbuk, V. L., and Keirim-Markus, T. B. 1977. Dosimetric criteria of canine mortality following total body nonuniform irradiation. *Radiobiologiia* 17(6): 936-938.

56. Lushbaugh, C. C., and Havier, J. 1969. Reestimation of the human LD_{50} radiation levels at Hiroshima and Nagasaki. *Radiat. Res.* 39: 526.

57. Martin, J. H. 1983. Human survival—Radiation exposure levels. *J. Soc. Radiolog. Protection* 3: 15-23.

58. Lushbaugh, C. C.; Comas, F.; and Hofstra, R. 1967. Clinical studies on the radiation effects in man: A preliminary report of a retrospective search for dose relationships in the prodromal syndrome. *Radiat. Res.* 7: 398-412.

59. Rotblat, J. 1986. Acute radiation mortality in a nuclear war. In *The Medical Implications of Nuclear War,* Institute of Medicine, National Academy of Sciences, 233-250. Washington, DC: National Academy Press.

60. Rider, W. D., and Hasselback, R. 1968. The symptomatic and haematological disturbance following total body irradiation of 300 rad gamma-ray irradiation. In *Guidelines to Radiological Health* [Public Health Service Publication No. 999-RH-33], 139-144. Washington, DC: U.S. Department of Health, Education, and Welfare.

61. Jammet, H. 1961. Treatment of victims of the zero energy research accident at Vinca. In *Diagnosis and Treatment of Acute Radiation Injury.* Proceedings of WHO Scientific Meeting, Geneva, October 1960, 85. Geneva: World Health Organization.

62. Hurst, G. S.; Ritchie, R. H.; Sanders, F. W.; Reinhardt, P. W.; Auxier, J. A.; Wagner, E. B.; Callihan, A. D.; and Morgan, K. Z. 1961. Dosimetric investigation of the Yugoslav radiation accident. *Health Phys.* 5: 179-202.

63. MacVittie, T. J. 1988. Unpublished information.

64. Jones, T. D. 1981. Hematologic syndrome in man modelled from mammalian lethality. *Health Phys.* 41: 83-103.

65. Scott, B. R.; Seiler, F. A.; and Young, R. W. Predicted deaths from bone marrow dysfunction after protracted radiation in a fallout field. Abstract presented at 36th Annual Meeting of Radiation Research Society, Philadelphia, April 1988.

66. Schull, W. J. Implications of the new dosimetry for risk estimates. In *New Dosimetry at Hiroshima and Nagasaki and Its Implications for Risk Estimates,* Proceedings No. 9 of the 23rd Annual Meeting of National Council on Radiation Protection, Washington, DC, 1987. In press.

Chapter 3

TRIAGE AND TREATMENT OF RADIATION-INJURED MASS CASUALTIES

ROBERT F. DONS, M.D.,* and T. JAN CERVENY, Ph.D.**

*Lieutenant Colonel, United States Air Force; Department of Experimental Hematology, Armed Forces Radiobiology Research Institute, Bethesda, Maryland 20814-5145
**Major, United States Air Force; Program Manager, Bioenvironmental Hazards, Air Force Office of Scientific Research, Bolling Air Force Base, Washington, D.C. 20332-6448

INTRODUCTION

The effective medical sorting of mass casualties (*triage*) and their subsequent treatment after a nuclear event have been considered extremely difficult or even impossible.[1] In the case of a major exchange of strategic nuclear weapons (500–5,000 MT), the triage of casualties using the remaining resources would certainly be futile and frustrating. Without transportation and tertiary medical-care facilities, the only benefit would be to identify persons who are capable of combat. Even the minimally injured casualty may receive little (if any) meaningful attention in such a situation.

However, if a nuclear event occurs, it is more likely to take place on a limited scale rather than as a strategic weapons exchange.[1] After a smaller-scale tactical detonation (0.1–2.0 kt) or a nuclear detonation by terrorists, hundreds or a few thousand casualties are more probable than millions[2] or billions.[3] Considerable medical resources may be intact and available for treating many of them. This chapter presents plans for the management of large numbers of casualties suffering either radiation injury alone or conventional trauma combined with radiation injury.

PRINCIPLES OF TRIAGE

In conventional triage, patients are assigned to one of the following priority categories, depending on the nature and extent of their injuries: *(a)* The *immediate treatment* group includes patients who have a high chance of survival if they are given immediate life-saving treatment or surgery that is relatively quick and uncomplicated. *(b)* The *delayed treatment* group includes patients who may need major surgery, but who can be sustained on supportive treatments until surgery is possible. *(c)* The *minimal treatment* group includes patients with relatively minor injuries who can care for themselves or who can be helped by untrained personnel. *(d)* The *expectant* category includes patients with serious or multiple injuries requiring extensive treatment, as well as patients with a poor chance of survival. This group should receive supportive treatments that are compatible with resources, including large doses of analgesics.

The speed of assessing and categorizing the status of patients is the key to effective triage. Any method is useful that gives the triage officer a quick, accurate idea of the extent of injury. When making the assessment rapidly based on anatomical findings, the probability of injury is related to the degree of estimated force on the body part. For example, a patient close enough to a nuclear explosion to be caught in the blast wind is assumed to have internal and possibly occult traumatic injury. Such a patient will most likely be in the expectant category (Table 3-1). A slower but more accurate method of assessment is to expose the injured area directly and perform an abdominal examination. Even with a relatively small number of casualties, this exam might be prohibitively time consuming in the critical moments shortly after a nuclear event.

Rapid assessment based on physiological status will permit the gathering of useful information on respiratory rate and systolic blood pressure in a large number of patients. In contrast, a determination of the Glasgow coma scale score[4] (although fairly rapid in experienced hands) is less useful than a brief neurological evaluation of the patient's degree of alertness, responsiveness to verbal and painful stimuli, and state of consciousness. Attention to other relatively obvious factors, such as extremes of age (under 5 years or over 55 years) and preexisting or recently induced cardiovascular or respiratory illness, will aid in establishing a patient's status as expectant.

Operational Considerations for Triage

Regardless of the findings from an anatomical or physiological assessment of the patient, the first priority of the military triage officer is to conserve the fighting force. Combatants in the expectant category, however, should not receive aid or resources that might be of greater benefit to less severely injured noncombatants, even if these re-

TABLE 3–1

PRIORITIES IN COMBINED-INJURY TRIAGE WHEN RADIATION DOSES ARE KNOWN*

Conventional Triage Categories if Injuries Are Only Trauma**	Changes in Expected Triage Category Following Whole-Body Radiation Dose (Gy)		
No radiation exists	<1.5	1.5–4.5	>4.5
T1	T1	T1	T4
T2	T2	T4	T4
T3	T3	T4	T4
T4	T4	T4	T4

*Decision based on whole-body radiation dose, assuming all casualties are wearing personal dosimeters.

**Conventional Triage Categories:
T1: Immediate treatment, high survival group
T2: Delayed treatment, patient can be sustained
T3: Minimal treatment, minor injury group
T4: Expectant, seriously injured—poor survival

Source: Adaptation from data in *NATO Handbook on the Concept of Medical Support in NBC Environments* (reference 15).

sources seem to be in adequate supply. In rare circumstances, a terminally injured unit commander might receive resources to permit continued functioning in a crucial command role.

This chapter pertains primarily to the management of acutely irradiated casualties following the detonation of a nuclear weapon. The military physician should recognize two essential facts in dealing with mass casualties during military triage in a declared war: *(a)* all medical resources fall under the jurisdiction of the military, and *(b)* peacetime triage practices are of limited use. However, in more limited events (such as a major nuclear reactor accident), the military may be asked to assist with the management of mass casualties under the constraints of peacetime disaster triage.

Peacetime Triage. In peacetime, a two-tiered system of care for the critically ill is assumed. Based on the triage decision, the patient goes either to the emergency room of the nearest community hospital or to the regional trauma center. This system depends on rapid, reliable transportation in which trained attendants monitor the patient with radio guidance from trauma staff at the hospital or center.[5]

In this scheme, the sorting of patients is based on a physiological trauma score in which the less-injured patient, with a score of 15–16, is in the de-

TABLE 3–2

ESTIMATION OF POSSIBLE RADIATION INJURY BASED ON SYMPTOMS

Symptoms	Unlikely	Probable	Severe
Nausea	(–)	(++)	(+++)
Vomiting	(–)	(+)	(+++)
Diarrhea	(–)	(±)	(± to +++)
Hyperthermia	(–)	(±)	(+ to +++)
Erythema	(–)	(–)	(– to ++)
Hypotension	(–)	(–)	(+ to ++)
CNS dysfunction	(–)	(–)	(– to ++)

layed category, a third priority. Patients with a trauma score of 3 or less are considered expectant (the fourth, or last, priority). Third- and fourth-priority patients would probably be sent to the local hospital emergency room. All patients with trauma scores of 4–10 (first priority) and some with scores of 11–12 (second priority) would go to the trauma center.[5]

Military Triage. Military triage contrasts starkly with that used in peacetime, but the two do have some elements in common. For example, military triage decisions would most likely be made at the level of the batallion aid or clearing station. The local community hospital might be equivalent to the second-echelon radiation decontamination center and field hospital. Only fixed medical-care facilities or existing tertiary-care facilities that are able to perform surgery would suffice as trauma centers for handling combined-injury casualties.

In wartime, it cannot be assumed that rapid and reliable transportation of wounded persons is possible, as it is in peacetime or might be in smaller, low-yield nuclear events. In the confusion of armed conflict, casualties with a wide variety of injuries might be expected to arrive at the nearest medical-care facility regardless of its capability. Extra effort will be needed to keep the patient moving forward in the system to an appropriate level of care. The greatest number of lives will be saved only by ensuring that time and materials are not allocated to hopeless cases or to those whose injuries are so minor or uncomplicated that definitive care can be postponed.

In a nuclear disaster, triage decisions cannot be made on the evidence or probability of conventional injury alone. When significant radiation exposure is combined with conventional injuries, there may be a dramatic shift of patients to the expectant category (Table 3-1). In order to make an appropriate decision, the triage officer must recognize the symptoms of ARS and understand the difficulties in estimating radiation exposure from clinical findings.

Signs and Symptoms of Radiation Injury

It will be difficult to assess the radiation doses of persons who have been injured in a mass-casualty disaster. Thus, a system has been devised to identify radiation exposure based on the symptoms of "unlikely," "probable," or "severe" radiation injury (Table 3-2).[6] These symptoms are nonspecific, and

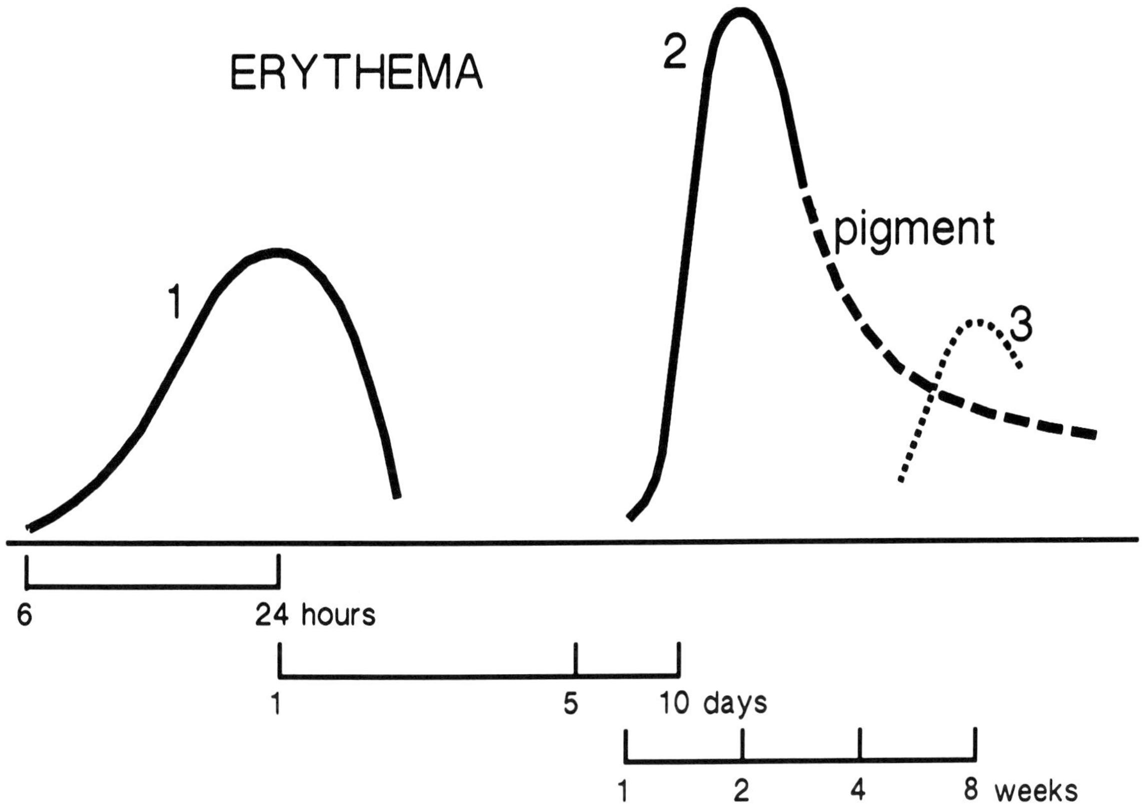

Fig. 3-1. Appearance of waves of erythema after irradiation of human skin. Dotted lines indicate pigmented lesions. Source: Redrawn from reference 6.

permit only the cursory screening of a large number of cases.

Cutaneous Phenomena. Information about the cutaneous changes after ionizing radiation exposure comes mainly from accidental or therapeutic high-dose local radiation exposures and, to a lesser extent, from studies of the victims of the 1986 nuclear reactor accident in Chernobyl, USSR, and the 1987 cesium-137 accident in Goiânia, Brazil. Skin injury in those events resulted from very intense local irradiation or direct contact of the skin with radioactive material. Burns among casualties at Hiroshima and Nagasaki in 1945 were caused by heat rather than radiation exposure.[3]

When extremely high doses of whole-body radiation (100 Gy) are delivered acutely, skin may have the sensation of tingling or being on fire even though no lesion immediately appears. Within the first 24 hours, there is the appearance of a characteristic transient erythema secondary to capillary dilation and the release of histamine-like substances. The initial erythema usually peaks within 24 hours, and then disappears for 1–3 weeks. Thereafter, it may reappear with pain and edema. Severe pain may occur if more radioresistant nerve tissue is surrounded by necrotizing tissues. Melanotic pigmentation (Figure 3-1) or ulceration may develop.[7] Pain from nerve compression may occur as healing and atrophy take place. Hair loss over the affected area occurs at the end of the second or third week. In contrast to erythema induced by high-dose beta radiation, skin injury from gamma radiation occurs only at doses that damage the bone marrow. Thus, if sufficient marrow is exposed, thrombocytopenia with cutaneous petechiae, purpura, and hemorrhage can be expected. In granulocytopenic patients, otherwise-noninvasive surface bacteria may colonize areas of wet desquamation and lead to suppurative lesions.

The threshold dose for gamma-radiation-induced erythema is about 3–5 Gy; for desquamation, it is about 10 Gy. Ulceration develops at doses of 20 Gy. At doses of more than 40 Gy, gangrenous radionecrosis can be confidently predicted, if the dose is well documented and can be confirmed on review of the evidence.[8] Different body areas may have different radiation sensitivities; a gradient from greater to lower resistance is observed for scalp, face and neck, trunk, ears, groin, and extremities. Exposure of the skin to temperatures greater than 42°C may enhance cutaneous radiosensitivity and increase the probability of a more severe injury.[7]

Beta-emitting isotopes from smoke and fallout can cause desquamation from high-dose local radiation delivered to exposed skin surfaces, but only if these isotopes are in contact with the skin for longer than 1 hour. Since beta radiation is not as penetrating as gamma radiation, dry desquamating skin lesions secondary to beta burns may not be as serious as wet desquamating lesions, which occur as the result of high-dose exposure and suggest that underlying structures are involved. The wet lesions may be complicated by secondary infection, and usually indicate a poor prognosis.

Gastrointestinal Phenomena. A sense of fatigue and malaise associated with nausea and loss of appetite is characteristic even of relatively low-dose radiation exposure (1–2 Gy). The abrupt onset of nausea and vomiting occurs with acute high-dose radiation in the range of 5–10 Gy. These initial symptoms may be followed by a short latent period of 1–2 days. The severity of initial symptoms, including diarrhea, serves as a useful index of probable outcome, as does the rapidity of onset or a delay in the appearance of symptoms. Following the latent period, an increase in vomiting, diarrhea, and anorexia, as well as dehydration and signs of infection, can be expected.[9]

An abrupt onset of bloody diarrhea after acute high-dose radiation indicates lethal exposure. If less-acute doses are received, diarrhea may not appear for several days or a week after exposure. The onset of diarrhea within a week of exposure is usually associated with death. However, patients have survived when the onset of radiation-related diarrhea was delayed for more than 1 week after protracted radiation exposure.[10]

Nausea and vomiting occur after exposure to doses greater than 2.5 Gy. Identification of the onset of these symptoms may be useful in the initial triage of a radiation-only casualty. However, in combined chemical-nuclear warfare environments, chemical agents may account for much of the nausea and vomiting.

Cardiovascular, Respiratory, Metabolic, and Neurological Phenomena. If a casualty has no conventional injuries or psychosomatic complaints, then cardiovascular, respiratory, metabolic, and neurological symptoms usually indicate terminal high-dose radiation exposure. Radiation-related hypotension, radiation pneumonitis, or ETI identify persons who may be expected to die within 2–3 days. This prognosis is certain, despite a variable period of transient improvement that occurs shortly after the event.

Initial symptoms of high-dose exposure may not be distinct from those of lower-dose exposures. Nausea and vomiting may occur even without direct exposure to the gut in patients who received high-dose local radiation to the head or chest.

Metabolic abnormalities can be expected after radiation of moderate to high doses, and include the consistent finding of nonbacteria-mediated hyperthermia with marked fever and shaking chills. A 25% drop in plasma glucose may occur within the first day, but a neuroglycopenic state of confusion has not been observed. Hemorrhagic coagulopathies, associated with disseminated intravascular coagulation and a reduction in noncellular clotting factors, are possible. Liver injury probably accounts for hypoglycemia and the coagulation factor deficiencies.[11,12] Cardiac arrhythmias associated with electrolyte imbalance (hyper- or hypokalemia) may occur.

In the later stages after lung exposure, the loud crepitus of radiation pneumonitis, which has been likened to the "thundering of a rain storm on an iron roof,"[10] is associated with tachypnea and severe hypoxemia.

ETI in primates (and its locomotor equivalent in rodents) is characterized by the complete but temporary cessation of motor function, and does not occur unless high-dose radiation is delivered acutely.[13] Transient loss of consciousness is not typical of ETI. Unconsciousness is more suggestive of conventional head injury.

Hematological Phenomena. The most useful and rapid method of assessing the degree of radiation exposure is to obtain serial total lymphocyte counts. Optimally, this should be done every 6 hours during the first 48 hours, or at least once every 24 hours after exposure. This estimate and its interpretation need to be standardized for the available laboratory methodology. To that end, a chart of blood cell morphology (Figure 3-2) and a nomo-

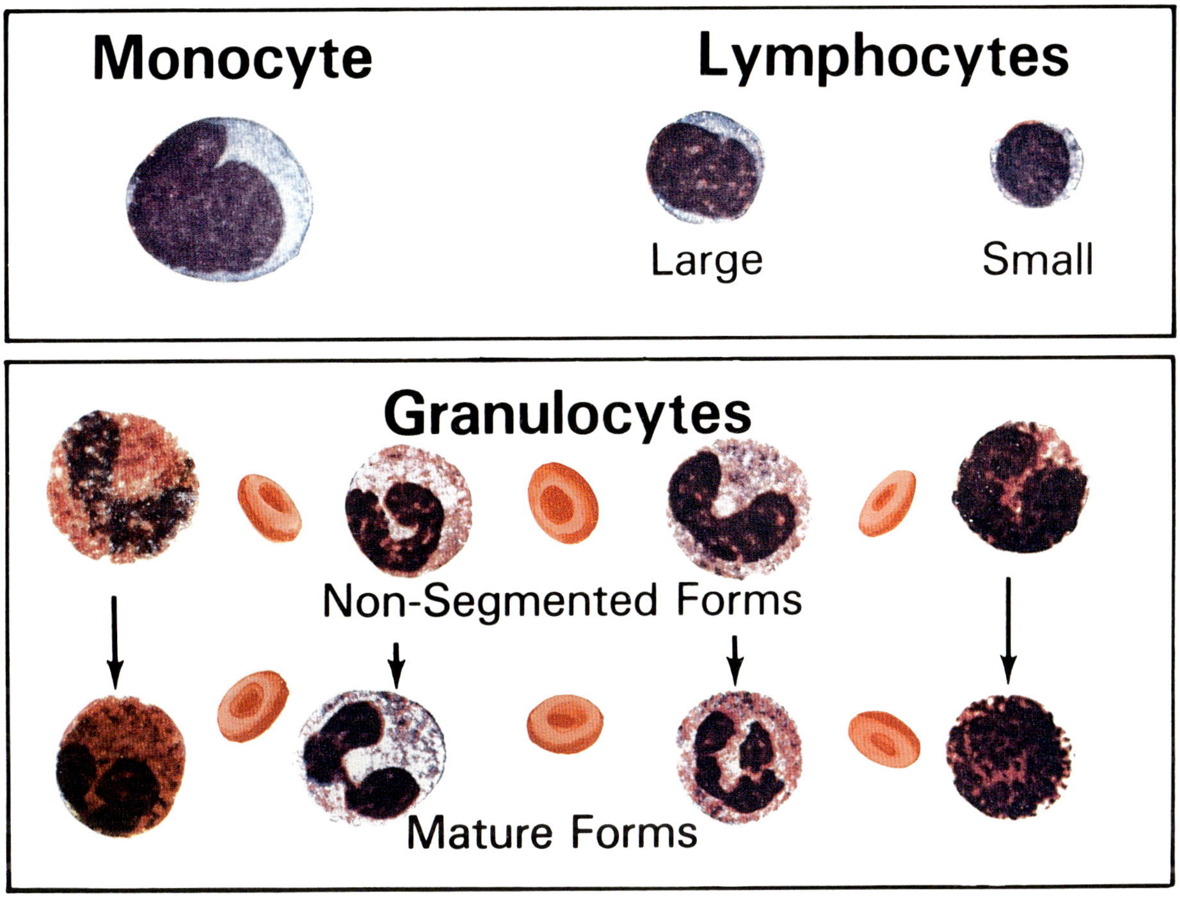

Fig. 3-2. Appearance of human mononuclear cells (lymphocytes and monocytes) compared to human granulocytic cells (eosinophils, neutrophils, and basophils) in their nonsegmented and segmented (mature) forms. Erythrocytes are shown for contrast in size.

gram of the acute radiation-induced change in lymphocytes/mm^3 (Figure 3-3) may be useful. A laminated copy of this nomogram should be included in the field kit of every medical officer. Changes in peripheral blood granulocytes do not give as clear a picture of the severity of radiation injury because their numbers are affected by stress and infection, fall more slowly, and vary widely.

Sophisticated methodology has become available that permits the rapid and quantitative determination of the total and differential leukocyte counts at DEPMEDS (Deployable Medical Systems) field hospitals. Using the QBC II assay methodology,[14] a total lymphocyte count requires only a fingerstick blood sample (rather than a phlebotomy) and can be performed by relatively inexperienced personnel. Effective suppression of electrical power surges and adequate supplies of special sample tubes would be needed to permit this operation on the nuclear battlefield at a field hospital.

A drawback of this method is that monocytes cannot be differentiated from lymphocytes unless a separate Wright-stained slide is prepared and interpreted. Such a determination done by hand would become prohibitively time consuming and labor intensive in a mass-casualty situation. However, with the QBC II methodology, the determination of the total granulocyte percentage and the mononuclear cell percentage is automated (although it still requires data transcription by hand).

Triage of the Combined-Injury Patient

Priorities in handling patients of conventional trauma are modified in cases of concurrent radiation injury. Triage priority is based on the conventional injury as well as the degree of radiation suffered by the combined-injury victim (Table 3-1).

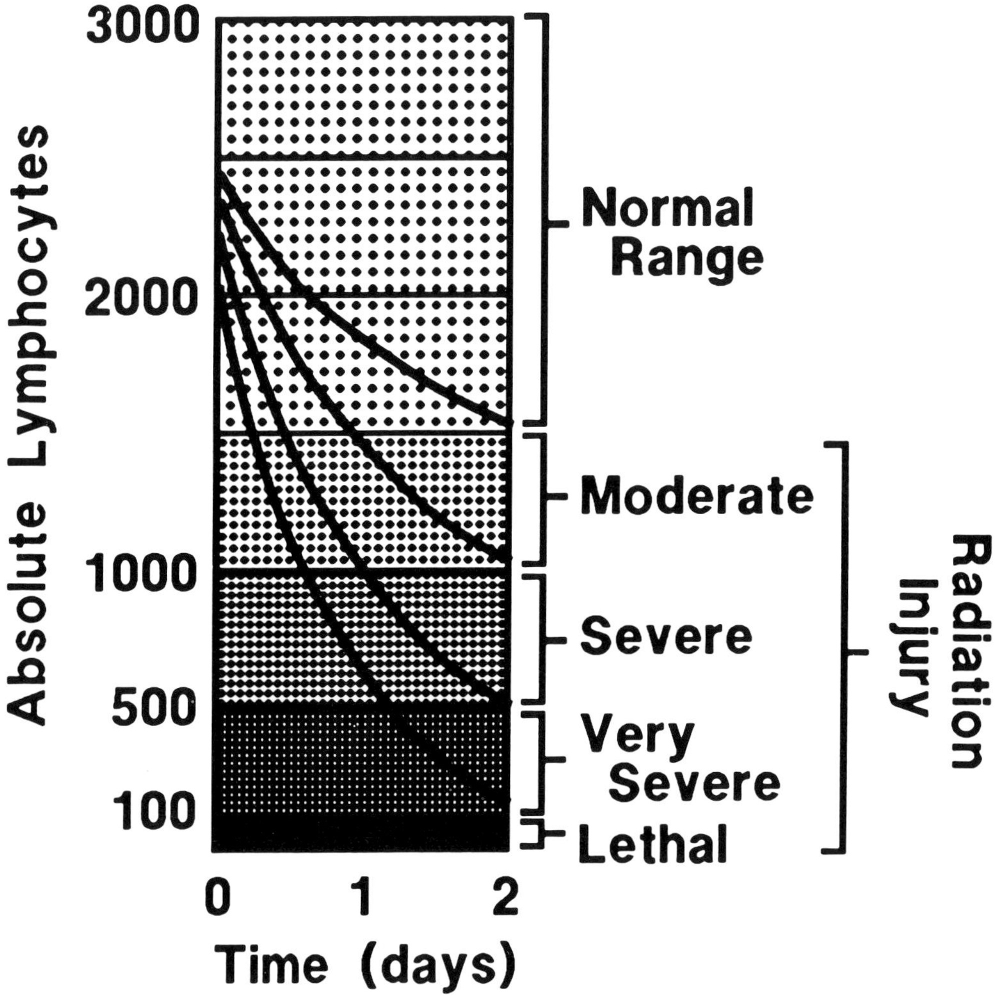

Fig. 3-3. To use a lymphocyte nomogram: *(a)* determine total lymphocytes/mm^3 every 6 hours; *(b)* because the absolute number of lymphocytes (Y axis) depends on technique, use standardized laboratory methodology; *(c)* because the ordinal scale (X axis) depends on acuteness of radiation exposure, do not use scale shown if exposure is protracted.

TABLE 3–3

PRIORITIES IN COMBINED-INJURY TRIAGE WHEN RADIATION INJURY IS POSSIBLE

Conventional Triage Categories if Injuries Are Only Trauma*	Changes in Expected Triage Category Following Possibility of Radiation Injury				
	Unlikely	Probable	Confirmed		
No radiation exists			Minimum**	Moderate	Severe
T3	T3	T3	T3	T3	T3
T2	T2	T2 /T4	T3	T4	T4
T1	T1	T3 /T4	T3	T4	T4
T4	T4	T4	T4	T4	T4

*Conventional Triage Categories:
T1: Immediate treatment, high survival group
T2: Delayed treatment, patient can be sustained
T3: Minimal treatment, minor injury group
T4: Expectant, seriously injured—poor survival

**Acute radiation dose of approximately 0.5 Gy

All patients exposed to more than 4.5 Gy are in the expectant category, as are those with exposure of 1.5–4.5 Gy who cannot be given care immediately. If exposure was less than 1.5 Gy, the nature of the conventional injury will dictate the treatment priority. Casualties who receive radiation exposure alone over a wide range of doses will need little if any treatment initially.[15]

Since an estimate of the exposure dose in the early phases of radiation-casualty triage will be almost impossible, a more practical triage scheme, based on symptoms of unlikely, probable, or severe radiation exposure, will be useful (Table 3-2). In the event of combined injuries, symptoms of probable or severe exposure may be confused with symptoms associated with conventional injury. In giving the benefit of the doubt to such patients, those with injuries treatable on an immediate basis should receive prompt attention. However, if radiation exposure does account for the observed symptoms, the patient in the conventional categories of immediate (Table 3-3) or delayed (Table 3-1) may actually be expectant. Even with severe symptoms of radiation exposure, patients with minimal traumatic injury may be capable of survival if evacuated for observation and advanced medical management. However, if transportation resources are limited, disposition of the minimally injured but heavily exposed patient should coincide with that of the casualty in the expectant category. Patients in the delayed category with probable radiation symptoms are expectant, unless adequate tertiary-care facilities are readily available. Regardless of the triage scheme used, it is probable that a number of combined-injury patients in the expectant category will receive treatment for more immediate and delayed conventional injuries.

Conventional injuries that are particularly relevant following a nuclear detonation include burn, blast, and eye trauma.

Burn Injury. The extent of a thermal burn may be rapidly estimated according to the "rule of nines."[4] Conventional thermal burns are predicted to be among the most frequent injuries to troops on the nuclear battlefield.[15] A more severe hematopoietic subsyndrome is likely if partial-thickness burns involve more than 10% of the body surface.[10]

Blast Injury. Dynamic overpressure from the explosion of a nuclear weapon will induce overt crush injuries and occult internal bleeding.[16] The triage officer should suspect occult traumatic injuries, which will likely place the irradiated patient in the expectant category.

Eye Injury. Eye injuries from a thermonuclear flash may be as minor as transient blindness (for a few seconds to minutes) or a permanent retinal scar in which peripheral vision is spared.[3,16] These are minimal injuries. However, permanent foveal damage with 20/200 visual acuity may occur if the victim focuses directly on the nuclear fireball. A variety of eye injuries resulting primarily from protracted high-dose radiation exposure was observed among firefighters at the Chernobyl reactor accident. These injuries will most likely lead to permanently impaired vision.[10] Clearly, if the corrected visual acuity of a patient is 20/200 or less after more than 1 hour from time of injury, the usefulness of that person as a combatant will be limited, and assignment to a category of delayed treatment is appropriate. Gross eye injuries, most likely from flying objects after a nuclear blast, may have a dramatic appearance, but they are frequently minimal and should not divert attention from more significant injuries.

MEDICAL MANAGEMENT OF THE COMBINED-INJURY CASUALTY

Patient management will focus on three issues. First, basic life-support concerns need to be quickly addressed for casualties in the immediate category; an airway, adequate ventilation, and circulatory function should be assured for patients whose injuries will permit them to survive. Concerns about internal or external contamination with radioactivity should be second priority. Finally, an effort should be made to retrieve data from any dosimeters carried by the military combat unit. Currently, radiation dosimeters cannot be relied on to accurately estimate the severity of an individual's radiation injury. Dosimeters do not account for partial shielding and do not reflect the delivery rate of a radiation dose, and so make only a small contribution to the diagnostic picture. Any data from physical dosimeters must be interpreted by the medical attendant in light of the observed physiological changes.

Because most of the radiation exposure likely to be encountered on the battlefield has no immediate life-threatening consequences, the medical attendant should first focus on conventional injuries. Needless risks, such as prolonged contact with contaminated clothing or wash water, must be avoided, but in emergency medical treatment, direct contact with a contaminated patient is usually not hazardous. No conclusive evidence exists that any attendant has ever been adversely affected by brief contact with a radiation casualty. On the other hand, in a nuclear attack that is combined with chemical or biological weapons (which may be more likely than a nuclear attack alone), the attendant will need to wear protective gloves, as well as a mask outfitted with an entire chemical ensemble, to manage these casualties safely.

Wearing this chemical ensemble will pose special problems in primary medical management. Even if the mask is equipped with a voice emitter, verbal communication over more than a few yards will be hampered. In the early phases of identification and triage, familiarity with a brief dictionary of sign language will be useful. The signs for "radiation casualty" and "chemical casualty" are illustrated in Figure 3-4.

Concerns in the Treatment of the Combined-Injury Patient

Once an airway, proper ventilation, and circulatory stability have been established, definitive care should be planned for the casualty who can survive. Treatment planning is based on the competent handling of conventional injury and the antici-

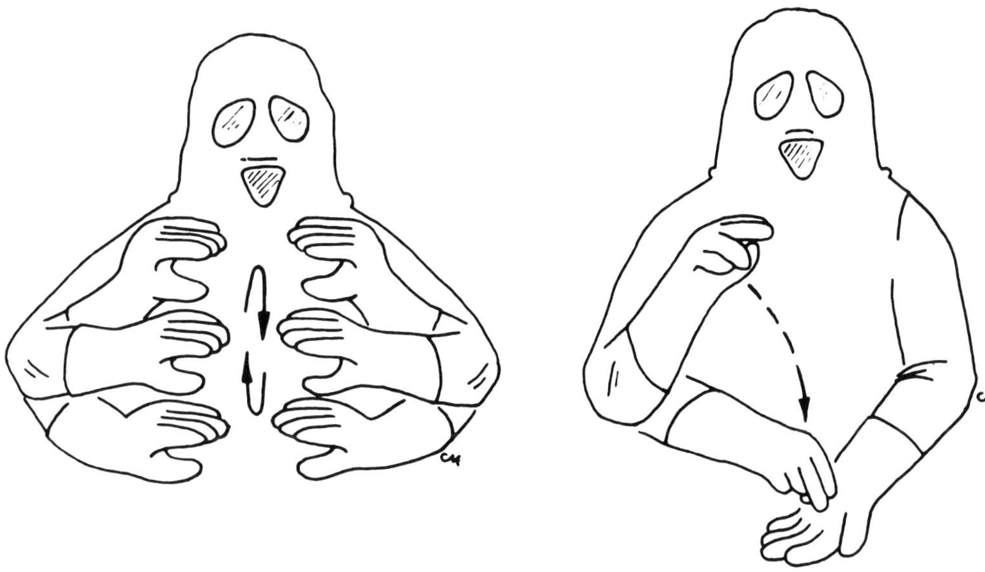

Fig. 3-4. To sign for "chemical," make a "C" with hands and move them in a circle away from lower thorax and toward shoulders. To sign for "nuclear," thrust second and third fingers toward open palm of opposite hand.

pation of predictable sequelae of radiation injury. In the following discussion, early placement of a peripheral intravenous catheter for infusion of adequate quantities of fluids and blood components is assumed. The use of central venous lines in protected sites for long-term infusions is also discussed.

The decision to apply any of these measures to the combined-injury patient will be a difficult one, and will have to be based on the availability of resources and the projected number of casualties. The prognosis for combined injury is markedly worse than for either traumatic or radiation injury alone. Patients with moderate or severe conventional injuries who arrive at tertiary centers that are capable of handling combined injuries will probably receive the maximum available care, unless they have received obviously massive doses of radiation (over 8 or 9 Gy). It will be hard to justify the decision to continue therapeutic interventions in a trauma patient whose dose of radiation is eventually determined to exceed 4 Gy. Continuing advanced life-support measures will not be in the best interests of a patient who will most likely suffer a protracted, terminal illness. Nor will less-injured patients benefit if their access to hospital resources is limited because of the excessive allocation to hopeless cases. On the other hand, the military organization should attempt to assure that the psychological support of casualties in the expectant category are augmented as much as possible by nonmedical personnel.

Specific Treatment Concerns

Surgery. Since exposure to doses of less than 5 Gy is of no immediate threat to health, conventional injury that is surgically remediable deserves priority treatment. Ideally, surgery should be initiated as soon as possible, or within 36 hours of radiation exposure,[3] and be completed before 48 hours.[17] Surgery after this time is contraindicated for at least 6 weeks, or until there is evidence that immunocompetence has returned and that incised tissue is able to revascularize. Clearly, the best candidate for surgery is the patient who requires only one procedure with no surgical revision. Patients who have been exposed to more than 1.5 Gy, who have extensive injuries, and who need multiple procedures and reconstructive surgery are classified as expectant. However, patients who have suffered severe conventional injury, who have had successful wound closure, and who then received radiation may actually be more radioresistant and better able to survive.[17] Decontamination of the radiation casualty should include prompt surgical debridement, if needed, and washing of the surgical area with mild antiseptic soaps. The skin should be cleansed before surgery to adequately reduce any radioactivity in the area of the incision. An important secondary concern is to cleanse crevice areas (nails, ears, and skinfolds) and orifices (particularly mouth and anogenital regions). To avoid abrading the skin, washing should be done gently with mild soaps and hair should be clipper-cut instead of shaved. These procedures will eliminate at least 95% of a patient's surface contamination with isotopes.

Anesthesia and Pain Control. In controlled trials with animals, the induction and recovery from anesthesia for irradiated subjects do not differ from those for nonirradiated subjects.[18] However, anecdotal experience in humans has suggested that the times of induction and recovery from anesthesia may be prolonged.[19] In irradiated animals and humans, there is a clear resistance to the effects of analgesics. However, care should be exercised to avoid overtreatment with sedative narcotics and anesthetics.[9]

In a local high-dose radiation injury (over 40 Gy) to an extremity, prompt amputation gives the patient the greatest pain relief and makes the most efficient use of resources. The use of nonsteroidal anti-inflammatory drugs and thrombolytic agents, as well as topical corticosteroids, has been claimed to delay the appearance of dermal necrosis and to lessen the pain of local skin damage.[20] However, topical corticosteroids are contraindicated in thermal burn injuries.

Control of Infections. A variety of measures has been advocated to reduce infections in the irradiated patient. These measures include meticulous hygiene of skin and orifices, aseptic skin punctures, reverse isolation, and prophylactic administration of immunoglobulin G. Difficulties associated with the strict maintenance of reverse isolation procedures are obvious. Laminar airflow rooms are in limited supply, constant surveillance is required for nosocomial infectious agents in plumbing fixtures and ice machines, and food must be free of gram-negative bacteria (no raw fruit, vegetables, or salad). The best result that might be achieved by these methods is a reduction in the appearance of new infections. Meanwhile, endogenous reinfection would be little affected unless antibiotics to eliminate opportunistic pathogens from the gut are effectively used. Although measures to control infection are prudent, their efficacy has not been clearly shown. Life-threatening infections remain a complication in the management of radiation casualties.

Maximum doses of two or three antibiotics of different classes should be infused empirically when specific signs of bacterial infection occur. These signs include the appearance of a sudden fever spike, usually in the presence of a depressed leukocyte count (that is, granulocytes fewer than $500/mm^3$). Prophylactic antibiotic treatment has given good results when used perioperatively in patients who have penetrating abdominal wounds.[21] The use of poorly absorbed oral antibiotics that selectively decontaminate the gut may be indicated as a preventive measure in patients known to have been exposed to moderate or high radiation doses. Even commonly used and widely available antibiotics (penicillins, streptomycins, and sulfas) may be useful with mass casualties, because sensitive and otherwise-noninvasive organisms usually become prominent pathogens in immunosuppressed radiation casualties.[10] Antifungal and antiviral agents are indicated when specific signs of these infections occur.

Antibiotics may rapidly become scarce in a mass-casualty radiation disaster and should be allocated to the victims most likely to survive. Such patients include *(a)* those with minimal injuries and evidence of localized infection, *(b)* those who require only one surgical procedure, and *(c)* those with contaminated wounds who have received lower doses of radiation.

Antiemetics and Antidiarrheals. The phenothiazine class of antiemetics, when used in the high doses needed to relieve a radiation victim's nausea and vomiting, has an unacceptably high incidence of extrapyramidal neurological side effects. Since the currently available antiemetic agents are of limited use, intense research efforts have been directed to finding new agents. Promising results have been obtained with the use of serotonin (5-HT3) blocking agents. This class of drugs significantly reduces radiation-induced emesis in the ferret, nonhuman primate, and human. However, some of the drugs may result in nausea.[22] Results of clinical trials of these relatively nontoxic agents are pending, as is their approval as agents potentially useful in the field by NATO forces. The goal in the use of any effective antiemetic is threefold: *(a)* to enhance patient comfort without drug side effects, *(b)* to reduce the risk of aspiration pneumonia, and *(c)* to conserve body fluid and electrolytes. It may be possible to prevent emesis by administering serotonin antagonists prophylactically or immediately after exposure.

Diarrhea from radiation damage to the gut may be controlled in part by a restricted-fiber diet and in part by medication. Drugs such as diphenoxylate HCl, codeine, or atropine have been advocated. If these are ineffective and the damage is localized to the large bowel, hydrocortisone enemas may help. The late complication of bowel stricture from local radiation damage is managed surgically.[23]

Fluids and Electrolytes. While adequate supplies of intravenous fluids are not likely to be available in a situation involving mass radiation casualties, the survival of patients with milder cases of fluid and electrolyte loss may be enhanced by replacement therapy. Careful measurement of the volume of losses will serve two purposes: *(a)* patients with severe degrees of fluid loss can be categorized as expectant, and *(b)* the proper volume of replacement can be given to patients who are capable of surviving. Measurement of the relative volumes of vomitus and diarrhea will help guide the fluid replacement. Those with more vomiting than diarrhea will suffer the greater loss of chlorides and may develop alkalosis, while those with secretory, cholera-like diarrhea may develop hypokalemia and hyponatremia with total-body salt depletion. The collection and measurement of excretions, including urine, serve another purpose: with the proper collection of serial specimens and access to radioanalysis equipment, estimates of internal radionuclide contamination can be made by measuring the radioactivity of the samples. In the event of combined-burn injury involving more than 10% of the body surface, crystalloid infusions are just as satisfactory as colloid, but a higher volume of infusate may be necessary.[24]

Placement of central venous catheters made of silicone elastomer (such as the Hickman or Broviac type)[25] should be considered a minor surgical procedure and be accomplished within the first 36 hours, if needed. Vascular obstructions and exotic infections increasingly complicate the use of these lines in immunocompromised patients,[26-28] and so they should be limited to the critically injured patients who need them most. However, a long-term illness following serious radiation injury will dictate that long-term venous access be maintained. The probability of wound-healing disturbances and the chronicity of phlebotoxic intravenous therapy involved in the care and treatment of any critically ill patient make central venous access preferable to peripheral intravenous access.

Using peripheral lines in the radiation casualty has further disadvantages: *(a)* placement is difficult if hemostasis is compromised and local hemorrhage develops, *(b)* placement is restricted to percutaneous insertion after 36 hours, even if a venous cutdown is otherwise desirable, *(c)* the lines are unsuitable for infusion of hyperosmolar solutions, and *(d)* the lines are at greater risk of becoming infected at the catheter tip if used longer than 72 hours. Long-term use of the percutaneous subclavian cannula made of polyethylene or polyvinyl chloride is contraindicated because of the high rates of infection, vascular occlusion, and thrombogenicity associated with these materials.

Blood Component Therapy. Impaired hemostasis after radiation injury is best related to the decline in platelet numbers that occurs several weeks after exposure. After protracted lower-dose irradiation, the decline in platelets may take more than 2 weeks. In the interim, autologous platelets can be harvested, cryopreserved, and stored for later reinfusion. This procedure was used successfully to aid the victims of the Chernobyl reactor accident. If bleeding develops, patients with reduced numbers of platelets secondary to marrow suppression benefit from platelet transfusion even if the count is greater than 20,000/mm^3. However, prophylactic platelet transfusions are indicated on a regular basis if the count falls below 20,000/mm^3, even in the absence of bleeding.

Platelets can be collected either by harvesting the platelet-enriched plasma obtained by centrifugation of fresh units of whole blood, or by using plateletpheresis. Although pheresis technology is complicated and expensive, each pheresis platelet concentrate provides the equivalent of platelets from five to eight whole-blood donations. Thus, a single pheresis unit is the usual transfusion dose and can be obtained in a single cost-effective procedure.[29]

Anemia develops rapidly in the critically injured radiation casualty. Maintenance of perfusion pressure and oxygen delivery to injured areas, better wound healing, and an enhanced sense of well-being will depend on preventing anemia through red-cell transfusions. As with patients suffering thermal burns alone, patients with radiation skin burns and those with combined injuries require more red-cell transfusions.[10] A recall system is essential for the large number of healthy blood donors needed to keep up with the demand for red cells for mass casualties.

Erythrocytes may be stored for up to 10 years using modern cryopreservation techniques. Critical government and military leaders should stockpile autologous blood for use in case of wartime emergency.

In the fight against infections, fresh heterologous granulocyte infusions, bone-marrow transplants, and even the use of recombinant leukocyte stimulatory factors, such as granulocyte-macrophage colony-stimulating factor (GM-CSF), have been advocated. Adequately controlled clinical investigations are needed to demonstrate the effectiveness and safety of these three therapies. Unfortunately, such a study was not performed during the clinical use of GM-CSF in the 1987 radiation disaster in Brazil.[30,31] Further research is needed if the preservation of granulocytes for autologous transfusion is to be made practical. A protocol has yet to be developed for the rational and balanced use of the many humoral hematopoietic stimulatory factors and the timing of their administration. The disappointing results from attempts to use conventional bone-marrow transplants in radiation victims have obviated the use of this procedure in the treatment of mass radiation casualties.[10]

Chelation Therapy. Chelator treatment of internal contamination is most effective when initiated within the first 2 hours, before the radionuclide leaves the vascular space and enters the cell. Currently available chelating agents are not lipophilic and will not cross the cell membrane. Ethylenediaminetetraacetic acid (EDTA) is widely available, but it is toxic regardless of the route of administration. The calcium disodium salt of EDTA is used to avoid hypocalcemic tetany. To avoid nephrotoxicity, the maximal total dose of intravenous EDTA should not exceed 550 mg/kg given as a dilute solution in divided doses over at least 4 days. Intramuscular EDTA (75 mg/kg three times daily) is very painful and should only be given with a local anesthetic. EDTA is contraindicated in renal and hepatic disease. EDTA is used to chelate lead, zinc, copper, cadmium, chromium, manganese, and nickel; none of these metals is related to nuclear weapons or reactor accidents. Its use in radiation accidents is largely confined to the treatment of contamination with the transuranic elements, plutonium and americium.

Diethylenetriaminepentaacetic acid (DTPA) is more effective than EDTA for the treatment of transuranic element contamination. This agent is particularly useful for plutonium, curium, californium, berkelium, and americium, which are commonly involved in nuclear weapons accidents. DTPA is administered intravenously or by external lavage as a dilute solution of the calcium or zinc trisodium salt in physiological saline or glucose. The recommended intravenous dose is 1,000 mg/day infused over 1 hour in 250 ml of solution for 4–5 days. Used as a solution for the irrigation of radionuclide-contaminated wounds, it will cause pain unless a local anesthetic (such as 2% lidocaine) is added.[32]

Nutritional Support. In combined-injury patients and in nonirradiated critically ill patients, heightened catabolic stress and impaired nutritional status may play pivotal roles in morbidity and mortality. The incidence of wound infections and sepsis has been reduced by correcting the indices of malnutrition in postoperative patients.[33] Malnutrition may also contribute to impaired wound healing, depressed immune response, prolonged postoperative ileus, bowel atrophy, increased respiratory infections and insufficiency, impaired ventilatory responses to hypoxia and hypercarbia, delayed weaning time for patients on ventilators, and prolonged hospitalization. Since many of the above phenomena or characteristics can be linked to radiation exposure alone, their accentuation in the malnourished radiation victim is highly probable.

Simple and reliable methods of nutritional assessment are not available, particularly in the irradiated patient, whose lymphocytes will be affected independent of nutritional status. However, parameters that can be used to assess nutritional status in critically ill patients are serum albumin, transferrin, body weight, allergic skin reactions, thickness of triceps skin fold, and direct assay or clinical evidence of micronutrient deficiencies.

In selecting the route of administration of nutrients in the radiation victim, the following considerations are important. The oral route is the safest, most economical, and most natural way to provide nutrients. However, some patients will be unable to consume sufficient quantities of nutrients because anorexia occurs over a wide range of radiation doses. If the alimentary tract has not been injured by radiation, and if inanition supervenes and persists, then nutrients can be infused by nasogastric, gastric, or intestinal feeding tubes. Fluid loss associated with the cholera-like diarrhea of the gastrointestinal subsyndrome may require that nutrients and fluids be administered by both the enteral and parenteral routes. With appropriate placement of an enteral feeding tube, the use of intravenous fluids can be reduced, and transition to enteral therapy alone will be facilitated.

The catabolic critically ill radiation casualty will require no less than 2,500–2,800 kcal/day. This requirement can be met by the infusion of a balanced mixture of glucose, amino acids or protein, and lipids. Based on ideal body weight, total protein or amino acid infusion should approach (but not exceed) 2 g/kg/day. Simple carbohydrates (3.5–6.0 g/kg/day) adequately supply most of the 30–40 kcal/kg of non-protein nutrients needed. Usually, a maximum of 30% of the total caloric requirement can be supplied as lipids. However, short-term peripheral infusion of up to 80% of total calories as lipids is acceptable if central venous access is unavailable.

The infusion of micronutrients, including vitamins, minerals, and trace elements, may need to be adjusted with long-term parenteral therapy. The usual daily replacement dosages of essential water- and fat-soluble vitamins, with the exception of vitamin K, are commercially supplied in a single vial. In thermal-burn-injury patients, the requirements for B-complex vitamins and vitamin C are increased. Vitamin K is given as a 10-mg intramuscular injection once a week. If renal impairment supervenes, the normal requirement for potassium (60–100 meq/day), magnesium (8–12 meq/day), and phosphorus (30–60 meq/day) may need to be reduced. Since sodium depletion may occur with diarrhea in the gastrointestinal subsyndrome, sodium infusion of over 150 meq/day may be needed. If chelation therapy with EDTA is undertaken, supplements of zinc (> 4 mg/day), copper (> 1.5 mg/day), chromium (> 15 µg/day), manganese (> 0.8 mg/day), and iron (> 2 mg/day) may be needed. The patient who receives multiple blood transfusions will not need iron supplements until after the blood count has stabilized. Trace element supplements, including iodine and selenium, should be considered if prolonged parenteral feeding becomes necessary.

SUMMARY

Triage

The degree of injury of a radiation casualty can be categorized by the symptoms of exposure. Casualties can be rapidly sorted on the basis of unlikely, probable, or severe radiation symptoms. This rapid sorting of victims allows the conventional traumatic injuries to receive appropriate attention.

Lymphocyte counts are the most necessary laboratory procedure in the first hours and days after exposure. Information from currently available physical dosimeters is of limited value and cannot be relied on entirely in making triage decisions.

Triage is greatly complicated if the patient has suffered combined injuries. A shift in priority to the expectant category is likely for a radiation casualty who requires more than one surgical procedure or who has received a surface burn of more than 10%.

Medical Management

In the first hours after radiation injury, the priority will be to treat the injuries that require immediate attention. Candidates for surgery must be carefully chosen. Only radiation victims who can be attended to within 36 hours and whose condition does not call for multiple procedures should go to surgery.

Decontamination of surface radionuclides is nearly always a second priority after the initial resuscitative support, and can be effectively done with lavage before surgery. Chelation therapy for internal radionuclide contamination can be safely accomplished with the experimental agent DTPA, but the effectiveness of this therapy with mass casualties remains uncertain.

The use of antiemetics and antidiarrheals may contribute significantly to patient comfort. Unfortunately, in effective doses, the currently available agents have major side effects that impair the patient's performance.

The prevention of infection and the appropriate use of antibiotics are important in the first few weeks after exposure. Within the first 7–10 days, selective gut decontamination should be used before leukopenia and sepsis occur. Two to 3 weeks later, if infection is indicated by fever and leukopenia, parenteral antibiotics should be initiated. To help prevent infection with new organisms, environmental control measures should be instituted as soon as possible.

Supportive therapy with blood components has

been shown to be extremely effective in combating hemorrhage and anemia following combined injury. However, granulocyte transfusions and bone-marrow transplants as currently used appear to be of little help. A combination of simple supportive measures, including fluids, electrolytes, antibiotics, adequate nutrition, and platelet transfusions, can significantly reduce mortality, as shown by studies of animal research models.

Effective triage will permit the use of limited resources to improve the greatest number of radiation casualties. Survival after either radiation injury alone or combined injury can be greatly enhanced by the application of currently available treatments. Research into new and experimental therapeutic agents for the treatment of radiation injury may be expected not only to benefit the civilian population, but also to enhance the survival of the fighting force.

REFERENCES

1. Walker, R. I., and Conklin, J. J. 1987. Military radiobiology: A perspective. In *Military Radiobiology,* edited by J. J. Conklin and R. I. Walker, 1-8. Orlando, FL: Academic Press.

2. Leaning, J. 1986. Burn and blast casualties: Triage in nuclear war. In *The Medical Implications of Nuclear War,* edited by F. Solomon and R. Q. Marston, 251-281. Washington, DC: National Academy Press.

3. Wiener, S. L., and Barret, J. 1986. Thermonuclear weapons. In *Trauma Management for Civilian and Military Physicians,* 497-506. Philadelphia: W. B. Saunders.

4. American College of Surgeons Committee on Trauma (D. D. Trunkey, chairperson). 1984. *Advanced trauma life support course for physicians.* Chicago: American College of Surgeons.

5. Champion, H. R., and Sacco, W. J. 1986. Triage of trauma victims. In vol. 2, *Current Therapy of Trauma,* edited by D. D. Trunkey, 5-12. Toronto: B. C. Decker.

6. Conklin, J. J., and Walker, R. I. 1986. Diagnosis, triage, and treatment of casualties. *Medical Bulletin of the U.S. Army, Europe* 43(7): 11-15.

7. Dutreix, J. 1986. Human skin: Early and late reactions in relation to dose and its time distribution. *Br. J. Radiol.* (Suppl.) 19: 22-28.

8. Lushbaugh, C. C.; Fry, S. A.; Ricks, R. C.; Hubner, K. F.; and Burr, W. W. 1986. Historical update of past and recent skin damage radiation accidents. *Br. J. Radiol.* (Suppl.) 19: 12-17.

9. Milroy, W. C. 1984. Management of irradiated and contaminated casualty victims. *Emerg. Med. Clin. North Am.* 2: 667-686.

10. Gus'kovaya, A. K., ed. 1987. *Early acute effects among the victims of the accident at the Chernobyl Nuclear Power Plant* [USSR Ministry of Health Order No. 4851]. Translated by U.S. Defense Intelligence Agency [LN 818-87]. Moscow: USSR Ministry of Health.

11. Murano, G.; MacVittie, T. J.; Conklin, J. J.; Casey L. C.; and Walker, R. I. 1985. Hemostatic changes in a canine model of combined injury. In *The Pathophysiology of Combined Injury and Trauma,* edited by R. I. Walker, D. F. Gruber, T. J. MacVittie, and J. J. Conklin, 105-110. Baltimore: University Park Press.

12. Cockerham, L. G.; Simpson, S. A.; Doyle, T. F.; and Gossett-Hagerman, C. J. 1984. Canine post-irradiation plasma glucose variations. *Life Sci.* 34: 2641-2646.

13. Landauer, M. R.; Ledney, G. D.; and Davis, H. D. 1987. Locomotor behavior in mice following exposure to fission-neutron irradiation and trauma. *Aviat. Space Environ. Med.* 58: 1205-1210.

14. Wardlaw, S. C., and Levine, R. A. 1983. Buffycoat analysis. *JAMA* 249: 617-620.

15. North Atlantic Treaty Organization. 1978. *NATO handbook on the concept of medical support in NBC environments* [AMed P-7 (A)]. Brussels: North Atlantic Treaty Organization.

16. Giambarresi, L. 1986. Nuclear weapons: Medical effects and operational considerations. *Medical Bulletin of the U.S. Army, Europe* 43(7): 7-10.

17. Streffer, C., and Messerschmidt, O. 1966. Untersuchungen uber Kombinationsschaden. Die Ausscheidung von Taurin und Harnstoff im Ur in wei er Mause bei einer Kombination von Strahtenbelastung und Hautwunde. *Strahlentherapie* 130: 285.

18. Hunt, W. Personal communication.

19. Conklin, J. J.; Walker, R. I.; and Hirsch, E. F. 1983. Current concepts in the management of radiation injuries and associated trauma. *Surg. Gynecol. Obstet.* 156: 809-829.

20. Messerschmidt, O. 1986. Treatment of subcutaneous radiation lesions. *Br. J. Radiol.* (Suppl.) 19: 122-137.

21. Fabian, T. C.; Hoefling, S. J.; and Strom, P. R. 1982. Use of antibiotic prophylaxis in penetrating abdominal trauma. *Clin. Ther.* 5: 38-47.

22. King, G. Personal communication.

23. Spiro, H. M. 1970. Inflammatory disorders other than ulcerative colitis. In *Clinical Gastroenterology*, 570-574. Toronto: Macmillan Co.

24. Kaplan, J. Z. Care of thermally injured victims of a thermonuclear explosion. In reference 11, 41-45.

25. Cormed, Inc. is located in Medina, NY.

26. Venezio, F. R., and O'Keefe, P. 1986. Infections of intravascular devices. *J. Nosocom. Infect.* 4: 10-26.

27. Kaufman, J. L. 1987. Venous catheter-related thrombosis and infection. *JAMA* 257: 2594.

28. Allo, M. D.; Miller, J.; Townsend, T.; and Tan, C. 1987. Primary cutaneous aspergillosis associated with Hickman intravenous catheters. *N. Engl. J. Med.* 317: 1105-1108.

29. Warkentin, P. I. 1987. Plateletapheresis: An invaluable blood resource. *Cleve. Clin. J. Med.* 54: 381-383.

30. Roberts, L. 1987. Radiation accident grips Goiânia. *Science* 238: 1028-1031.

31. Butturini, A.; Gale, R. P.; Lopes, D. M.; Cunha, C. B.; Ho, W. G.; Sanpai, J. M.; De Souza, P. C.; Cordiero, J. M.; Neto, C.; De Souza, C. E.; Tabek, D. G.; Burla, A.; and the Navy Hospital Radiation Team. 1988. Use of recombinant granulocyte-macrophage colony-stimulating-factor in the Brazil radiation accident. *Lancet* 2 (August 27): 471-475.

32. Durakovic, A. Internal contamination with medically significant radionuclides. In reference 1, 241-264.

33. Schmitz, J.-E.; Ahnefeld, F. W.; and Burri, C. 1983. Nutritional support of the multiple trauma patient. *World J. Surg.* 7: 132-142.

Chapter 4

TREATMENT OF INTERNAL RADIONUCLIDE CONTAMINATION

T. JAN CERVENY, Ph.D.*

*Major, United States Air Force; Program Manager, Bioenvironmental Hazards, Air Force Office of Scientific Research, Bolling Air Force Base, Washington, D.C. 20332-6448

INTRODUCTION

Military and civilian providers of medical care must be prepared to deal with the medical aftermath of a nuclear detonation or accident. With the earth's increasing nuclear arsenal and the growing use of nuclear energy systems, our biosphere is threatened by the production and release of large quantities of radioisotopes. The accidents at Chernobyl, USSR, in 1986 and at Goiânia, Brazil, in 1987 have stressed the importance of knowing how to manage the radioactive contamination of persons in military and civilian settings. Such management requires knowledge of the metabolism of various radionuclides in humans and methods to increase their elimination from the body.

Many aspects of medical management are based on judgments and evaluations that are difficult to instruct. Treatment information is sparse and often subjective. This chapter discusses difficult treatment decisions, with the understanding that considerable latitude exists in medical evaluation.

In a nuclear explosion, over 400 radioactive isotopes are released into the biosphere.[1] About forty are considered to be potentially hazardous to humans because of either their organospecificity or their long half-life. Both early and delayed radioactive fallout will be deposited in our external environment, which could result in internal contamination with radionuclides.

INITIAL MANAGEMENT

The medical staff providing the initial management of radionuclide-contaminated patients will have varying responsibilities, depending on the isotopes involved, radiation-monitoring capabilities, location, and available facilities. Thorough evaluation and estimates of internal contamination may take days or weeks, however, so these decisions may have to be based only on historical information and superficial measurements. Medical personnel must proceed quickly to obtain information and make treatment decisions based on available early estimates of possible exposure. Treatment risks must be weighed against the presumed risks of untreated exposure. Damage from the latter may not be manifested until 20–30 years after internalization.

Initial management may be divided into four applications: *(a)* uptake and clearance, *(b)* sampling of radioactivity, *(c)* on-site management, and *(d)* hospital management.[1-3]

Uptake and Clearance

Internal contamination occurs by three main routes (listed in order of importance): *inhalation, ingestion,* and *wound contamination.* A fourth and infrequent route is *percutaneous absorption*, which applies almost exclusively to the radioisotope tritium and its association with water. The uptake and retention of a radionuclide are influenced by its portal of entry, chemistry, solubility, metabolism, and particle size.[1-4] Of the three main routes, inhalation poses the biggest threat, especially in a fallout environment.[1-3,5,6] The size of the radioactive particle determines if it will be deposited in the lungs, because particles greater than 10 microns in diameter cannot pass by the nasal hairs. *Clearance time* (time required for particles to be removed from the lungs) depends on which respiratory compartment receives the deposit,[1-3] and time will be an important factor in treatment decisions. Times for respiratory clearance into the next higher compartment are as follows: trachea, 0.1 hour; bronchi, 1 hour; bronchioles, 4 hours; and alveoli, 100–1,500 or more days.[1,3] Soluble particles that are deposited into the alveoli may be systemically absorbed at the alveolar-blood interface, and may thereby become incorporated into target organs. Insoluble particles also pose a threat, especially if plutonium from unspent fuel or industrial accidents is present. Prolonged exposure of the alveolar epithelium to high-LET alpha emitters, like plutonium, has been related to increased incidence of malignancy.[2,6]

In 1955, the International Commission on Radiological Protection adopted a model for evaluating the hazards of inhaled radioactive particles.[6] According to this model, 25% of inhaled radioactive particles are immediately exhaled, and the remaining 75% are deposited along the respiratory tree. About half of the particles are deposited in the upper bronchial tree, where they are moved by the ciliary epithelium to the nasopharynx. In the nasopharynx, they are propelled by the mucociliary swallowing reflex into the digestive tract, where they enter the gastrointestinal path.[2]

Ingestion is usually secondary to inhalation and the mucociliary swallowing response. However, in a fallout environment, direct ingestion from contaminated foodstuffs is also probable. The degree of intraluminal gastrointestinal exposure depends on transit time through the gut, which will vary widely from person to person.[1,3] The mean clearance times of the human digestive tract are stomach, 1 hour; small intestine, 4 hours; upper large intestine, 13–20 hours; and lower large intestine, 24 hours, resulting in a total mean emptying time of 42 hours. The much slower rate of movement in the large intestine places its luminal lining at higher risk for damage from nonabsorbable radionuclides. Gastrointestinal transit time may be shortened by use of emetic and/or purgative agents.

Some relatively soluble radionuclides may not be absorbed due to acidic or caustic properties that fix them to tissue proteins.[1,2,7,8] Systemic absorption through the intestine varies widely, depending on the radioisotope and its chemical form. Clear differences exist between radioiodine, which is rapidly and completely absorbed, and plutonium, which is almost nonabsorbed (0.003%). Furthermore, nonabsorbable alpha emitters apparently do not cause gastrointestinal injury, even in large amounts. Nevertheless, the gastrointestinal tract is the critical target organ for the many insoluble radionuclides that travel its length almost unabsorbed.

Wounds contaminated by fallout and shrapnel may provide continuous irradiation of surrounding tissues and increase the likelihood of systemic incorporation.[1,3,5,9-11] This hazard remains until the contaminant is removed by cleansing, surgical debridement, or radionuclide decay. The last process may take a few days or millions of years, depending on the contaminant.

Sampling of Radioactivity

Since the identification of radionuclide contaminants is important for treatment, it may be necessary to know whether beta-gamma or alpha emitters are present. Health-physics personnel should be able to provide this information even with limited radiation-detecting equipment. Separate swabs of the nares should be taken to determine radioactivity and possible inhalation contamination before decontaminating the skin by showering or washing. The nasal swab should be taken at the site and sent in a sealed, clean container to higher-care facilities along with the patient. Although skin decontamination should be done as quickly as possible, the stability of an injured patient is vital, and first aid must be the primary concern.

On-Site Management

Contamination of the skin with radionuclides is usually not immediately life threatening to either the patient or medical personnel, unless the contamination is from a gamma emitter and the dose rate is several Gys per hour. Partial or complete emergency decontamination should be done at the site before a patient is transported to a higher-care facility. Discarding contaminated clothing will remove up to 85% of external contaminants; following this with showering or washing will remove more than 95% of surface contamination.[1,3,5] A combined nuclear-chemical war may present many problems for decontamination procedures. A light wash-down and vacuuming or brushing of protective clothing may be all that can be done.

Hospital Management

Hospital emergency plans should provide for the proper management of incoming contaminated casualties. The National Council on Radiation Protection and Measurements provides a universal outline guide that can be adapted for most facilities.[1] A designated decontamination area should be prepared, and traffic in this area should be one-way to prevent contaminating "clean" areas of the facility. Ideal decontamination facilities should have equipment to wash ambulatory and injured patients, shielding to use with high-level beta-gamma contamination, and a floor plan that minimizes cross-contamination of clean areas.[1-3] Medical personnel should be rotated through the decontamination area to ensure that their radiation exposure is kept to a minimum. Clothing and other contaminated materials should be discarded at a contained location away from the health-care facility. At many hospitals, the morgue or autopsy room is an excellent decontamination area. It has contained liquid systems, a table easily adapted to wash a contaminated patient, and often a heavily lined area that can be used to store contaminated materials. Other possibilities include physiotherapy areas and cast rooms. Table 4-1 lists the supplies that are recommended for a decontamination room.[1]

The initial evaluation of a patient should include

TABLE 4-1

CHECKLIST OF SUPPLIES FOR DECONTAMINATION AREA

Category	✓	Items
Radiation Equipment and Supplies		
	☐	Personal dosimeters (ionization chamber, self-reading type; 200 mR and 20 R scale levels)
	☐	Portable beta-gamma ray survey meters
	☐	Dosimetery badges (TLD type)
	☐	Radiation tags
	☐	Radiation area signs, including "Do Not Enter"
	☐	Respirators for team personnel
Contaminated Tissue and Specimen Collection		
	☐	Prelabled urine containers
	☐	Prelabled fecal containers
	☐	Tissue and contaminated material specimen containers
	☐	Disposal bags (large plastic) for contaminated materials
	☐	Formalin-containing specimen containers (for use if freezing equipment is not available)
Sterile Supplies		
	☐	Surgical gloves
	☐	Suture sets with 2 extra scissors, 4 forceps, 1 scalpel, and 6 hemostats
	☐	Applicators
	☐	Assortment of dressings
Clothing and Protective Wear		
	☐	Surgical scrub suits or coveralls
	☐	Surgical caps (disposable)
	☐	Surgical gloves (plastic or rubber; reuseable)
	☐	Aprons (plastic or rubber)
	☐	Shoe covers (plastic)
	☐	Socks
	☐	Patient gowns (long) or coveralls
	☐	Blankets
General Supplies		
	☐	Two bandage scissors
	☐	Safety razor (with extra blades)
	☐	Aerosol shaving cream
	☐	Masking tape (2 inches wide)
	☐	Pens (felt type; black and red)
	☐	Pencils
	☐	Notebooks
	☐	Paper

a complete history of the contamination incident, a physical examination to uncover conventional injuries (but which usually provides no evidence of radionuclide contamination), and laboratory tests, including a complete blood count with platelets and a routine urinalysis. The incident history should provide some background for predicting possible internalization of radionuclides. The internalization may be from fallout; handling a damaged, undetonated nuclear weapon; accidental ingestion of (or external contamination by) a specific radioactive substance; or radionuclide-contaminated wounds. The patient should then be placed into the emergency-plan triage system and treated accordingly.

MEASUREMENT OF RADIOACTIVE CONTAMINATION

Generally, health physicists at large medical facilities will be responsible for radiation monitoring. However, all medical personnel should be aware of the various monitoring techniques in order to understand their reliability, limitations, and sources of possible error. The determination of surface contamination will require monitoring for alpha and beta-gamma emissions.

Alpha particles have limited penetration, and a patient will be protected by an intact epidermis. Alpha contamination does not become hazardous unless it is internalized through inhalation, ingestion, or wounds.[1,6,11] Alpha particles are the most difficult radiocontaminant to detect, and negative monitoring results are not always reliable. Due to the high absorption of alpha particles even in air, it is important to keep the radiation monitor close to the measured surface. Direct contact readings are preferred. Proportional counters are the most common device for detecting alpha radiation in the laboratory, and they are capable of discriminating between alpha and beta-gamma emitters. However, the counters are not yet available for military field use. Scintillation counters are currently used for determining radioactivity contamination while in the field, but they are less sensitive than proportional counters. Surface monitoring with swipes may also be used to test for transferable alpha material. Textured paper (such as filter paper) is wiped across the test surface and then measured in a laboratory scintillation counter. Results may identify contamination with transferable alpha (plutonium) or weak beta (tritium) radiation. The nose swipe is also used for alpha emitters. A cotton swab or narrow strip of filter paper moistened with distilled water is gently wiped around the naris opening (one per naris). After the swab or paper is dry, the radioactivity is determined.

Beta and gamma radiations are often emitted simultaneously by decaying radioisotopes. These types of radiation present internal and external hazards. Instruments for measuring either type of radiation are similar, but the Geiger-Mueller (GM) counter is the most common detection device. Unfortunately, high radiation levels can saturate GM counters and give false or even zero readings. Ionization chambers can measure higher dose rates. Both are sensitive to extremes of heat and humidity, and both may fail in a corrosive chemical environment. Shielding the probe of the detection device will provide a relatively pure reading of the gamma component, and the difference between the shielded and unshielded readings provides the beta (and often soft gamma) component.

All medical personnel need to be alert to possible mixed external-internal contamination. A patient may have inhaled contaminated steam or dust during the cleanup of an accident, as happened in the 1986 nuclear reactor accident at Chernobyl.[12,13] If the internalized materials are beta- or gamma-emitting substances, they may provide radiation readings on the monitoring devices used for external decontamination. Of course, internalized alpha particles will not register on monitoring devices, but their presence may be suggested by the incident history or by the detection of external alpha particles.

If patients are few and there is a need to know (or closely estimate) the total internal radiation dose, all body effluents must be collected for an extended time. Careful measurements of all excreted radiation will provide data for calculating a close estimate of the total internal body burden.[1] Depending on the radioisotope involved and its physicochemical characteristics, the collections may have to be made for months.

Many pitfalls exist in the interpretation of excretion data analyses. Variations in excretion rates from person to person will interfere, and the time of exposure, possible interim therapy with chelators, and data on the excretion of inhaled contaminants may complicate the estimate.

A nuclear detonation or accident may result in alpha, beta, gamma-ray, X-ray, and neutron emissions. Devices that are available to detect exposure to gamma, X, and neutron radiations include dosimeters, film badges, and thermoluminescent detectors.

TREATMENT DECISIONS

Early information on the history of the exposure incident may identify the major isotopes involved and provide some dosimetry information. Patients will likely present with no clinical symptoms other than possible conventional trauma. Therefore, critical decisions on the initial treatment may have to be based on knowledge of human physiology, the pharmacology of agents to be used, the metabolism of the radioisotopes, and the historical information. Treatments for internal contamination should begin within hours of exposure.[1-5,7,14] Emergency planning will pay off by reducing the time for dosimetric evaluations and will result in more informed initial decisions. After the initial treatment, there will generally be time to assess the situation as data from monitoring become available. Later, dose estimates will determine if further treatment and evaluation are needed, or if the treatment involves risks.

Usually no immediately life-threatening hazard is associated with radiation contamination, especially after the removal of clothing and washing. The probability that a patient will incur radiation-induced health problems is low, and any incidence may be decades in the future. Risky decontamination procedures (such as lung lavage or surgery) that could lead to internalization should be carefully evaluated, and a decision may require assistance by expert consultation.[1,15]

Physicochemical properties of radiocontaminants play a significant role in determining treatment. The solubility of the material containing the contaminant may determine its distribution within the body, or even its accessibility into the body. As no material is completely insoluble, some small fraction may rapidly become internalized from the lung or through a wound. In contrast, normally soluble materials may be present in an insoluble form, or may be made insoluble under systemic physiological conditions. Therefore, treatment begun as early as possible after exposure will significantly increase the probability of successful internal decontamination.[1-3,5,7,10]

Medical personnel should be aware of the possible presence of *mixed-fission products* (MFP), which are groups of radionuclides likely to be found together after nuclear reactor or detonation incidents. The appropriate treatment regimen is based on the time of exposure after the nuclear event. Some MFP groups are plutonium with associated americium, curium, and neptunium, and uranium with thorium, radium, and their decay products. Treatment is determined by the particular radioisotopes.

In a complete nuclear detonation, over 400 radionuclides are released. However, only about forty of these are potentially hazardous to humans.[1-3] The most significant radioisotopes from unspent nuclear fuel are tritium, plutonium, and uranium. Of particular interest are the radioisotopes whose organo-specificity and long half-lives may result in irreversible damage or induction of malignant alterations. Radioisotopes of immediate medical significance are listed in Table 4-2, with descriptions of properties, target organs, and treatment.

THERAPEUTIC MANAGEMENT

Skin decontamination has two goals: *(a)* to remove radiocontaminants and thereby reduce the total dose, and *(b)* to prevent possible internalization. If done appropriately, skin decontamination will also contribute to a more accurate determination of the internal contamination. If the radioactive contaminant is resistant to an initial washing with soap or detergent and water, further decontamination should be supervised by a physician. The physician needs to understand the basic physical and physiological principles involved. The contaminant's half-life, energy level, and dose rate must be weighed against continued and harsher decontamination procedures, which may abrade the intact skin or decrease the distance to the important dermis basal layer. Because the skin regenerates every 10–14 days, contamination would eventually be shed naturally. Signs of excessive decontamination

TABLE 4-2

SIGNIFICANT RADIONUCLIDE INFORMATION

Radionuclide	Radiation Type	Critical Body Site	Contamination Mode*	Treatment Agent
Americium	α, γ	Bone	I/W	DTPA†
Californium	γ, α, n	Bone	I/W	DTPA
Cerium	β, γ	GI, lung	I/GI	DTPA
Cesium	β, γ	Total body	I/S/GI	Prussian blue£
Curium	α, γ, n	Bone	I/GI	DTPA
Iodine	β, γ	Thyroid	I/GI/S	KI (sat.)¥
Plutonium	α, γ	Bone	I/W	DTPA
Polonium	α	Lung	I	Dimercaprol‡
Strontium	γ	Bone	I/GI	$AlPO_4$**
Tritium	β	Total body	I/S/GI	Forced H_2O§
Uranium	α, β, γ	Bone	I/S/W	$NaHCO_3$***

* I: contamination by inhalation
GI: contamination by gastrointestinal absorption
S: contamination by skin absorption
W: contamination by wound absorption

** The antacid aluminum phosphate in gel form used as a gastrointestinal adsorbent for radiostrontium

*** Sodium bicarbonate to maintain alkalinity of urine used in conjunction with diuretics

† Diethylenetriaminepentaacetic acid used as a tissue chelation agent forming stable complexes which may be excreted by the kidney (approved by the FDA as an investigational new drug)

‡ A mercury poisoning chelation agent (very toxic)

¥ An agent blocking radioiodine absorption in tissues resulting in dilution of the isotope

§ Simple forced intake of water, resulting in isotope dilution

£ A dye used as an ion exchanger (not yet approved by the FDA)

efforts will be more evident 24 hours later, and two or three less intensive decontamination efforts are less traumatic to the skin than one major effort. If necessary, further cleansing may include mild abrasives, chelating agents, and bleach. Chemical techniques are rarely needed.

After first aid to control hemorrhage and shock, the next steps are to determine if wounds are contaminated and then to locate any other contamination.[1-5,10,11,14] Alpha emitters and possibly weak beta emitters are difficult to locate around wounds. A simple film of irrigation fluid, blood, or tissue fluid can entirely mask this contamination, which then may internalize via the circulatory or lymph systems. Once the surface contaminant is located, irrigation should be sufficient to remove it, although some wounds may need debridement that is deeper than conventional injuries require. This debridement involves a certain risk of translocation or absorption (especially when working with possible alpha emitters, like americium or plutonium); therefore, the chelating agent DTPA should be given systemically and the wound should be irrigated with DTPA before debridement.

If limb wounds have high concentrations of beta-gamma contaminants, medical personnel must limit their exposure by frequently rotating shifts or by working with shields. Amputation of the limb may have to be considered if *(a)* the wound is highly contaminated and decontamination attempts cannot be made or are not successful, *(b)* the contamination is so intense that extensive radiation-induced necrosis is likely, or *(c)* the injury is so severe that functional recovery is unlikely.

TREATMENT OF INTERNAL CONTAMINATION

The goals of internal decontamination are to reduce absorption and to enhance elimination and excretion. Treatment is most effective if it is started as soon as possible after exposure.

Clearance of the Gastrointestinal Tract

Gastric absorption can be reduced by stomach lavage, emetics, purgatives and laxatives, ion exchangers, and aluminum antacids. Other less effective treatments are alginates, barium sulfate, and phytates, which currently are not recommended for internal decontamination of radionuclides.

Stomach lavage is useful only if the ingested dose is known to be large, and if the intake is recent and still in the stomach. Lavaged material must be monitored for radioactivity and the patient must be kept in a head-low position to prevent aspiration.

The most common emetic agents are apomorphine (5–10 mg, subcutaneous) and ipecac (1–2 g in capsule or 15 ml in syrup), which should be given concomitantly with 200–300 ml of water. Caution should be used not to induce emesis in an unconscious patient.

Laxatives or purgatives (such as castor oil) will stimulate intestinal motility, and saline cathartics will increase water movement into the intestine and induce removal of contents within 3–6 hours. The selection of purgatives or laxatives should be based on their speed of action (slowly acting drugs, like bulk-forming and wetting agents, are not appropriate). These agents are contraindicated if the patient has abdominal pain of unknown origin, or if surgery is a possibility.

Prussian blue, an ion exchanger, was used to treat victims in the 1987 cesium-137 contamination incident in Goiânia[16] and has been well tolerated in humans (1 g given orally with water three times per day).[1,2] It may be continued for 3 weeks or longer, as indicated. However, Prussian blue is not approved by the Food and Drug Administration (FDA), and emergency approval for an investigational drug would have to be obtained. Ion-exchange resins, like sodium polystyrene sulfonate (for adults, 15 g, 4 level teaspoons of resin suspension), have an assumed but untested usefulness for inhibiting the uptake of radionuclides in the gut.

Aluminum antacids are an effective treatment for reducing the uptake of radioactive strontium. A dose of 100 ml of aluminum phosphate gel, given immediately after exposure, decreases the absorption of radioactive strontium in the gut by about 85%. Aluminum hydroxide, given in a single dose of 60–100 ml, reduces uptake by about 50%. Both forms are nontoxic. This is the treatment of choice for contamination with radiostrontium.[1,2]

Prevention or Reversal of Radionuclide Interaction with Tissues

Blocking and Diluting Agents. Blocking and diluting agents decrease the likelihood of absorption by decreasing the availability of the radionuclide. A blocking agent, such as potassium iodide (300 mg/day for 7–14 days) for radioiodine, blocks the uptake of a radioisotope by significantly increasing the availability of the stable isotope. Diluting agents simply dilute the radioisotope, which statistically decreases the opportunity for absorption. Water is a diluting agent in the treatment of tritium contamination. For maximum efficacy, the stable isotopes that are used as the blocking or diluting agents must be as rapidly absorbed or metabolized as the radioisotopes are.

Mobilizing Agents. Mobilizing agents are compounds that enhance and increase the natural turnover processes and thereby induce the release of radioisotopes from tissues. They are most effective when given immediately, but they may retain some effectiveness for up to 2 weeks after exposure. Included in this group are antithyroid drugs, ammonium chloride, diuretics, expectorants and inhalants, parathyroid extract, and corticosteroids. These agents require experienced consultation, treatment, and management.[1,9]

Chelating Agents. Chelators are substances that bind with some metals more strongly than others to form a stable complex that, when soluble, can be more readily excreted by the kidneys. The effectiveness of chelation therapy is influenced by many physiological factors, including plasma proteins, blood pH, enzymes, and even nucleic acids. The most commonly known chelating agent is EDTA, normally given as the calcium salt. However, for treatment of the heavy-metal multivalent radionuclides expected from a nuclear yield, the powerful chelator DTPA is generally more effective. DTPA-chelated complexes are more stable than EDTA complexes, and are therefore less likely to release the radionuclide before excretion. The calcium and zinc forms of DTPA have both been approved by the FDA as investigational new drugs (IND) for the chelation of plutonium, berkelium, californium, americium, and curium. Physicians finding a need for DTPA should contact the Radiation Emergency Assistance Center/Training Site (REAC/TS) to become a coinvestigator (see address in reference note).[17] REAC/TS usually responds to nuclear accidents and incidents and will arrive at the site within 48 hours. It is doubtful that DTPA will be available in combat.

DTPA is administered as an intravenous solution of 1 g dissolved in 250 ml of saline or 5% glucose, infused over 1 hour per day for up to 5 days.[1,15] As an irrigation solution, 1 g CaDTPA and 10 ml of 2% lidocaine are dissolved in 100 ml normal saline for plutonium and americium contamination.[5] If the contaminants have an atomic number greater than uranium's 92, the treatment is simple: DTPA is used for all contaminants except uranium. The use of DTPA is contraindicated for treatment of uranium contamination because of the added risk of renal damage.[18] Uranium contamination has been treated with oral sodium bicarbonate, regulated to maintain an alkaline urine pH, and accompanied by diuretics.[1]

Other chelating agents are dimercaprol, penicillamine, and deferoxamine (DFOA). Dimercaprol is a highly toxic chelator that has been effective in treating mercury poisoning. Penicillamine and CaEDTA are significantly less toxic and more effective for mercury poisoning. (Radiomercury, however, is not a likely hazard of nuclear detonation.) Penicillamine is an amino acid derived from penicillin, but it has no antibacterial properties. It has been used to treat contamination with many metals, mainly copper, mercury, and lead. It does not appear to be especially promising for the treatment of internal radionuclide contamination. DFOA has been used to treat iron poisoning. In combination with DTPA, it has an increased affinity for iron. DFOA appears to be more useful than DTPA in treating plutonium contamination, but until it is approved by the FDA for this purpose its use cannot be recommended.

Lung Lavage. Lung lavage has been successful in decreasing radiation-induced pneumonitis in laboratory animals.[1] It has been used in human therapy for chronic obstructive lung diseases.[19] However, the procedure requires general anesthesia, and a careful risk-benefit assessment must be made before it is used for radionuclide decontamination. Endoscopy is the procedure most similar to lung lavage, and it has a mortality rate of 0.08%–0.85% in patients judged to be in good condition. Considering that the risk from lung lavage is immediate and that the possible effects from internal radionuclides are decades away, medical personnel will have to weigh the benefit to the patient carefully. Unless the lung burden is so great that it will result in acute radiation injury, lung lavage is not recommended.[1-3]

SUMMARY

A plan for medical care must be available to deal with the contingency of a nuclear event. The first priority is basic first aid, followed by decontamination in a predesignated area. The level and type of radiation exposure must be caculated as accurately as possible. Contamination may be internalized via inhalation, ingestion, and absorption through wounds and skin. Treatment is determined by the particular radiation to which the patient has been exposed. Internal decontamination must be started in the first few hours after exposure if radionuclides could have been internalized.

REFERENCES

1. National Council on Radiation Protection and Measurements. 1980. *Management of persons accidentally contaminated with radionuclides* [NCRP Report 65]. Washington, DC: National Council on Radiation Protection and Measurements.

2. Durakovic, A. 1987. Internal contamination with medically significant radionuclides. In *Military Radiobiology*, edited by J. J. Conklin and R. I. Walker, 241-264. Orlando, FL: Academic Press.

3. Cerveny, T. J., and Cockerham, L. G. 1986. Medical management of internal radionuclide contamination. *Medical Bulletin of the U.S. Army, Europe* 43(7): 24-27.

4. International Commission on Radiological Protection. 1955. Recommendations of International Commission on Radiological Protection. *Br. J. Radiol.* (Suppl. 6).

5. Conklin, J. J.; Walker, R. I.; and Hirsch, E. F. 1983. Current concepts in the management of radiation injuries and associated trauma. *Surg. Gynecol. Obstet.* 156: 809-829.

6. Biological effects of inhaled radionuclides. *Ann. ICRP* 31(1980): 4(1/2).

7. Moskalev, Y. I., ed. 1974. *Distribution, biological effects and accelerated excretion of radioactive isotopes* [AEC-TR-7590]. Translated from the Russian by the U.S. Atomic Energy Commission. Springfield, VA: National Technical Information Service.

8. Butler G. C. 1976. *Metabolic excretion and retention patterns of incorporated radionuclides in reference man* [STI/PUB/411], 3. Vienna: International Atomic Energy Agency.

9. Lushbaugh, C. C.; Andrews, G. A.; and Hubner, K. F. 1976. *REAC/TS: A pragmatic approach for providing medical care and physician education for radiation emergencies* [STI/PUB/411], 565. Vienna: International Atomic Energy Agency.

10. Ohlenschlager, L. 1970. First aid measures in radiation accident with special reference to wounds contaminated with radioactivity. *Atompraxis* (Ger.) 16(4): 236.

11. Foreman, H. 1963. Medical management of radioactively contaminated wounds. In *Proceedings of the Scientific Meeting on the Diagnosis and Treatment of Radioactive Poisoning*. Vienna: International Atomic Energy Agency.

12. USSR State Committee on the Utilization of Atomic Energy. 1986. *The accident at the Chernobyl Nuclear Power Plant and its consequences. Part II, Annex 7.* Vienna: International Atomic Energy Agency Experts' Meeting.

13. Gus'kovaya, A. K., ed. 1987. *Early acute effects among the victims of the accident at the Chernobyl Nuclear Power Plant* [USSR Ministry of Health Order No. 4851]. Translated by U.S. Defense Intelligence Agency [LN 818-87]. Moscow: USSR Ministry of Health.

14. Cosgriff, J. H., Jr. 1987. Guidelines for the emergency management of radiation injury. *Internal Medicine (for the Specialist)* 8: 170-180.

15. Program Update: DTPA chelation drugs. *REAC/TS Newsletter* (Winter/Spring, 1987).

16. Roberts, L. 1987. Radiation accident grips Goiânia. *Science* 238: 1028-1031.

17. Radiation Emergency Assistance Center/Training Site (REAC/TS) is located in Oak Ridge, TN. The telephone number is (615) 576-3086.

18. Update on chelation therapy: Chelators should not be used for uranium or neptunium. *REAC/TS Newsletter* (April, 1981)

19. Klystra, J. A.; Rausch, D. C.; Hall, K. D.; and Spock, A. 1971. Volume controlled lung lavage in the treatment of asthma, bronchiectasis, and mucoviscidosis. *Am. Rev. Respir. Dis.* 103: 651.

Chapter 5

INFECTIOUS COMPLICATIONS OF RADIATION INJURY

RICHARD I. WALKER, Ph.D.*

*Captain, United States Navy; Director, Enteric Diseases Program, Naval Medical Research Institute, Bethesda, Maryland 20814-5055 and Armed Forces Radiobiology Research Institute, Bethesda, Maryland 20814-5145

INTRODUCTION

Infection with normally harmless indigenous microorganisms is a major cause of morbidity and mortality when normal host defenses have been compromised. These opportunistic pathogens are responsible for hundreds of thousands of serious infections in injured and immunosuppressed patients in the United States annually, and the mortality rate for these infections can range from 50% to 70%.[1,2] Advances in surgical and resuscitation techniques are increasing the immediate survival of victims of severe trauma, but many die later from overwhelming infections. In trauma victims who survive the first few days after the event, sepsis is the second major cause of death (with head injury the first).

The nature of the postinjury events that are responsible for infection is illustrated in Figure 5-1. Both radiation and trauma can cause damage to or destruction of tissues. The insult triggers an inflammatory response which, via mediators, activates significant physiological and immunological processes, including disturbances of permeability in the intestine. Leakage of endotoxin from the intestinal lumen can occur, and facultative anaerobic flora increase in numbers in the gut. As this happens, macrophages and other cells contribute to a suppression of the immune system. This early immunosuppression may be beneficial and not pose a serious hazard because mucosal bacterial populations are not excessive at this time.

If the physiological and immunological deficiencies associated with trauma or radiation exposure are not resolved, then suppression of immunity persists. Subsequently, mucosal microorganisms, such as those in the intestine, multiply dramatically and may translocate to other tissues. Many enteric flora find their way to wound surfaces, where they begin to predominate. The best management of opportunistic infections is to use interventions that interrupt or compensate for these processes, thereby preventing overwhelming infection and shock.

INFECTIONS ASSOCIATED WITH CONVENTIONAL INJURIES

Incidence and Type of Pathogens

The nature of the microbial agents responsible for most opportunistic infections has changed since antibiotics were first used, but the incidence of infection has changed relatively little. For example, data from early World War II show a 6% incidence of infections in soft-tissue wounds in 926 patients, a 14% incidence of serious infections with compound fractures in 674 patients, and a 22% incidence of burn infections in 591 patients.[3] The incidence of infection was not much different for soldiers injured in the 1973 Yom Kippur War in Israel (Table 5-1). The overall incidence of infection was 22% in 420 patients.[4] Of those, 49 burn patients had a 35% incidence of infection; 99 patients with fractures, 18% incidence; 178 patients with soft-tissue injuries, 6%; and 53 patients with penetrating abdominal wounds and perforated colon, 30%.

With the increased use of antibiotics, organisms such as *Clostridium perfringens* (which causes gas gangrene) have become less important. Others have become more troublesome, especially gram-negative organisms such as the *Pseudomonas* or *Klebsiella* species or *Escherichia coli*. Other important opportunistic pathogens are *Streptococcus fecalis* and *Staphylococcus aureus* as well as the *Enterobacter* and *Bacteroides* species. However, many other microorganisms have also been implicated in opportunistic infections.

Because gram-negative bacteria can live in soil, they have evolved ways to adapt to the antibiotics produced naturally by other soil microorganisms, and they maintain this ability to adaptively resist the antibiotic drugs that are used to fight infection. Thus, gram-negative organisms are serious threats in a hospital environment. Hospitals are contaminated with antibiotics, so only resistant organisms can colonize that environment. In studies of infections among tornado casualties in Lubbock, Texas, in 1970, seventy-eight isolates of gram-negative bacteria were obtained from twenty-four hospitalized patients, versus eleven isolates in twenty-three victims treated as outpatients. These results suggest that many of the organisms were acquired in the hospital.[5]

A low incidence of infection was seen among British soldiers injured in the Falkland Islands War in 1982.[6,7] One reason may have been that the patients were treated either on a makeshift hospital ship, the HMS *Uganda*, or in an abandoned icehouse at Ajax

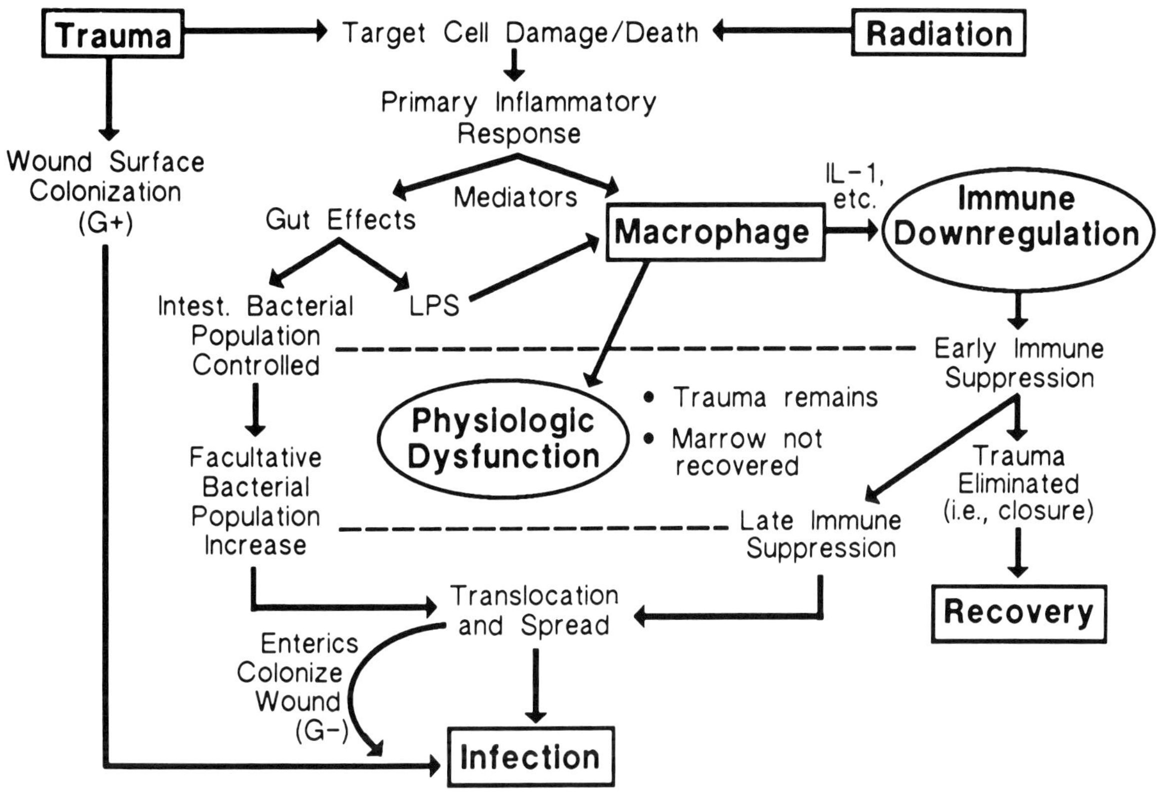

Fig. 5-1. Overview of postinjury events that contribute to development of infectious complications

Bay. Neither facility had been used previously as a hospital and thus did not contain antibiotic-resistant bacteria.

Causes of Opportunistic Infections

Immunosuppression is a consequence of injury and is an underlying cause of many infectious complications. Four other factors also contribute to post-trauma infections. In decreasing order of importance, they are *(a)* the presence of foreign bodies in wounds; *(b)* the time lag between injury and surgery; *(c)* the number, location, and extent of wounds; and *(d)* the virulence of the organism.

The influence of a foreign body on infection is seen in studies of the minimum dose of *C. perfringens* spores required to cause lethal infections in guinea pigs.[8] The dose required when spores were injected alone was 1×10^6. If the spores were inoculated into crushed muscle, then only 1×10^3 spores were needed. When sterile dirt was added to the spores injected into crushed muscle, then one spore instead of one million was required for lethality. Similarly, $1–5 \times 10^6$ injected staphylococci caused a lesion in humans, but if the organisms were introduced on a buried silk suture, as few as 1×10^2 bacteria produced spreading cellulitis.[9]

This effect of foreign material or damaged tissue on the development of infections demonstrates the need for early surgical management and debridement of wounds. Even the placement of originally sterile materials into the body of a patient can provide a focus for infection. Inert biomaterials, such as catheters and other invasive devices, can become covered with biofilms in which indigenous bacteria move onto the surface and become surrounded by exopolysaccharides and the host's accreted macromolecules.[10] These biofilms also form on detritus and dead tissue. Bacteria in these colonies cannot be cultured by usual means, and they are more resistant to antibodies, phagocytes, and antibiotics. For example, *P. aeruginosa* in a biofilm can withstand forty times the concentration of tobramycin that kills floating cells. Therefore, the best intervention is the early removal of material that can support the development of biofilm. Because only living tissue resists

TABLE 5-1

INCIDENCE OF WOUND INFECTION IN 1973 YOM KIPPUR WAR IN ISRAEL

Type of Injury	Number of Patients		Infection (%)	
Overall	420		22	
Soft tissue	178		6	
Fracture	99		18	
Involving femur		20		40
Not involving femur		79		15
Penetrating abdomen	53		30	
Colon perforated		19		58
Colon not perforated		34		14
Burn	49		35	
<25%		37		14
>25%		12		100

the formation of a biofilm, debridement is an important treatment. Artificial devices, such as catheters, should be used carefully.

Resistant biofilms have a greater chance to develop on dead tissue and detritus if the time interval between injury and surgical resolution is prolonged. In a study of gas gangrene, 511 patients (162 of whom became infected) had a 15% increased incidence of infection for each day between injury and debridement.[11] These data from World War I are relevant today because a similar situation could develop with mass casualties in a modern conventional or nuclear war.

The incidence of infection is also influenced by the nature of the wounds. Data from the 1973 Yom Kippur War in Israel (Table 5-1) show that burns of less than 25% of the body surface were rarely complicated by infection, but all burns of more than than 25% of the body surface were associated with infectious complications.[4] Perforation of the colon was more often associated with infection than was abdominal penetration without perforation of the colon. Fractures involving the femur were also frequently associated with infection.

In general, it is the failure of normal host barriers and defense mechanisms that permits infection by opportunistic pathogens. Once these deficiencies develop, a variety of otherwise harmless microorganisms can take over. Their uncontrolled multiplication in tissues of compromised hosts leads to the accumulation of both toxic microbial products and the products of host responses, which causes shock and death.

Little is known about the lethal mechanisms of most bacteria. Gram-positive organisms, such as *S. aureus*, produce a variety of extracellular protein toxins. Gram-negative organisms can produce extracellular toxins, but they also have a lipopolysaccharide (LPS) cell wall component known as endotoxin which, if present in sufficient quantities, can induce a variety of toxic host responses that mimic many of the responses associated with overwhelming bacterial infections. However, microbial pathogenesis is probably not due to a single factor. For example, although C3H/HeJ mice are low responders to endotoxin effects, they are easily infected with doses of gram-negative bacteria that cannot be established in other mouse strains.[12] The C3H/HeJ mice die with numbers of organisms in their tissues similar to numbers seen at death in other strains of mice challenged with higher doses of bacteria. Other data illustrating the importance of multiple virulence factors can be taken from a survey of twenty-four *Aeromonas* isolates that were grouped according to high virulence and low virulence for mice challenged intraperitoneally.[13] The high-virulence group of bacteria was more often positive for a variety of factors (Table 5-2) not found among the low-virulence strains. The shock syndrome resulting from the accumulation of lethal numbers of gram-positive bacteria in host tissues is similar to the syndrome involving gram-negative bacteria.[14]

INFECTIONS ASSOCIATED WITH RADIATION INJURY

Importance of Infection

Opportunistic pathogens are not only a major complication of conventional injuries, but also a major cause of morbidity or mortality in radiation-associated injury. Histological specimens of spleen, liver, lymph node, intestinal wall, and other tissues were taken from patients dying from the effects of the atomic blasts over Hiroshima and Nagasaki in 1945. Many specimens revealed microscopic bacterial colonies of both gram-positive and gram-negative bacteria growing freely in the tissues. There is a relationship in animals between infections and deaths after whole-body radiation doses in the midlethal range.[15] A curve based on mouse data depicting increased incidence of infection can be drawn parallel to but preceding the mortality curve. All mice that developed bacteremia after irradiation died, whereas those with no bacteremia survived. Studies such as these show that infection is an important cause of death during the hematopoietic subsyndrome.

Infection and Combined Injury

More recently, data from severely injured victims of the 1986 Chernobyl disaster also illustrate the serious threat of infections for radiation victims. Of twenty-nine deaths (not counting the two persons killed by the explosion), most were caused by infections associated with burns and hematological injury due to radiation exposure. This type of combined injury is predicted to be the most common trauma problem that will be seen in nuclear warfare. Insults that are sublethal or minimally lethal when occurring alone will act synergistically when occurring together. For example, almost 100% mortality occurred in rats given both 2.5 Gy of gamma radiation (no mortality when given alone) and a burn wound over 33% of their body surface area (50% mortality when given alone).[16]

A role for endogenous microorganisms in deaths following combined injury has been established by determining survival in germ-free rats and conventional rats undergoing combined radiation exposure and wound injury.[17] No mortality was seen in germ-free rats exposed to 8.0 Gy of total-body radiation compared to 55% mortality in conventional rats. If a 3-cm wound was also inflicted, mortality was 17% and 100% in germ-free and conventional animals, respectively.

As suggested in Figure 5-1, opportunistic infections do not occur until days or weeks after the injury. A chart from a Chernobyl victim (Figure 5-2) shows that elevated temperature, indicating infection, was not recorded until more than 3 weeks after injury. In laboratory animals given lethal radiation, infections are detected at about 9 days after exposure, and death occurs between days 11 and 15.[18]

TABLE 5-2

AEROMONAS INFECTION:

ASSOCIATION OF VARIOUS CHARACTERISTICS WITH VIRULENCE FOR MICE

Potential Virulence Factors	Number of Positive Cultures per Total	
	High Virulence	Low Virulence
Cytotoxin	15/15	0/9
Protease	15/15	0/9
Lipase	13/15	1/9
Elastase	11/15	7/9
Pili	9/15	2/8
Hemolysin	8/9	1/7

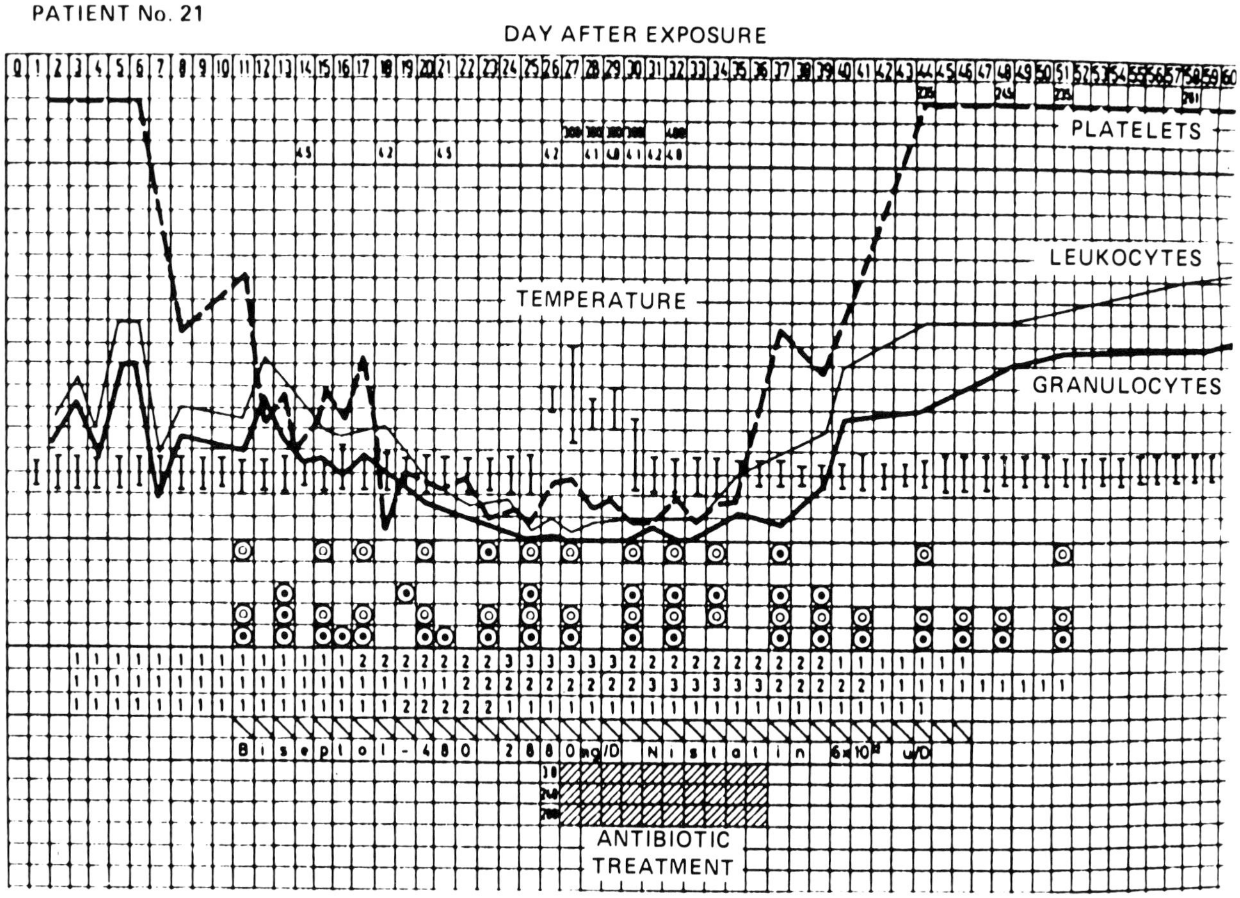

Fig. 5-2. Medical chart of a victim of the Chernobyl reactor disaster, illustrating occurrence of infection associated with granulocytopenia

FACTORS PREDISPOSING TO POSTIRRADIATION INFECTIONS

Impaired Inflammatory Response

Postirradiation infections are associated with neutropenia. In normal persons, inflammatory responses control many microorganisms that penetrate normally sterile tissues (Figure 5-3). Humoral components of inflammation, such as complement, interact with the microbial antigens and become activated to induce cellular responses, such as vasoconstriction and exudation of polymorphonuclear leukocytes. These cells phagocytose and kill many microorganisms. Later, macrophages enter the inflammatory site where they contribute to the removal of microorganisms and debris, and secrete factors that promote tissue repair.

Microorganisms are also removed from the circulation by the reticuloendothelial system (RES). In the presence of proper opsonins, RES macrophages, such as those in the liver and spleen, sequester and kill microorganisms and also secrete mediators that help augment host defenses. Failure in systemic host defenses after trauma may be caused in part by a deficiency of circulating opsonic protein (plasma fibronectin). The infusion of this substance into persons depleted by trauma has been associated with enhanced RES activity.[19] Since macrophages are relatively long-lived, they can be used to augment the host's resistance to infection after radiation exposure.

In traumatized subjects, an adequate inflammatory response is often not achieved because of immunosuppressive factors and the loss of functional cells. For example, the mortality rate from infection varies directly with the degree of granulocytopenia. Dogs given gentamicin plus granulocytes survived longer and cleared *P. aeruginosa* better than dogs given the antibiotic alone.[20] Although granulocytes are undoubtedly important in controlling gram-negative sepsis, it is questionable whether transfusion with these cells is essential for effective therapy.

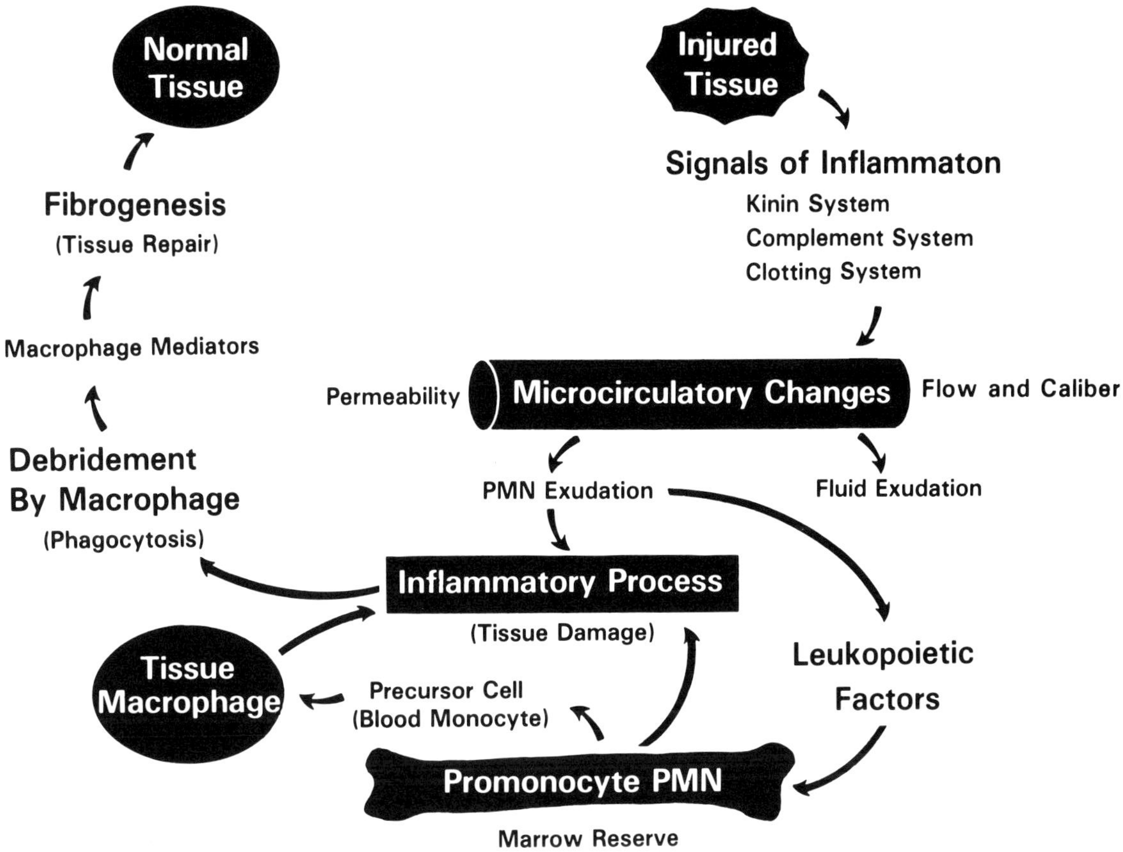

Fig. 5-3. Overview of essential components of the inflammatory response

Antibiotics are available, and safer and more realistic agents are being developed for use in mass-casualty situations.

Other cells and humoral agents are also lost due to trauma and radiation exposure. Fibronectin and immunoglobulin G are depleted in trauma victims, and lymphocytes are directly injured by irradiation. In addition, some injuries (such as burns) produce immunosuppressive factors that may impair the function of macrophages or other surviving cells.[21]

There are several examples of increased susceptibility to systemic infection after irradiation. When mice were challenged with *K. pneumoniae*, the LD_{50} was 1 x 10^6. Radiation alone reduced the LD_{50} to 1 x 10^3, and radiation plus a 3-cm dermal wound reduced the LD_{50} still further to 1 x 10^2. Similarly, the inoculation of *E. coli, S. aureus*, or *S. pyogenes* into muscles of mice exposed to 6.5 Gy of gamma radiation resulted in increased numbers of microorganisms in their tissues 5 days later, compared to normal mice. When *S. aureus* was injected into the local wounds of mice exposed to 7.0 Gy of gamma radiation, fewer bacteria were required to produce a lesion or death than in nonirradiated animals.[22]

Postirradiation infections are often polymicrobial, and it has recently been found that the complexity of infection in mice increases with increasing doses of radiation.[23] While *S. aureus* was more often recovered at 9.0 Gy and below, *E. coli* and anaerobes were isolated most frequently in mice receiving a dose of 10 Gy.

Changes in Resident Microbial Populations

Various deficiencies in host defenses can increase the susceptibility to infection, but changes in the microbial populations on body surfaces are also important. Such population shifts can occur when protective coatings on epithelial cells are lost and when indigenous flora, which resist colonization by exogenous pathogens, are reduced in number. These events allow pathogens to colonize mucosal surfaces, from which they may spread to ordinarily sterile sites in the body.

Recent evidence suggests that epithelial surfaces

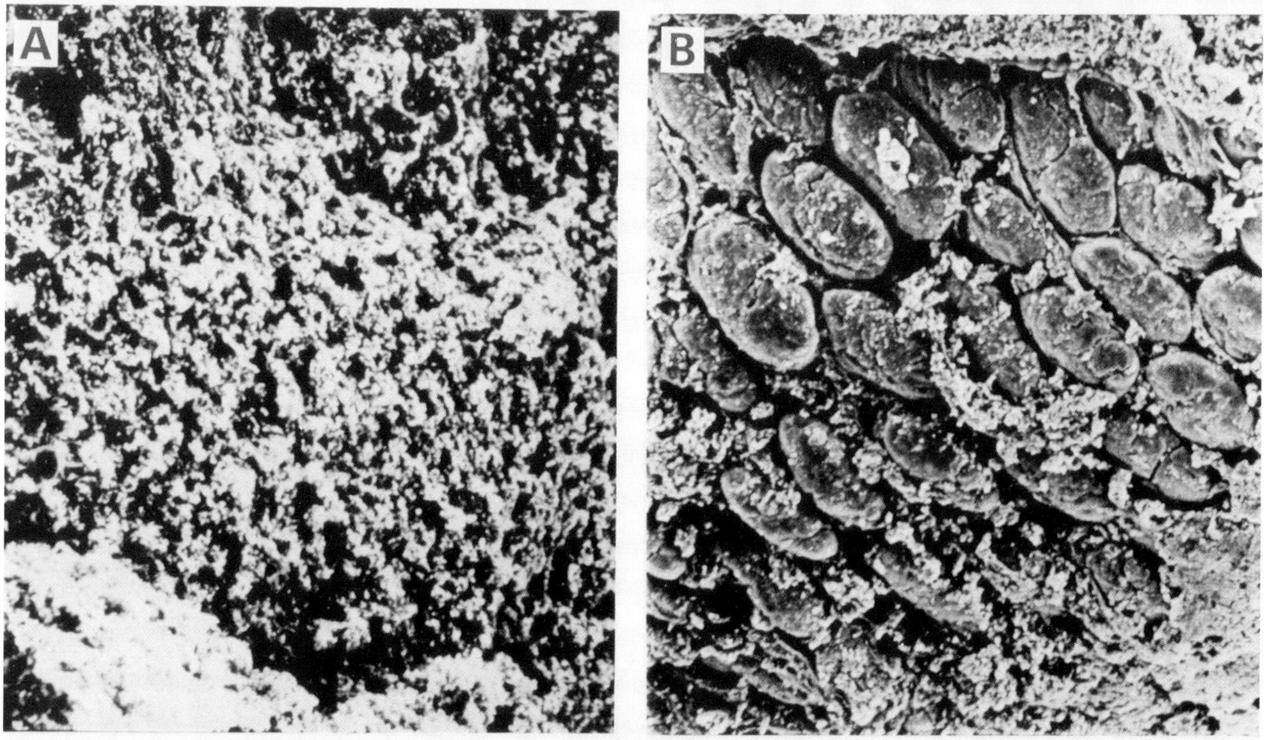

Fig. 5-4. Loss of mucous barrier over epithelium of mouse ileum after exposure to 9-Gy cobalt-60 radiation. Normal ileum has intact blanket of mucus covering the villi (A). The blanket is lost by 3 days after irradiation, exposing the villi (B).

in the oropharyngeal cavity of trauma victims can lose cell-surface fibronectin and become prone to attachment by gram-negative bacteria, such as *P. aeruginosa*.[24] This may also occur after irradiation and may enhance the possibility that pathogens will successfully colonize the host.

Microorganisms in the intestine increase in numbers distally and provide a focus for abnormal colonization, which can lead to overwhelming infections when systemic host defenses have also been compromised. This phenomenon can be found in rats given sublethal or lethal radiation exposures.[25] The ileum of a normal rat is colonized by unusual bacteria, known as segmented filamentous microflora (SFM), which cannot be cultivated but whose numbers can be easily discerned with scanning electron microscopy. These organisms are intimately associated with the epithelium of the intestine. Their precise role in the intestine is unknown; however, because they are associated with well-being, SFM can be used as indicator organisms, demonstrating that an injury (which could alter bacterial populations) has occurred in the intestine. Twenty-four hours after sublethal exposure to 5 Gy of gamma radiation, SFM disappeared from the rat ileum. However, by day 4, SFM populations were back to normal. In rats given a lethal radiation dose (10 Gy), SFM did not return at day 4 and were still absent from the ileum at day 11. Potential opportunistic pathogens, measured by the cultivation of dilutions of intestinal homogenates, declined in numbers shortly after exposure to 5–10 Gy. At the lower radiation dose, their numbers began to increase after the return of SFM, but they were still subnormal at day 11. In contrast, rats given 10 Gy showed increasing numbers of facultative flora after the first few days following irradiation, and by day 11 these organisms had colonized the ileum in numbers far above normal. This event correlated with systemic infection and preceded death.

It is apparent that an event associated with exposure to higher doses of radiation is responsible for abnormal colonization preceding infection. Little is known about the pathophysiology of this injury. Intestinal epithelial cells are almost as sensitive to radiation as are marrow cells, and even doses of radiation below the gastrointestinal-subsyndrome level can cause injuries that affect bacterial colonization.

Since most intestinal microorganisms are found in the 450-micron mucin layer at the epithelial surface, any injury that produces changes in this structure can contribute to significant alterations in patterns of microbial colonization in the intestine. Evidence for the loss of the intestinal mucous barrier has been found in mice that received 10 Gy of cobalt-60 radiation.[26] When procedures were used that stabilized the mucous gel for electron microscopy, a progressive loss of this material was observed between irradiation and day 3 (Figure 5-4). Prior to irradiation, villi were not visible beneath the mucus, but by day 3, major sections of villi were completely uncovered.

Loss of the mucous barrier and other ecological and immunological changes in the intestine enable opportunistic pathogens to overgrow on the mucosal surface and subsequently to translocate to other tissues. Translocation from the intestine has been well correlated with conventional disturbances of mucosal ecology and also systemic trauma.[27] This process can lead to infections when defense mechanisms are also suppressed.

MANAGEMENT OF INFECTIONS

Opportunistic infections that are a consequence of trauma in conventional warfare have been difficult to control. This will also be true in persons with radiation injuries or combined injuries. In seriously injured Chernobyl victims (Table 5-3), the number of patients with radiation and thermal burns was greater with higher radiation doses, and mortality rose with the severity of combined injuries. Of the twenty-nine deaths, most were directly attributable to infectious complications. It is clear from the Chernobyl experience that bone-marrow transplants in persons who received uneven radiation exposures (in whom stem cells may have survived) can be dangerous.

If bone-marrow transplantation is not practical in treating radiation victims, the management options are those used in conventional injury: antibiotics, surgery, and supportive therapy.

Antibiotics

New antibiotics are continually being developed. Figures 5-5 and 5-6 describe the different groups of antibiotic agents and indicate their usefulness against different kinds of infections. Some newer antibiotics, such as ceftazidime or the quinolones, may be useful as monotherapy, but most antibiotics seem more effective when used in synergistic combinations. Today, the effectiveness of some antibiotics may be enhanced by the use of inhibitors of bacterial enzymes (such as clavulanic acid) which inhibit beta-lactamase activity and thereby preserve the function of penicillin derivatives.

Antibiotic effectiveness may also be enhanced by ensuring that therapy is directed against all components of an infection. For example, *Bacteroides* species and facultative gram-negative microorganisms often occur together. One of these organisms may produce capsular material that protects the other organism from phagocytosis, as well as beta-lactamase for protection against antimicrobial therapy. Also, one organism could create an anaerobic environment that is essential to the other organism, or could produce nutritional growth factors. Many slowly growing and fastidious pathogens, which are important in infections of severely compromised patients, may still be unrecognized. Further studies of these organisms will be necessary for better selection of antimicrobial therapy.

It is important that initially avirulent bacterial populations may become more virulent if allowed to persist in mixed infections. Nonabscess-forming cultures, when inoculated into mice along with capsular material or other pathogens, may convert to encapsulated populations that are capable of establishing abscesses on their own.[28]

Antibiotics can also be used to reduce the colonization of intestinal mucosa by opportunistic pathogens. Total intestinal decontamination is difficult to achieve, and it creates further vulnerability to colonization by antibiotic-resistant pathogens. However, selective decontamination with oral antibiotics has already been tested clinically, and it offers promise for the management of mass casualties who have been exposed to midlethal radiation. The oral administration of specific antibiotics eliminates opportunistic pathogens but leaves intact the relatively benign intestinal flora.[29,30] These benign flora increase resistance to colonization by occupying binding sites and creating an environment that is inhospitable to pathogens. This approach eliminates the need for elaborate methods of isolation. In patients

TABLE 5-3

MORTALITY OF 203 COMBINED-INJURY PATIENTS IN THE CHERNOBYL NUCLEAR ACCIDENT

Combined-Injury Classification	Radiation Dose (Gy)	Burns	Reported Deaths	Number of Patients			Survival Time (days)
				Total	Moscow	Kiev	
4th Degree (extremely severe injury)	6–16	In all cases*	21	22	20	2	4–50
3d Degree (severe injury)	4–6	6 out of 7 deaths	7	23	21	2	14–49
2d Degree (moderate injury)	2–4	Almost none	1	53	43	10	—
1st Degree (slight injury)	1–2	None	0	105	31	74	—

*40%–90% of body surface area

with aplastic anemia, leukemia, or burns, selective decontamination with antibiotics (such as oral nalidixic acid, cotrimoxazole, or amphotericin B) significantly reduces the number of infectious episodes.

The importance of the presence of colonization-resistant flora after irradiation and the hazard of using systemic antibiotics are indicated by experimental studies in mice. After exposure to 10 Gy of gamma radiation, mice treated with metronidazole, which reduces the intestinal anaerobe population, died about 5 days earlier than did the untreated irradiated mice.[31] In contrast, gentamicin did not affect colonization-resistant flora in the intestine and did not shorten the survival times.

Antimicrobial therapy was reasonably effective against infections in those Chernobyl victims who suffered from ARS only, but was not as effective if the ARS was complicated by burns, radiation enteritis, or acute secondary illness due to bone-marrow transplantation. Patients were treated prophylactically with a selective decontamination procedure that called for the daily administration of six tablets of biseptol 480 and 5×10^6 units of nystatin.

If fever appeared, the Chernobyl victims were given intravenous therapy with two or three antibiotics, including an aminoglycoside, cephalosporin, or semisynthetic penicillin with antipyocyanic action. If no effect was seen after 24–48 hours, intravenous gamma globulin (Sandoglobulin) was given in three or four doses of 6 grams every 12 hours. If the fever persisted after 1 week, amphotericin B (1 mg/kg/day) was administered.

A number of Chernobyl patients became infected with herpes simplex. In these cases, acyclovir was used as a topical treatment.

Supportive Therapy

Antibiotics will undoubtedly be a basic part of any infection management after radiation exposure. This supportive therapy, in combination with fluids and platelets, has been shown to increase resistance to infection. Dogs receiving this treatment showed an $LD_{50/30}$ (LD_{50} at 30 days after exposure) increase from 2.6 to 3.3 Gy after exposure to cobalt-60, and from 1.5 to 1.8 Gy after exposure to mixed neutron-gamma radiation.[32] These increases in resistance to radiation are significant, considering the steepness of the survival curve between an LD_5 and an LD_{95} dose of radiation.

ANTIBIOTIC AGENTS

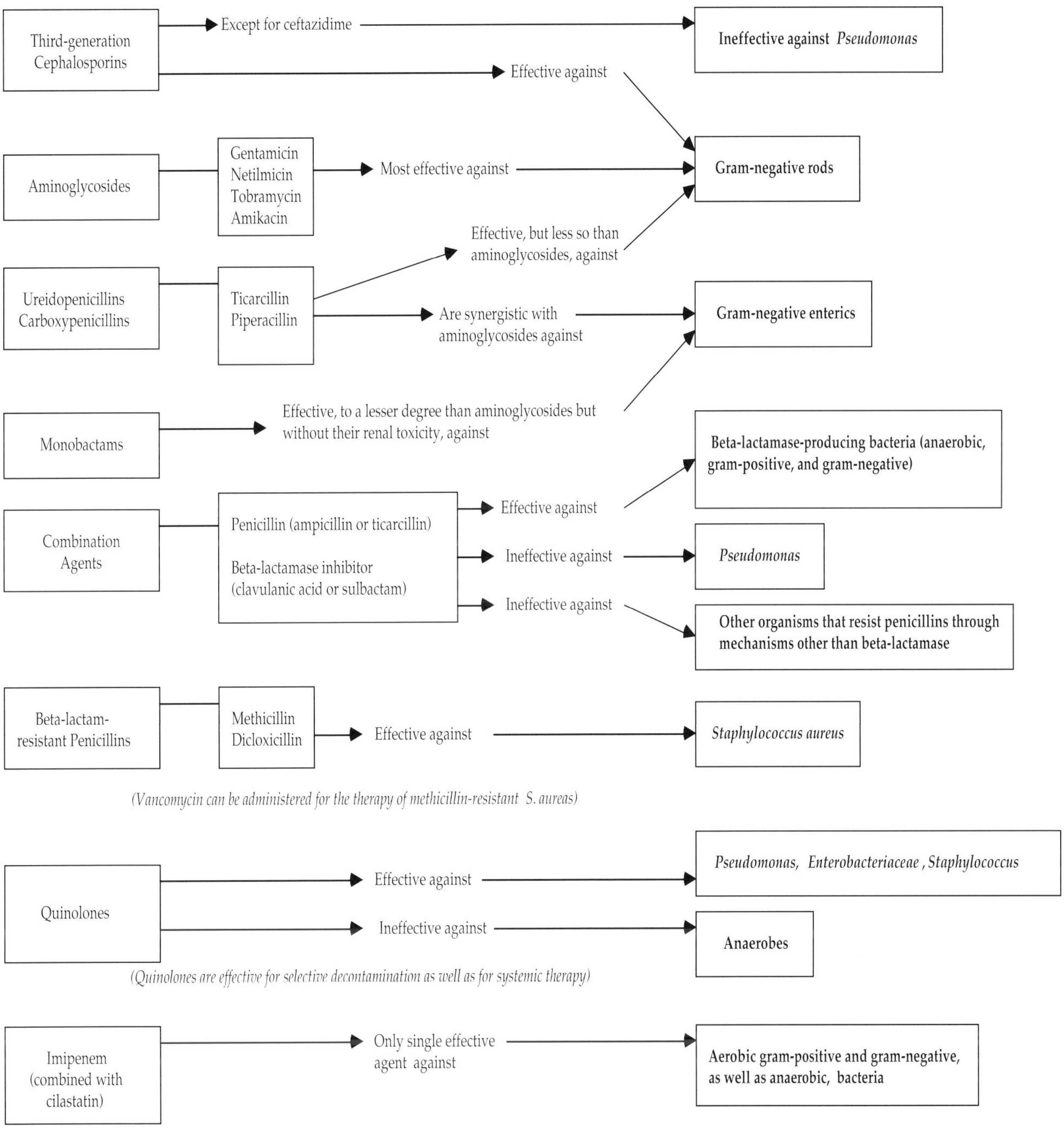

Fig. 5-5. Types of agents used in antibiotic therapy of irradiated host

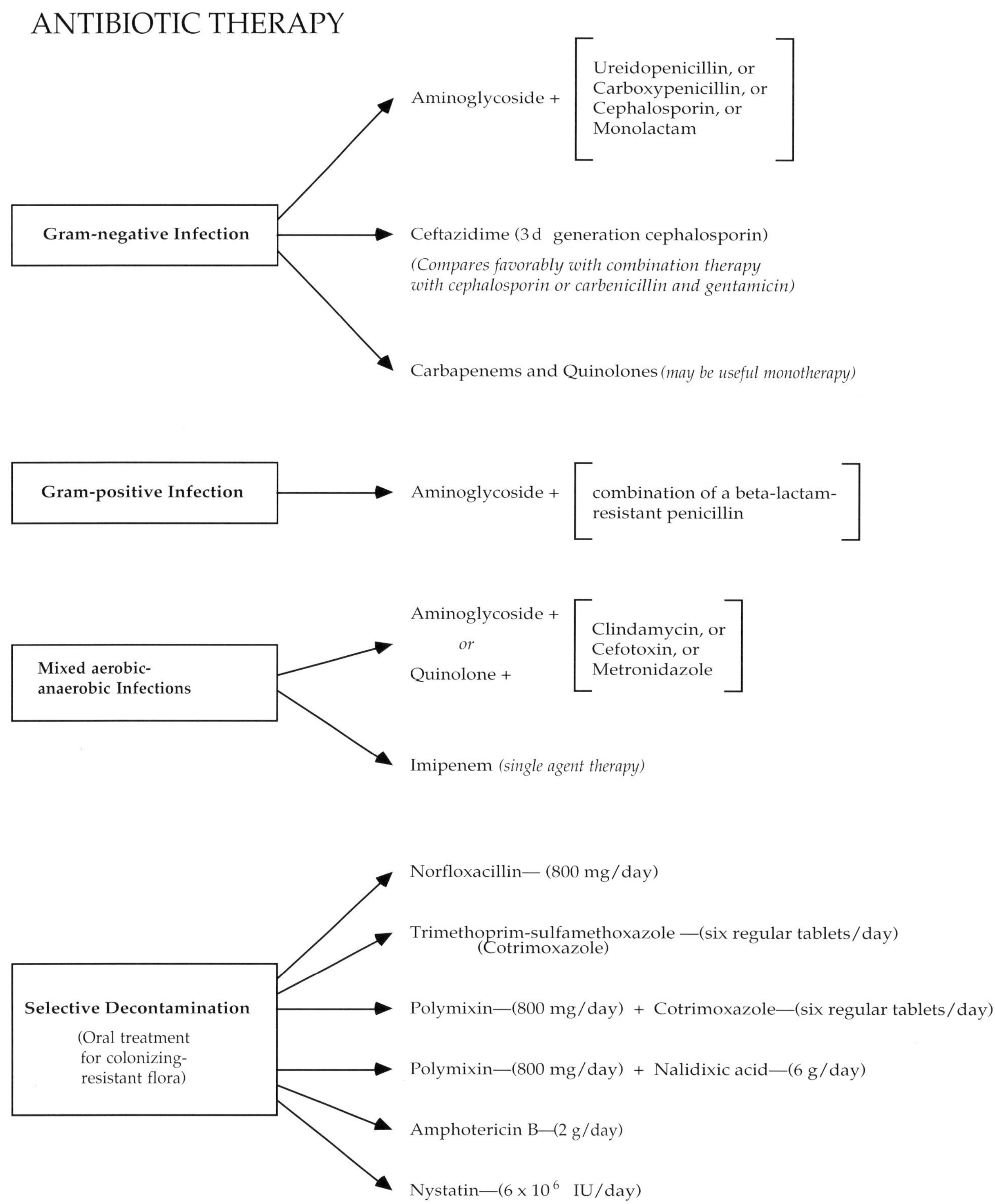

Fig. 5-6. Suggested therapies for specific infections

Another supportive therapy that may be useful against gram-negative infections in irradiated persons is immunoglobulin. Immunoglobulin will act against some portion of the LPS component of the cell wall of gram-negative bacteria. Most experience with anti-LPS antibody preparations has been in nonirradiated research models.[33-35] Clinically, antiserum prepared from the J5 mutant of *E. coli* has been used to reduce deaths from 39% to 23% in patients with bacteremia, and from 77% to 44% in those with profound shock.[33] Various immunoglobulin preparations have been used to protect experimental animals against infection.[34]

The development of human monoclonal antibodies opens new possibilities for passive immunization against microbial infections. Passive antibody therapy was widely used in the pre-antibiotic era to treat infectious diseases. Although this therapy may be effective in specific instances, appropriate stocks of specific antibodies with high-affinity constants are expensive and difficult to prepare in large amounts by conventional methods. Further, since such antibodies are usually obtained from animals, particularly horses, humans often have immune reactions to the injection of these immunoglobulins. This results in serum sickness, which prevents further use of the specific therapy in that patient. The new technique of producing antibodies *in vitro* by somatic cell fusion (hybridoma technology) has the potential of generating the desired amounts of high concentrations of pure human-specific antibody preparations, which can be used against opportunistic pathogens in host tissues.

Active vaccination against specific antigens of gram-negative bacteria does not appear to be a good option for controlling infection. It is questionable whether an immunosuppressed person can evoke or maintain an immune response. Moreover, the large number of potential opportunistic pathogens makes it unlikely that a sufficient number of different vaccines can be developed in the near future.

TABLE 5-4

CONTRIBUTORS TO INFECTION

- Colonization of oropharyngeal respiratory tree
- Colonization of intestinal tract
- Contamination of wound
- Profound immunosuppression
- Invasive treatment devices
- Environmental pathogens

Surgery

In combined-injury victims, surgery is expected to be an important adjunct to supportive therapy, but will be complicated by impairments in wound healing that are manifested shortly after exposure to radiation. In contrast to trauma without radiation, the period of opportunity for reparative surgery following irradiation is very short (1 to 2 days), followed by a period of several weeks in which surgery should not be attempted if it can possibly be avoided (Figure 5-7).

As indicated in Figure 5-1, the closure of wounds can eliminate late immunosuppression and other synergistic effects of combined injury. This is illustrated by experiments conducted in mice.[36] Exposure to 5.1 Gy of radiation resulted in 26% mortality, and the same exposure combined with an open wound resulted in 90% mortality. When the wound was closed, the percentage of mortality dropped and was similar to that from radiation alone. This suggests that a deleterious signal or mediator was interrupted. Unfortunately, excision and closure are not always easily achieved. Closure, if done prematurely, will promote the occurrence of systemic sepsis from microbial colonization of necrotic tissue or detritus. Early debridement should be followed by an inspection of the wound 48 hours later, and if the wound seems free of infection or nonliving material, closure can be considered.

Although this approach has not been fully tested for radiation victims, surgical experience suggests that full-thickness burns should be primarily excised and grafted, and partial-thickness burns should probably be treated by aggressive topical therapy and avoidance of nosocomial sepsis. Prophylactic topical management of burn wounds may be accomplished with mafenide acetate (sulfamylon) or silver sulfadiazine (silvadene).[37] Antibiotics are used for prophylaxis only in traumatic cutaneous wounds, selective decontamination, and early surgery.[38]

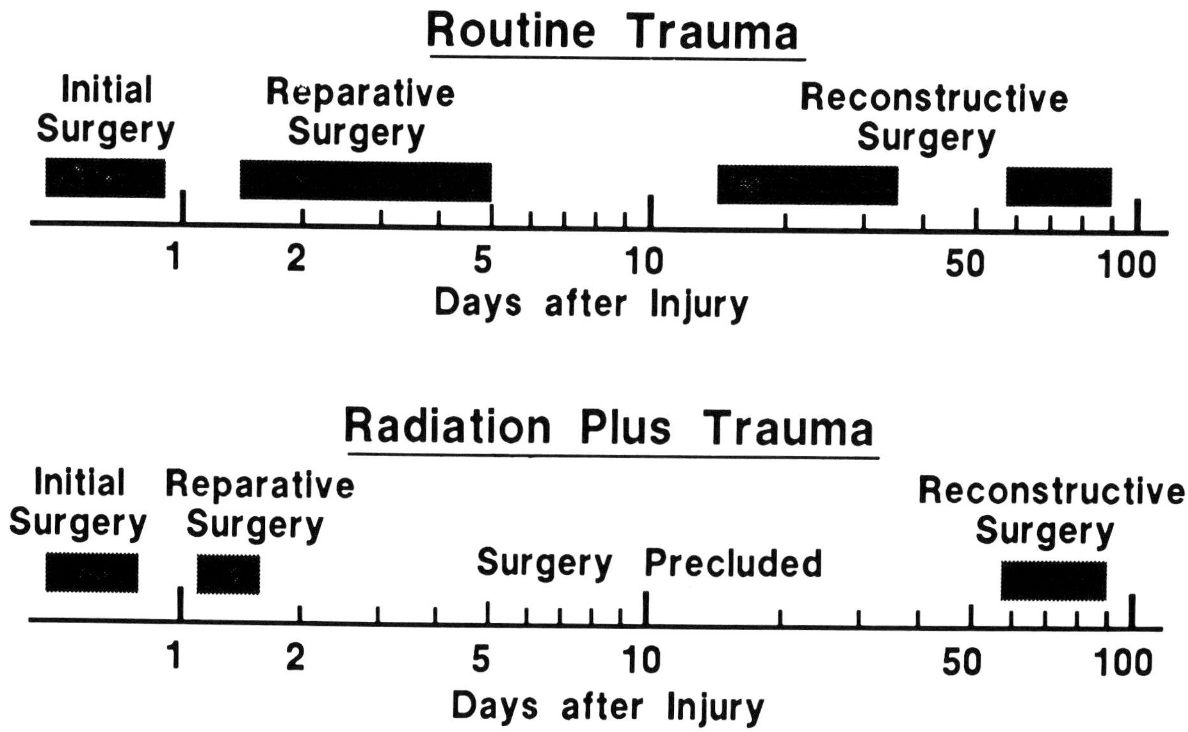

Fig. 5-7. Comparison of timing for surgical management of combined injuries in routine trauma victims and in those exposed to radiation

SUMMARY

A number of conditions may allow opportunistic infections to occur (Table 5-4). Changes in epithelial cell surfaces can enhance colonization of the oropharyngeal-respiratory tree. Frequently, wound contamination, first by skin flora and later by gram-negative flora from the intestine, can also lead to overwhelming infections. Antibiotic-resistant pathogens in the environment can be particularly troublesome if they colonize wounds on vulnerable mucosal surfaces. Artificial invasive devices also subject susceptible surfaces to colonization by pathogens. Finally, if all these events are accompanied by decreased host defenses, then uncontrolled multiplication by opportunistic pathogens can quickly lead to shock and death.

It should be noted that more virulent organisms can also be a problem after a nuclear detonation. Mild immunosuppression in nonhospitalized personnel working in an environment with poor hygiene can lead to epidemics of respiratory and enteric infections.

General principles of patient management (Table 5-5) and current technology can be used in treating postirradiation infections.

TABLE 5-5

PRINCIPLES OF PATIENT MANAGEMENT

- Treat conventional injuries first, since radiation injuries will not be immediately life threatening.
- Evaluate the extent of trauma and initiate resuscitation procedures.
- Begin corrective procedures, such as surgery and fluid administration, based on the triage assessment of conventional injuries.
- Prevent infection until immunocompetence is regained.
- Take steps to reduce the foci of infections from colonizing artificial devices or damaged tissues.
- If infection is suspected, use empiric therapy with broad-spectrum antibiotics to complement these physical interventions.
- Take steps to improve immunocompetence and physiological well-being of the patient.

REFERENCES

1. Zimmerman, J. J., and Dietrich, K. A. 1987. Current perspectives on septic shock. *Ped. Clinics N. A.* 34: 131-163.

2. Cavanagh, D.; Knuppel, R. A.; Shepherd, J. H.; Anderson, R.; and Rao, P. S. 1982. Septic shock and the obstetrician/gynecologist. *South. Med. J.* 75: 804-810.

3. Meleney, F. L. 1945. A statistical analysis of a study of the prevention of infection in soft part wounds, compound fractures and burns with special reference to sulfonamide. *Surg. Gynecol. Obstet.* 86: 263-296.

4. Klein, R. S.; Berger, S. A.; and Yekutiel, P. 1975. Wound infection during the Yom Kippur war: Observations concerning antibiotic prophylaxis and therapy. *Ann. Surg.* 182: 15-21.

5. Gilber, D. N.; Sanford, J. P.; Kutscher, E.; Sanders, C. V. J.; Luby, J. P.; and Barnett, J. A. 1973. Microbiologic study of wound infections in tornado casualties. *Arch. Environ. Health* 26: 125-130.

6. Beeley, M. 1983. Hospital ship HMS *Uganda*—At war in the South Atlantic. *J. R. Naval Med. Serv.* 69: 21-25.

7. Jolly, R. T. 1983. Ajax Bay. *J. R. Naval Med. Serv.* 69: 35-39.

8. Altemeier, W. A., and Furste, W. L. 1949. Studies in virulence of *Clostridium welchii*. *Surgery* 25: 12-19.

9. Elek, S. D., and Cohen, P. E. 1957. The virulence of *Staphylococcus pyogenes* for man. A study of the problems of wound infection. *Br. J. Exp. Pathol.* 38: 573-586.

10. Costerton, J. W.; Marrie, T. J.; Gristina, A. G.; and Moody, M. R. 1987. The role of bacterial biofilms in the etiology, persistence, and antibiotic resistance of wound infections. In *The Pathophysiology of Combined Injury and Trauma: Management of Infectious Complications in Mass Casualty Situations,* edited by D. Gruber, R. I. Walker, T. J. MacVittie and J. J. Conklin, 165-190. New York: Academic Press.

11. Petit, R. T. 1919. Infections of wounds of war with special reference to gas gangrene. *JAMA* 73: 494-496.

12. MacVittie, T. J.; O'Brien, A. D.; Walker, R. I.; and Weinberg, S. R. 1982. Inflammatory response of LPS-hyporesponsive and LPS-responsive mice to challenge with gram-negative bacteria *Salmonella typhimurium* and *Klebsiella pneumoniae.* In *Macrophages and Natural Killer Cells: Regulation and Function,* edited by S. J. Normann and E. Sorkin, 325-334. New York: Plenum Press.

13. Daily, O. P.; Joseph. S.; Coolbaugh, J.; Walker, R. I.; Merrell, B. R.; Seidler, R.; Rollins, D.; Lissner, C.; Kaper, J.; and Colwell, R. 1981. Association of *Aeromonas sobria* with human infection. *J. Clin. Microbiol.* 13: 769-777.

14. Natanson, C.; Danner, R. L.; Elin, R. J.; Hosseini, J. M.; MacVittie, T. J.; Walker, R. I.; and Parrillo, J. E. 1989. The role of endotoxemia in cardiovascular dysfunction and mortality: *E. coli* and *S. aureus* challenges in a canine model of human septic shock. *J. Clin. Invest.,* in press.

15. Miller, C. P.; Hammond, C. W.; and Tompkins, M. 1950. The incidence of bacteria in mice subjected to whole-body X-radiation. *Science* 3: 540-551.

16. Alpen, E. L., and Sheline, G. E. 1954. The combined effects of thermal burns and whole-body X-radiation on survival time and mortality. *Ann. Surg.* 140: 113-118.

17. Donati, R. M.; McLaughlin, M. M.; and Stromberg, L.-W. R. 1973. Combined surgical and radiation injury. VIII. The effect of the gnotobiotic state on wound closure. *Experientia* 29: 1388-1390.

18. Walker, R. I.; Ledney, G. D.; and Galley, C. B. 1975. Aseptic endotoxemia in radiation injury and graft-versus-host disease. *Radiat. Res.* 62: 242-249.

19. Saba, T. M., and Jaffe, E. 1980. Plasma fibronectin (opsonic glycoprotein): Its synthesis by vascular endothelial cell and role in cardiopulmonary integrity after trauma as related to reticuloendothelial function. *Am. J. Med.* 68: 577-594.

20. Love, L. J.; Schimpf, S. C.; Schiffer, C. A.; and Wiernick, P. H. 1980. Improved prognosis for granulocytopenic patients with gram-negative bacteremia. *Am. J. Med.* 68: 643.

21. Ninnemann, J. L. 1983. Immune depression in burn and trauma patients: The role of circulating suppressors. In *Traumatic Injury, Infection and Other Immunologic Sequelae,* edited by J. L. Ninnemann, 33-35. Baltimore: University Park Press.

22. Elliott, T. B., and Brook, I. 1986. Ionizing radiation and infected wounds. In *Abstracts of 86th Annual Meeting of American Society for Microbiology* [#B123], 44. Washington, DC: American Society for Microbiology.

23. Brook, I.; Walker, R. I.; and MacVittie, T. J. 1986. Effect of radiation dose on the recovery of aerobic and anaerobic bacteria from mice. *Can. J. Microbiol.* 32: 719-722.

24. Wood, E. E.; Straus, D. C.; Johanson, W. G., Jr.; and Bass, J. A. 1981. Role of fibronectin in the prevention of adherence of *Pseudomonas aeruginosa* to buccal cells. *J. Infect. Dis.* 143: 784-790.

25. Porvaznik, M.; Walker, R. I.; and Gillmore, J. D. 1979. Reduction of the indigenous filamentous microorganisms in the rat ileum following radiation. *Scan. Electron Microsc.* 3: 15-22.

26. Walker, R. I.; Brook, I.; Costerton, J. W.; MacVittie, T. J.; and Myhal, M. L. 1985. Possible association of mucous blanket integrity with postirradiation colonization resistance. *Radiat. Res.* 104: 346-357.

27. Deitch, E. A., and Bridges, R. 1987. Effect of stress and trauma on bacterial translocation from the gut. *J. Surg. Res.* 42: 536-542.

28. Brook, I.; Gilmore, J. D.; Coolbaugh, J. C.; and Walker, R. I. 1983. Pathogenicity of encapsulated *Bacteroides melaninogenicus* group, *Bacteroides oralis* and *Bacteroides rumincola* in abscesses in mice. *J. Infect.* 7: 218-226.

29. Reeves, D. S. 1986. The effect of quinolone antibacterials on the gastrointestinal flora compared with that of other antimicrobials. *J. Antimicrob. Chemother.* (Suppl. D) 18: 89-102.

30. Mulder, N. H.; Nieweg, H. W.; Sleijfer, D. T.; de-Vries-Hospters, H. G.; van der Waaij, D.; Fidler, B.; and van Saene, H. K. F. 1979. Infection prevention in granulocytopenic patients by selective decontamination of the digestive tract. In *New Criteria for Antimicrobial Therapy: Maintenance of Digestive Tract Colonization Resistance,* edited by D. van der Waaij and J. Verhoef, 113-117. Amsterdam: Exerpta Medica.

31. Brook I.; Walker, R. I.; and MacVittie, T. J. 1988. Effect of antimicrobial therapy on the gut flora and bacterial infection in irradiated mice. *Int. J. Radiat. Biol.* 53: 709-716.

32. MacVittie, T. J.; Monroy, R. L.; Vigneulle, R.; Nold, J.; Patchen, M.; Zeman, G. Treatment of the radiation induced hemopoietic syndrome in canines. Paper presented at the NATO Research Study Group 11, Lyon-Bron, France, October 20–23, 1986.

33. Ziegler, E. J.; McCutchan, A.; Fierer, J.; Glauser, M. P.; Sadoff, J. C.; Douglas, H.; and Braude, A. I. 1982. Treatment of gram-negative bacteremia and shock with human antiserum to a mutant *Escherichia coli. N. Engl. J. Med.* 307: 1225-1230.

34. Pollack, M. 1983. Antibody activity against *Pseudomonas aeruginosa* in immune globulins prepared for intravenous use in humans. *J. Infect. Dis.* 147: 1090-1098.

35. Braude, A. I.; Ziegler, E. J.; and Douglas, H. 1985. Treatment of gram-negative bacteremia, endotoxemia, and shock with antibody to core glycolipid. In *The Pathophysiology of Combined Injury and Trauma: Radiation, Burn, and Trauma,* edited by R. I. Walker, D. F. Gruber, T. J. MacVittie, and J. J. Conklin, 201-208. Baltimore: University Park Press.

36. Messerschmidt, O. 1976. Kombinationsscheaden als Folge nuklearer explosion. In vol. 4 of *Chirurgie der Gegenwert,* edited by R. Zenker, M. Deucher, and W. Schink, 1-102. Munich: Urban und Schwarzenborg.

37. Pruitt, B. A., Jr. Opportunistic infections in the severely injured patient. In reference 10, 53-77.

38. Shack, R. B. 1987. Factors affecting the success of antibiotic treatment of traumatic cutaneous wounds. *Internal. Med.* 8: 154-170.

RECOMMENDED READING

Hathorn, J. W.; Rubin, M.; and Pizzo, P. A. 1987. Empiric antibiotic therapy in the febrile neutropenic cancer patient: Clinical efficacy and impact of monotherapy. *Antimicrob. Agents Chemother.* 31: 971-977.

Walker, R. I.; Gruber, D. F.; MacVittie, T. J.; and Conklin, J. J., eds. 1985. *The pathophysiology of combined injury and trauma: Radiation, burn, and trauma.* Baltimore: University Park Press.

Gruber, D.; Walker, R. I.; MacVittie, T. J.; and Conklin, J. J., eds. 1987. *The pathophysiology of combined injury and trauma: Management of infectious complications in mass casualty situations.* New York: Academic Press.

Chapter 6

BIOLOGICAL ASSESSMENT OF RADIATION DAMAGE

THOMAS L. WALDEN, Jr., Ph.D.* AND NUSHIN K. FARZANEH, M.S.**

*Radiation Biologist, Radiation Biochemistry Department, Armed Forces Radiobiology Research Institute, Bethesda, Maryland 20814-5145
**Radiation Biologist, Radiation Biochemistry Department, Armed Forces Radiobiology Research Institute, Bethesda, Maryland 20814-5145

INTRODUCTION

Biological dosimetry involves measuring a given physiological response to a known or estimated exposure dose of a toxin (in this case, ionizing radiation). Reliable biological dosimeters of radiation injury are needed *(a)* to perform casualty triage, *(b)* to determine probable exposures when *physical dosimeters* (external indicators of radiation that are used in the field) are absent, *(c)* to confirm physical dosimetry, and *(d)* to monitor the progress of radiotherapy. This chapter deals with biological dosimetry relating to accidental exposure or nuclear warfare, rather than the clinical monitoring of radiotherapeutic progress, although similarities exist. The armed forces presently issue physical radiation dosimeters to groups rather than to individuals; shielding differences may affect individual doses. Variations in age, gender, health, and genetic background may greatly affect the biological responses to a given radiation dose. Careful monitoring through biological dosimetry can provide more reliable indicators of exposure, which will be used in formulating prognoses on treatment and survival.

Damage from ionizing radiation occurs at both the local and systemic levels. Biological indicators are diverse and may include changes in levels of tissue enzymes,[1-13] metabolites,[14-22] and cell populations (such as lymphocytes[23-25] or sperm[26]); changes in individual behavior;[21,22] and a general onset of malaise.[21,23-27] Both early and late responses to radiation injury may be reflected. Elevations in serum amylase levels may occur within hours to days,[2-8] and elevated levels of lactate dehydrogenase[11,28] or zinc protoporphyrin[29] are observed several weeks after irradiation. The ideal biological dosimeter should be reliable, able to detect 0.1–10.0 Gy, linear in response regardless of dose or quality of radiation, simple to use, preferably noninvasive, sensitive to radiation occurring during the first hours or days after exposure, and preferably radiation specific.

A combination of five indicators (Table 6-1) may provide a reliable gauge of radiation exposure: *(a)* the physical symptomatology of the prodromal stage of ARS, *(b)* lymphocyte numbers, *(c)* serum components (diamine oxidase and serum amylase), *(d)* urinary components, and *(e)* chromosomal aberrations.

PHYSICAL SYMPTOMATOLOGY AT THE PRODROMAL STAGE

The most reliable method of biological dosimetry is the physical symptomatology at the prodromal stage of ARS,[21,24] which occurs within minutes to 1 day after irradiation and includes nausea, vomiting, anorexia, diarrhea, and general malaise. The severity, duration, and time of onset of these symptoms are related to the dose and quality of the radiation received. A dose-dependent latent period occurs between the end of the prodromal symptoms and the onset of later hematopoietic or gastrointestinal complications (Table 6-2). The onset and latency are inversely related to the dose, whereas the duration and severity are directly related and vary for individuals. The median acute gamma radiation doses have been estimated for anorexia (0.97 Gy), nausea (1.4 Gy), fatigue (1.5 Gy), vomiting (1.8 Gy), and diarrhea (2.3 Gy).[25,27] Protraction of the dose over 1 to 7 days results in doubling the median doses.

Several early physiological responses are associated with exposure to radiation doses in the high-lethality (greater than 5.5 Gy) range (Table 6-3). These symptoms usually reflect an unfavorable prognosis for survival without adequate hospitalization and extraordinary lifesaving measures, such as bone-marrow transplantation.[21,24,25] At still higher radiation doses, even these measures would not be effective.

Erythema and epilation are two other indicators of clinically significant radiation exposure. Erythema has a threshold of 3–4 Gy, depending on the area of irradiated skin, with a median dose estimate of 6 Gy.[25,30] Erythema occurs in two phases: an early phase, appearing within several to 24 hours after irradiation, and a later "main erythema," reappearing 2–3 weeks after irradiation and persisting for several weeks.[31] Erythema also depends on the type of radiation and the skin condition. Epilation occurs approximately 2 weeks after radiation doses larger than 2–3 Gy.[30]

TABLE 6-1

BIOLOGICAL INDICATORS OF RADIATION INJURY

SERUM	URINE
Acid phosphatase	Amino acids, particularly metabolites of tryptophan
Acid deoxyribonuclease	Amylase
Amylase	Beta-aminoisobutaric acid
A-T phosphatase	Creatine and creatinine
Beta-glucuronidase	Deoxyribonuclease
Beta-galactosidase	Histamine
Catalase	Indoxy sulfate
Calcium	Nucleic acids (pseudouridine)
Diamine oxidase	Prostaglandins
Factor XXII	Taurine
Fluorescence and/or chemiluminescence	
Free amino acids:	SALIVA
phenylalanine	Albumin
leucine	
proline	CELL COUNTS AND MORPHOLOGY
tyrosine	Peripheral blood: reticulocyte, granulocyte (chromosome aberration—micronuclei test)
Glucose	Sperm
Histamine	Sperm abnormality
Immunoglobulins	
Iron incorporation into erythrocytes	PHYSICAL PARAMETERS
Lactate dehydrogenase	Early transient incapacitation
Lipids:	Epilation
triglycerides	Erythema
phospholipids	Prodromal stage symptoms: nausea, vomiting, diarrhea
cholesterol	
Lipoproteins	ANALYSIS OF ACTIVATED ELEMENTS
Lysylaminopeptidase	Neutron exposure and/or activation in body tissues
Nucleic acids	
Plasma-free hemoglobin	
Plasma-free haptoglobin	
Prostaglandins	
Zinc protoporphyrin	

HEMATOLOGICAL DOSIMETERS

Peripheral blood lymphocytes are extremely sensitive to ionizing radiation. They may succumb to interphase death after exposure to a dose of only 0.05–0.15 Gy.[30] The decrease in the number of blood lymphocytes at 24–48 hours after irradiation can be a useful indicator of radiation exposure (Table 6-4).[21,23,24] The radiation doses listed in Table 6-4 are based on exposure to gamma radiation, but the lethality patterns should be similar for a neutron or mixed-field pure radiation exposure as determined from the lymphocyte counts. A lymphocyte count of 1,200–1,500/mm^3 at 24 hours after irradiation is a reduction of 50%. It indicates a potentially lethal exposure, requiring immediate medical attention.[23] Monitoring for the onset of hematological problems at the end of the latency period (which may last several weeks) is advised for persons whose lymphocyte counts reflect a lower but potentially lethal level of exposure. Lymphocyte counts drop to zero in persons

TABLE 6-2

TIME OF PRODROMAL STAGE AS A FUNCTION OF RADIATION DOSE*

Dose (Gy)	Onset (hours)	Duration (hours)	Latency
0.5–2.0	Absent to 6	<24	Absent or 3 weeks
2.0–3.5	2–6	12–24	2–3 weeks
3.5–5.5	1–2	24	1.0–2.5 weeks
>5.5	Minutes to 1	48	2–4 days

*With larger radiation doses, prodromal stage may persist until death.

TABLE 6-3

EARLY SYMPTOMS AFTER HIGH-LETHALITY EXPOSURE*

Coma
Fever
Dizziness
Convulsion
Disorientation
Severe headache
Mild to severe hypotension
Lymphocyte count 0–300 /mm^3
Severe fluid loss and/or electrolyte imbalance

*0–24 hours after exposure

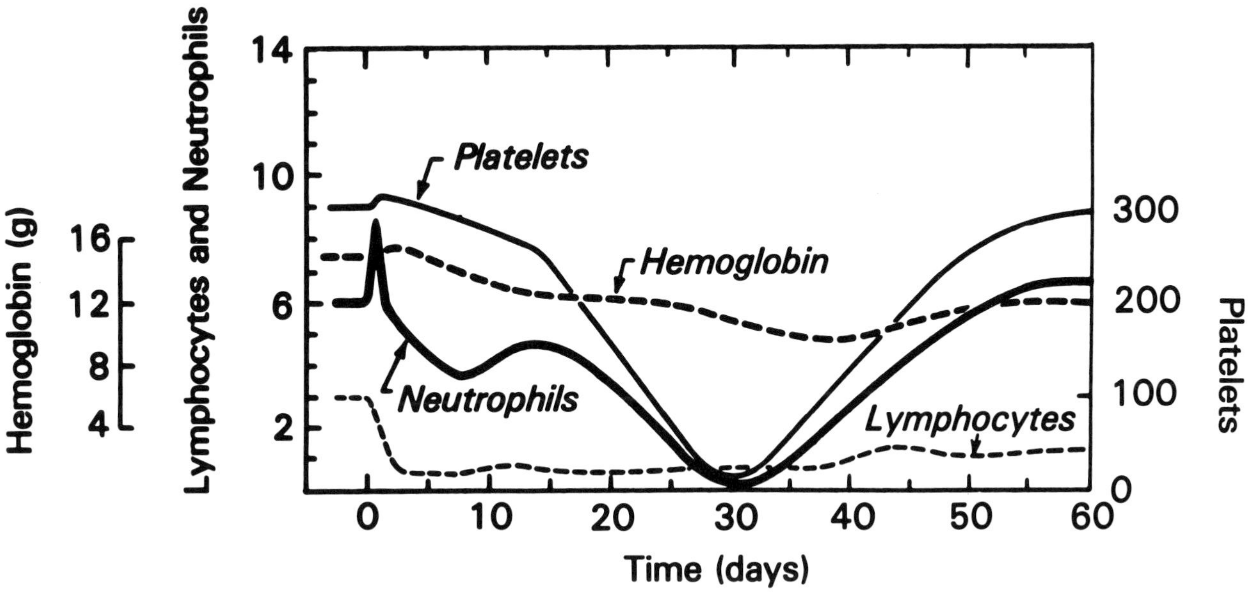

Fig. 6-1. Estimated changes in human blood-cell numbers after irradiation with 3 Gy of gamma rays
Source: used by permission, reference 77.

TABLE 6-4

LYMPHOCYTE COUNT IN HUMANS AT 24–48 HOURS AFTER RADIATION

Lymphocyte Count ($x1000/mm^3$)	Dose Range (Gy)	Lethality (%)
3.0	0–0.25	—
1.2– 2.0	1–2	<5
0.4–1.2	2.0–3.5	<50
0.1–0.4	3.5–5.5	50–99
0–0.1	>5.5	99–100

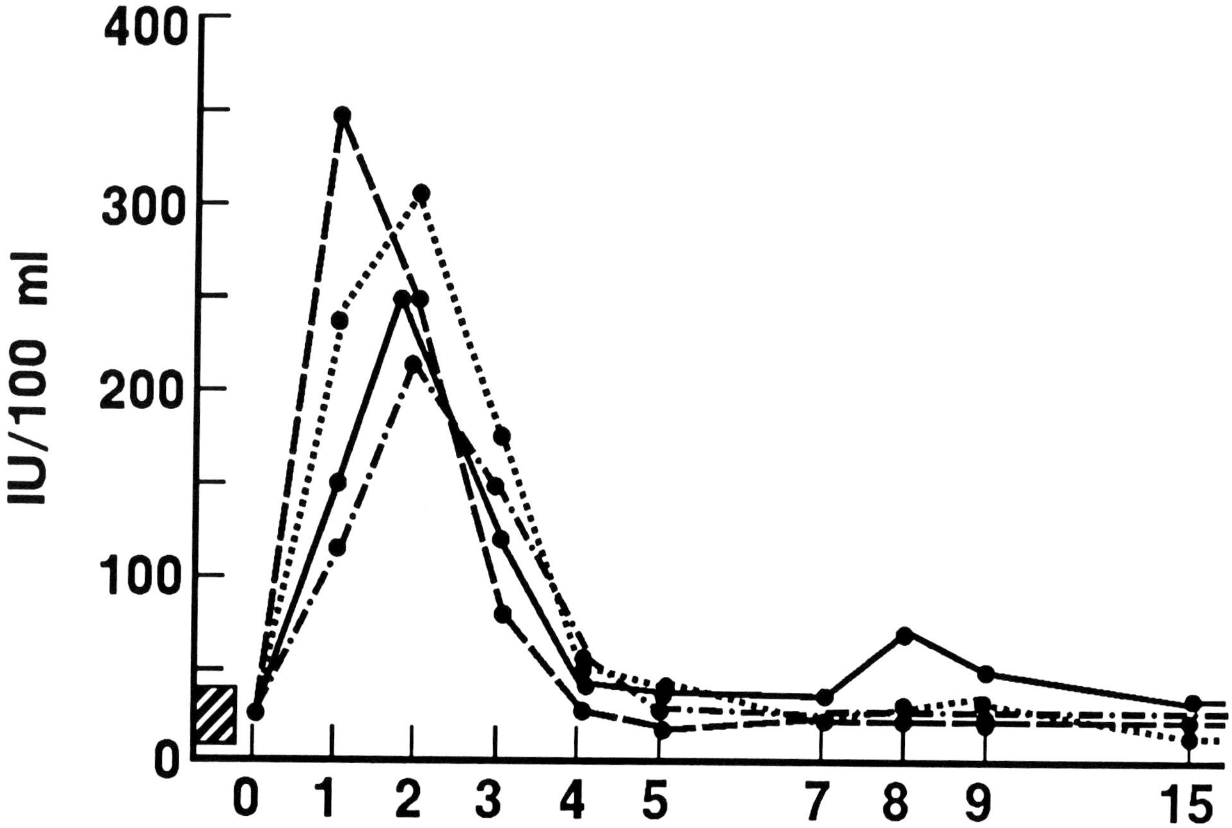

Fig. 6-2. Elevation of serum amylase levels in humans receiving fractionated radiotherapy. Four different fractionation protocols were used: patients receiving 2 Gy/day (•---•); three fractions per day of 2 Gy, each fraction separated by 3–4 hours (•–•–•–•); three fractions per day of 1 Gy, each separated by 3–4 hours (•——•); and two fractions per day of 2 Gy (• • • • •), separated by 7–8 hours. Control values are represented by shaded region.
Source: redrawn; used by permission, reference 2.

who received doses greater than 5.5 Gy.

Granulocytes, platelets, reticulocytes, and erythrocytes are also affected by radiation (Figure 6-1). In particular, lymphocyte and granulocyte counts proved to be valuable biological dosimeters after the 1986 reactor accident in Chernobyl, USSR.[32] Blood cell effects may be detectable in humans after exposure to 0.5–1.0 Gy of gamma radiation. These responses reflect interphase cell death and also the mitotic delay or destruction of the hematopoietic stem cells of the bone marrow.[33] Hematopoietic depression may result either directly from radiation damage to the hematopoietic stem cells, or indirectly from damage to the stromal stem cells that are responsible for maintaining the microenvironment of the bone marrow. Hematopoietic precursor cells in later stages of development are less sensitive to radiation damage than are the stem cells. In an abnormal process called *maturation-depletion,* these more mature differentiated cells may continue to develop without other precursor cells differentiating to take their place. This same process may be observed in the irradiated testes, where radiation exposure is followed by temporary aspermia.[26]

The length of the latency period between the radiation exposure and the decrease in blood cell numbers depends on the degree of damage and on the normal lifetime of that particular class of blood cells. Human platelets have a life span of 4–5 days, and because they decrease by attrition without replacement, hemorrhage will occur. Radiation-induced mortality after a dose of 2–12 Gy results from hemorrhage and other hematopoietic problems. These symptoms are called the hematopoietic subsyndrome. Physical examination and blood cell counts are readily obtainable, although other technologies may be too time consuming or otherwise not presently feasible for large-scale field use.

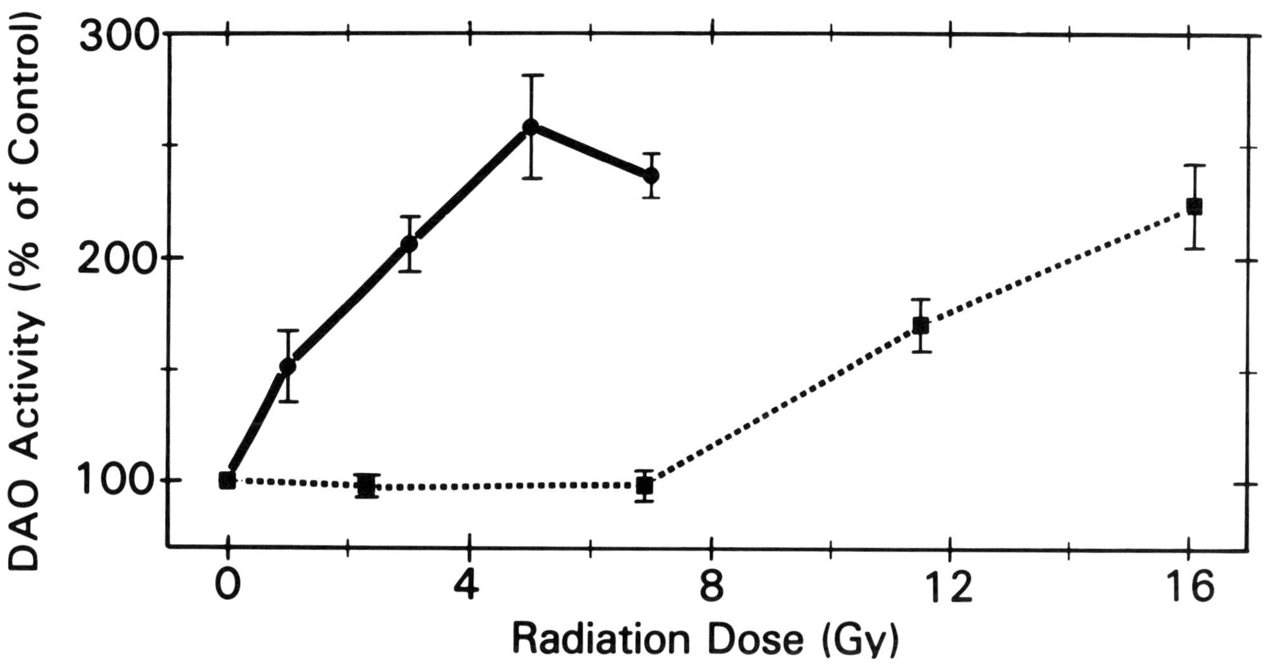

Fig. 6-3. Plasma levels of diamine oxidase in mice as a function of radiation dose. Plasma levels of diamine oxidase were determined in mice on day 4 after irradiation with either cobalt-60 gamma (•- - -•) or fission neutron (•——•) radiation. Source: used by permission, reference 1.

BLOOD SERUM DOSIMETERS

Although a number of serum factors may be useful biological dosimeters, none has received widespread verification or acceptance. However, two show potential: serum amylase [2-8] and diamine oxidase (DAO).[1,13] Serum amylase (Figure 6-2) becomes elevated in humans who receive radiotherapy when the parotid gland is included in the field of exposure.[2,4] This response is an early indicator of damage, and elevation can be seen within hours after irradiation. Amylase levels increase almost tenfold, peaking at 24–36 hours after exposure to 1 Gy.[2] A linear correlation exists for the peak serum elevation and the radiation dose received; the peak response occurs slightly earlier with increasing doses.[2,4] Radiotherapeutic fractionated doses of 1–2 Gy/day result in the further destruction of the parotid gland and a reduction in serum amylase by the end of the first week. The response depends on exposure of only the salivary glands (levels of pancreatic serum amylase are not altered in response to radiotherapy).[5] Interestingly, the elevation of serum amylase in response to radiation has been reported only in humans; it cannot be reproduced in rodent research models.[7] The effect of neutron radiation or of combined injury on the elevations of serum amylase has not been determined.

DAO is another serum enzyme that is a potential biological dosimeter of radiation injury.[1,13] DAO is produced primarily by intestinal villi during cell proliferation and differentiation. In humans, DAO levels have been used to monitor the effects of chemotherapy on the gut, but the response following irradiation has not been determined.[34] Plasma levels of DAO (Figure 6-3) increase in a dose-dependent manner in mice on days 2–4 following exposure to cobalt-60 gamma or neutron radiation.[1] This initial increase may not be associated with gut damage but may reflect a more systemic injury.[1] If the human response is consistent with the mouse model, patients who receive radiotherapy that does not involve the gut should have changes in DAO levels related to the radiation exposure. The mouse model also indicates that the DAO response may not be reliable in combined injuries involving radiation and burns.[1]

Other changes in serum enzymes have been reported; however, they are not as indicative as those in serum amylase and DAO. Serum alkaline phosphatase in rats decreases after irradiation in a dose-dependent manner.[10] The decrease occurs primarily in the intestinal and liver isozymes, and may be useful for dosimetry on days 2–4 after irradiation. The intestinal isozyme decreases on day 3 by 77% after a 5-Gy radiation dose, and by 90% after an 8-Gy dose. The responses of these isozymes in humans have not been confirmed.

Other serum indicators have been examined in humans receiving radiotherapy, but results are sometimes difficult to interpret because of interactions between the chemotherapy, cancer, and long fractionation schedules. Changes in the levels and classes of immunoglobulins in association with immunosuppression after radiotherapy do not appear to be useful in biological dosimetry.[35] Serum lactate dehydrogenase increases during the first week of radiotherapy, with even higher levels at weeks 4–5 in a majority of patients, but these increases may be influenced by other factors, including infection.[11] Levels of plasma hemoglobin and haptoglobin increase up to 40%, but not until week 4 of radiotherapy in cancer patients.[36] Haptoglobin is produced by the liver and hemoglobin is produced by hematopoietic precursors. The elevation of hemoglobin is probably associated with recovery of the hematopoietic system, and the dose dependency (not yet determined) will be associated with increased delay of elevation.

URINARY DOSIMETERS

Lacking metabolic enzymes, urine provides relatively stable biological indicators. It can also be obtained noninvasively. After irradiation, urine contains more creatine,[18,19,28] histamine,[17] taurine,[16] amylase,[5] and prostaglandins.[15]

Postirradiation elevation of creatine occurs during the first 3 days after exposure of rats to less than 0.25 Gy of X radiation.[18] The average urinary creatine-creatinine ratio during this period is dose dependent for 0.25–6.5 Gy. Creatinuria occurs in humans after irradiation, but because it may also be affected by exercise, muscular atrophy, trauma, or starvation,[28,37] it cannot be considered specific to radiation injury.

Elevations of histamine occur in the blood of patients receiving radiotherapy.[20] The maximal elevation of histamine in the urine of rats occurred on the first day after exposure to 9 Gy of cobalt-60 gamma radiation.[17]

Taurine is an amino acid that is excreted in large concentrations from rats in the first 3 days after irradiation.[16] Elevated taurine levels have been reported in exposed humans,[38] and may be attributed to altered excretion patterns from kidney damage, altered synthesis, and increased release from damaged tissues (particularly lymphoid tissue).[39]

Glycine and hydroxyproline are also excreted in increased amounts (up to ten times normal levels) in the urine of humans during the first week after receiving 25–180 rem.[38] Elevations of prostaglandins have been detected in the plasma of patients receiving radiotherapy[14] and in the urine of laboratory mice receiving cobalt-60 gamma radiation or neutron radiation.[15]

The development of biological dosimetry kits based on urinalysis would be hindered by *(a)* biphasic responses, such as occur with prostaglandins[15] and taurine;[39] *(b)* diurnal variations, as with creatine;[37] *(c)* reductions in urinary volume following irradiation;[15] and *(d)* problems with 24-hour urine collection.

CHROMOSOMAL DOSIMETERS

Although the most widely used biological dosimeter of radiation injury is prodromal symptomatology as revealed by physical examination, the most precise method is the determination of chromosomal aberrations in human blood lymphocytes.[40] Such chromosomal analysis has been used to determine the radiation doses received after industrial accidents,[41-43] the occupational expo-

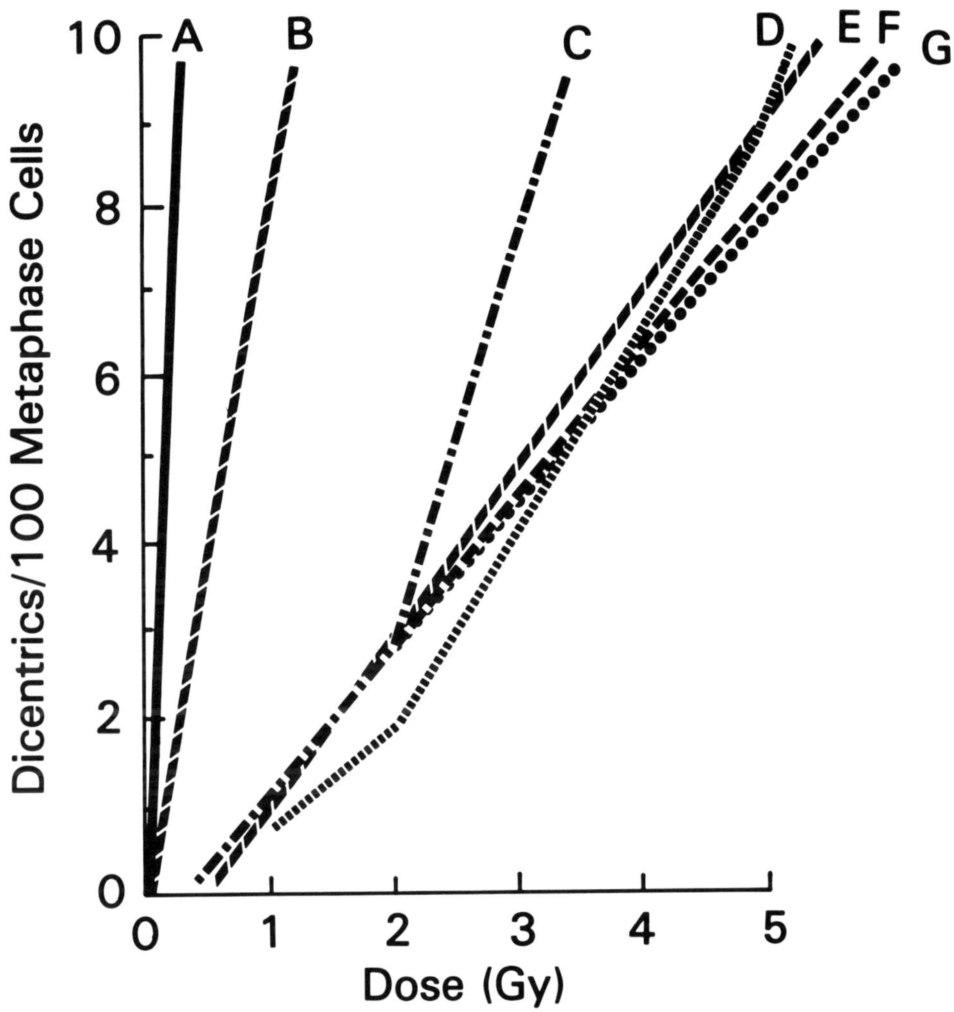

Fig. 6-4. Dicentric chromosome yield as a function of radiation dose. Yields of dicentric chromosome formation per 100 lymphocytes in metaphase are shown for the following conditions: (A) alpha radiation, (B) neutron radiation, (C) high-dose-rate X radiation, (D) low-dose-rate gamma radiation, (E) high-dose-rate gamma radiation, (F) high-dose-rate gamma radiation, and (G) low-dose-rate gamma radiation. Differences between laboratories are apparent in comparisons of curves D and G showing low-dose-rate gamma radiation and of curves E and F showing high-dose-rate gamma radiation.

Source: redrawn; used by permission from references 57 and 59.

TABLE 6-5

COMPARISON OF CHROMOSOMAL ASSAY SYSTEMS

Assay Type	Volume of blood required (ml)	Assay time (hours)	Lowest radiation dose
Phytohemagglutinin-stimulated peripheral blood lymphocytes	5.0	48	4.0 rads (X rays) 20.0 rads (gamma rays) 0.2 rads (neutrons)
Premature chromosomal condensation method (PCC)	0.5	2	6.0 rads (X rays)
Micronuclei technique	5.0	48	Linear: 0–400 R (gamma rays) 0–80 R (neutrons)

sures received by uranium miners,[44] and the radiation exposure of the atomic-bomb survivors of Hiroshima and Nagasaki.[45] A correlation of chromosomal damage with the radiation dose has been confirmed with *in vitro* experiments and with patients receiving radiotherapy.[46] Response curves have been prepared for the various types of radiation (Figure 6-4), and for the three assay methods in use (Table 6-5): *(a) cultured peripheral blood lymphocyte technique,*[40-47] *(b) premature chromosomal condensed chromosome (PCC) technique,*[48-50] and *(c) micronuclei technique* with lymphocytes or erythroid precursors.[51-54]

Cultured Peripheral Blood Lymphocyte Technique

Typically, blood lymphocytes are nondividing cells that have progressed to the G_0 stage of the cell cycle. They may be stimulated into mitosis with phytohemagglutinin. This culturing process requires about 48 hours to obtain a sufficient number of lymphocytes in mitosis, at which time the chromosomes have become condensed and the damage is visible.[40,55] The number of dicentric aberrations, ring structures, or total number of aberrations per mitotic cell are tabulated and recorded. Dicentric (Figure 6-5) and ring chromosomes are formed from asymmetrical interchromosomal exchanges, in which one of the resulting chromosomes contains two centromeres. The formation of dicentric chromosomes is linearly related to the radiation dose (Figure 6-4), although the response may vary with the type of radiation (and also between laboratories).[56-58] These differences can be seen in curves D (curvilinear) and G (linear) of Figure 6-4, which are low-dose-rate gamma radiation exposures from two laboratories.

In addition, Figure 6-4 shows a difference between high-dose-rate X radiation (C) and high-dose-rate gamma radiation (E and F), although the RBE for gamma and X radiation is usually similar. Irradiation with high-LET alpha particles (curve A) or medium-LET neutrons (curve B) is more damaging than irradiation with low-LET radiation, such as X rays and gamma rays (curves C-G). To assess the dose accurately, the type of radiation must be known. Beta radiation exposure may produce skin damage of medical consequence, but it would not be accurately reflected in this assay.

An average assay requires one workday for a trained technician to count about 10,000 lymphocytes to obtain 200 cells in metaphase.[58-59] Lower radiation doses produce lower aberration yields, and require that even more cells be counted for statistical accuracy. Several problems are associated with the standardization of this technique, including variations in tissue culture conditions between laboratories, the percentage of cells in first mitosis at 48 hours, variations in health and age of

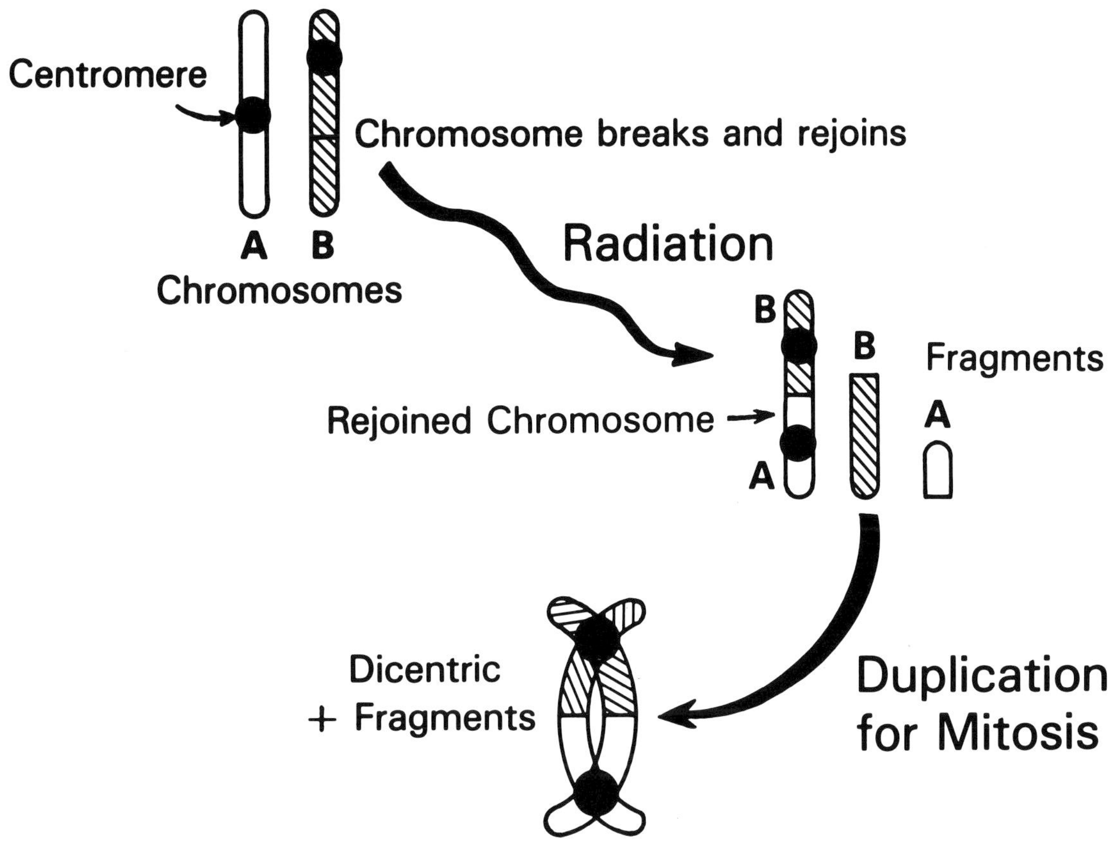

Fig. 6-5. Formation of dicentric chromosomes. Dicentric chromosomes are formed when two chromosomal fragments (A and B), each containing a centromere, rejoin to form a new chromosome containing two centromeres. During mitosis, when chromosomes are separated by spindle fibers attached to the centromere, the new chromosome may be pulled from each pole (in a different direction) and may fail to separate properly, stopping the mitotic process. Additional chromosomal information is lost at this time in the fragments that do not contain centromeres and are unable to migrate to either pole.

persons examined, whole-body versus partial-body exposure, and radiation effects resulting from different types of radiation (low versus high LET) and dose rates.[47,48,56,58,60-63] The normal incidence of chromosomal aberrations increases with the increasing age of the individual and previous exposure to carcinogens.[52,64] The time interval at which the sample was collected after irradiation can also affect the results because the damage may have a chance to repair.[47] A program coordinated by the International Atomic Energy Agency found a 15%–36% difference in the scoring of a standard test sample among fourteen test laboratories.[56] A previous study found an eightfold difference, which was attributed mainly to differences in culture conditions and in the time of first mitosis.[56,65] When all laboratories examined the same slides, the differences were greatly reduced. A computer system has been applied to the analysis of chromosomal aberrations using parallel image processing,[66] but the preparation of samples still requires a specialized laboratory and is not feasible for a military or civilian field hospital.

Premature Condensed Chromosome Technique

The PCC technique eliminates many of the inherent problems of mitotic peripheral blood lymphocyte cultures.[48-50] In this method, human lymphocytes are fused to mitotic Chinese hamster ovary (CHO) cells using polyethylene glycol. The mitotic CHO cells cause the individual lymphocyte chromosomes to condense and become visible.[62,63] After staining, the human chromosomes and those from CHO cells will be different colors.[62,63] The damage is assessed by determining the number of human chromosomal fragments in excess of the normal forty-six. Samples for PCC

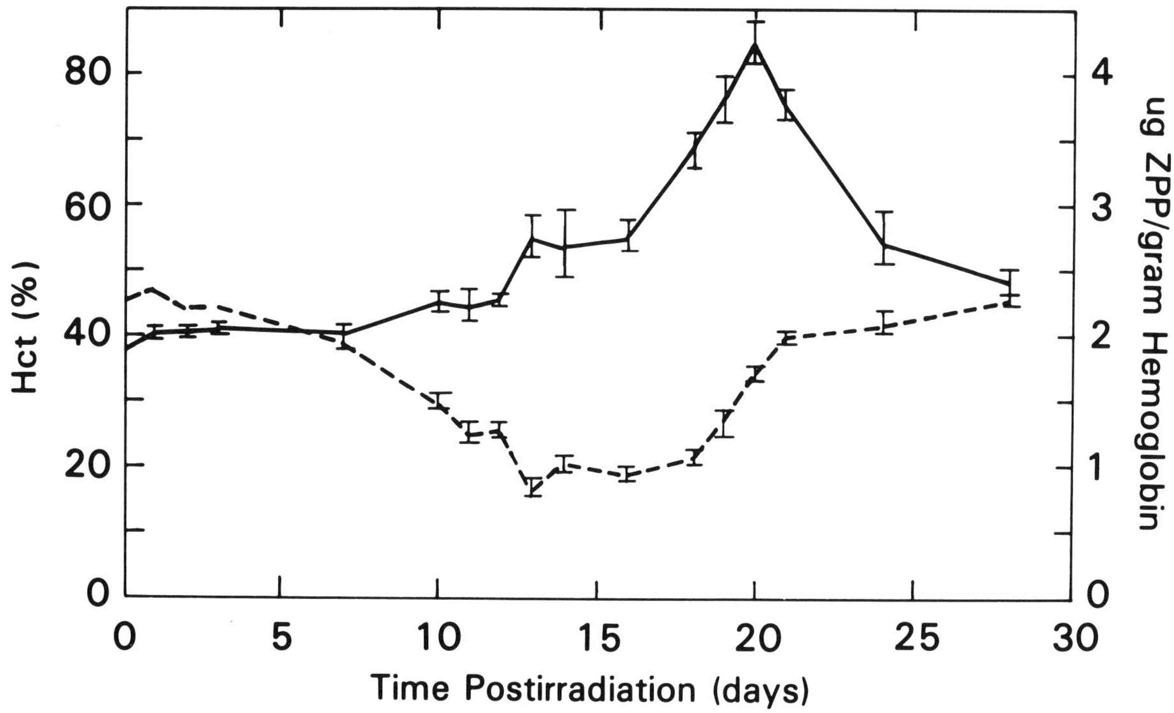

Fig. 6-6. Radiation-induced elevation of zinc protoporphyrin (ZPP) in mouse erythrocytes. ZPP (---) becomes elevated in mice receiving 5.5 Gy of X radiation. ZPP is measured by fluorescent detection from a drop of whole blood. Its elevation occurs after irradiation in association with recovery of hematopoiesis, as indicated by an increase in the hematocrit level (–) at the same time. It may be possible to develop dedicated spectrofluorometers for other fluorescent biological indicators in blood.
Source: used by permission, reference 29.

analysis require less than 2 hours for preparation time, eliminate variations due to culture conditions, and may be analyzed quickly because 200 lymphocytes with visible chromosomes are easier to locate and count.[48-50,63] As with chromosomal aberration analyses of cultured lymphocytes, assay-sampling time after irradiation remains a concern, because repair can reduce the aberration yield.[48,49] The effects of dose rate, radiation quality, and LET on the reliablity of this technique have not been investigated, nor have the possible alterations from combined injury. Future research may focus on the development of a nuclease-free homogenate from mitotic cells that will induce the premature condensation of chromosomes. This would eliminate the requirement of specialized tissue-culture laboratories for fresh mitotic cells and would permit the development of a standardized assay kit. Even with computer analysis, the assay may still be too time consuming for use with mass casualties.

Micronuclei Technique

Micronuclei are chromosomal fragments that lack centromeres. As a result, they are not incorporated into the new nucleus during mitosis but form a smaller satellite structure. As with other chromosomal aberrations, the rate of micronuclei formation depends on the dose rate and the LET. Therefore, neutrons have an RBE of 4.4 in mouse bone-marrow cells compared to a lower RBE of cobalt-60 gamma radiation.[54] Micronuclei are easier to detect in the bone-marrow normoblasts because the micronuclei remain after the main nucleus has been eliminated. Control values for this assay are about 1–2 micronuclei/1,000 cells, based on an average screening of 2,000 cells.[54] The assay may also be performed on mitotically stimulated peripheral blood lymphocytes, extending the analysis time by the standard 48-hour culture period, or it may be performed on cells obtained from a bone-marrow transplant.

OTHER DOSIMETERS

Fluorometric Immunoassay

Fluorometric assays or immunoassays have been developed for specific biological indicators present in blood or urine. During the late 1970s, increased emphasis was seen in the Soviet literature on fluorescent and chemoluminescent changes in blood cell and serum components after irradiation.[67-70] Fluorescent techniques permit the development of dedicated fluorometers for use in screening blood samples rapidly for changes in specific components. Dedicated field-portable fluorometers are currently used by the U.S. Public Health Service for detection of zinc protoporphyrin (ZPP) from a drop of blood.[71] Elevation of ZPP is a diagnostic indicator for lead poisoning and for iron deficiency anemia.[72] ZPP also becomes elevated in the blood of mice following whole-body exposure to ionizing radiation (Figure 6-6).[29] This elevation is associated with the recovery of the hematopoietic system at 10–18 days after irradiation, and is not observed in animals dying from the hematopoietic subsyndrome. The elevation of ZPP occurs too late to be useful in general screening or triage; however, it may be feasible to develop a field-portable dedicated fluorometer for other biological dosimeters.

Immunoassay offers another promising technique for field-dosimeter assay kits. A fluorescent immunoassay has been developed at the Lawrence Livermore National Laboratory to detect changes in the determinants of the MN antigens located on the surface of red blood cells.[73,74] The M and N blood-group antigens are heterozygous forms of glycophorin A. Like those antigens of the AB blood group, persons may be homozygous MM or NN, heterozygous MN, or hemizygous NO and MO. The general population is predominantly MN, and MN-antibody-labeled human blood cells fluoresce red and green when exposed to laser light. Blood cells from MN-heterozygous humans exposed to ionizing radiation have a greater variant frequency or proportional alteration in the MN blood antigen (MM, NN, MO, NO).[73] These abnormal cells (nonheterozygous) fluoresce red or green, reflecting the presence of one antigen; they do not reflect both colors as do normal cells. This assay has been used on blood samples from the atomic-bomb survivors in Japan[73] and the more recent victims of the nuclear-reactor accident in Chernobyl.[74] The change in the MN blood-group antigen occurs in the stem cells of the bone marrow, and its earliest appearance in the recovering marrow will be 2–3 weeks after irradiation. It would not be useful as an early triage indicator during the first few days.

Determination of Whole-Body Radionuclides

The degree of internal contamination from most radionuclides can also be determined by the use of physical dosimeters, such as whole-body radiation scanners. Iodine-131, a radioactive isotope with a half-life of 8 days, is usually released in large quantities after a nuclear accident or explosion. It is usually either inhaled or ingested. It enters the food chain when it is deposited on grass, which is eaten by dairy cows who, in turn, produce milk for human consumption. Once internalized, iodine-131 collects in the thyroid, where sufficient concentrations may lead to hypothyroidism, organ ablatement, or increased incidence of thyroid cancer. The levels of iodine-131 can be determined with an external thyroid scan.

A neutron dose can be calculated either by measuring the presence and concentration of sodium-24 in the plasma or by using a whole-body scan. Exposure to neutrons results in the conversion (neutron activation) of sodium-23 (the nonradioactive, abundant isotopic form of sodium) to sodium-24. Sodium-24 is a radioactive isotope with one more neutron than sodium-23. It has a half-life of 15 hours and decays to nonradioactive magnesium-24, releasing both beta and characteristic gamma radiation. Sodium-24 should be determined from plasma samples rather than from whole blood, because it appears mainly in plasma rather than in red cells.[75] The presence of sodium-24 above background levels indicates a neutron exposure,[75] and the radiation dose can be calculated from the levels of sodium-24 present.

PROBLEMS

Problems exist in the use of biological dosimeters, including their potential unreliability in combined-injury situations.[23,47,48,61-63] For example, the value of a lymphocyte count becomes questionable in a combined injury involving infection or burn. Additional problems include the following:

- Collection, contamination, stability, and reproducibility of the sample
- Variable changes in a biological response, according to the dose of radiation received and the time elapsed between exposure and examination
- Length of time required for assay (48–72 hours for some chromosomal analyses), which makes its feasibility for field use questionable
- Lack of an appropriate research model system (Some biological changes observed after radiation exposure in humans, such as serum amylase, do not occur in laboratory animals.)
- Radiation variables: dose, dose rate, quality, type, and mixed-radiation fields (Fission neutrons have an RBE of 18 compared with X radiation for the production of dicentric chromosomal aberrations.[57] The possibility exists for a significant error in measurement if the type of radiation or proportion of mixed-field radiation is not known.)

Many of these problems might be overcome by using more than one biological indicator (for example, using one as a screening agent and another as confirmation). Lymphocyte and granulocyte cell counts, combined with chromosomal aberration assays, provided biological dosimetry for the Chernobyl patients, in order to minimize the unreliability from burn indicators alone.[32] Biological indicators for use during different time periods after irradiation need to be identified. For example, one set would be used at 1–3 days and another set at 1–2 weeks after exposure. Indicators from the different status groupings in Table 6-6 should be used jointly to provide a more complete picture of the damage and the biological response.

SUMMARY

The levels of a number of biological compounds become altered in body tissues after radiation exposure. These changes occur *(a)* as a direct result of the radiation damage, or *(b)* in response to mobilization for repair, regeneration, and cell proliferation. In some cases, the degree of alteration is proportional to the dose of radiation, and those degrees may serve as diagnostic aids in the triage of casualties and in the monitoring of radiotherapy. With the exception of neutron activation of the elements in tissues, none of the biological indicators is unique to radiation injury.

Several problems are associated with the use of most biological dosimeters, particularly in a mass-casualty situation. Many biological indicators have not been completely characterized in humans. In addition, many indicators (including lymphocyte counts) may not be reliable with injuries involving radiation combined with burn or infection. Combinations of nonlethal doses of radiation, burn, or infection may result in mortality.[76] Immunosuppression induced by radiation exposure may increase the likelihood of succumbing to infection or neoplasm,[77] and the degree of immunosuppression is an important prognostic indicator. At present, we have no reliable measurement of that degree (Table 6-6). Future research needs to address the detection of immunosuppressive factors that are released in blood and tissue fluids after injury.

The most reliable indicator for mass casualties is the characterization of early symptoms of the prodromal stage of ARS: nausea, vomiting, and diarrhea. Greater accuracy may be obtained with a lymphocyte chromosomal analysis that can detect radiation exposure as low as 0.03–0.06 Gy. However, this procedure must be performed by a tissue culture laboratory, and it is time consuming. Table 6-6 shows biological indicators of post-irradiation damage in patients. For instance, blood-cell counts may indicate the need for a bone-marrow transplant, but indicators of gut status may show possible gastrointestinal cell death, which would contraindicate the transplant.

Two serum enzymes, amylase and diamine oxidase, show promise as biological dosimeters. Each has drawbacks: the salivary glands must be in the field of exposure for elevations of serum amylase to occur, and the response of DAO has not been characterized in irradiated humans. Portable fluorometers for specific biological compounds and the development of specific immunological assays also hold promise for the future of biological dosimetry.

TABLE 6-6

BIOLOGICAL INDICATORS OF POSTIRRADIATION DAMAGE IN PATIENTS

DOSE-RESPONSIVE CLINICAL INDICATORS
Prostaglandins (?)
Diamine oxidase (?)
Serum amylase
STATUS OF BONE MARROW
Granulocytes
Platelets
Reticulocytopenia
INTESTINAL INJURY
Diarrhea
Bloody stool
Diamine oxidase
DIRECT CELLULAR DAMAGE
Lymphocytes
Cytogenetics
IMMUNOSUPPRESSION
Unknown

REFERENCES

1. DeBell, R. M.; Ledney, G. D.; and Snyder, S. L. Quantification of gut injury with diamine oxidase activity: Development of a fission neutron RBE and measurements with combined injury in mouse models. *Radiat. Res.*, in press.

2. Becciolini, A.; Porciani, A.; Lanini, A.; Chiavacci, A.; and Cellai, E. 1987. Effects of irradiation with conventional and multiple daily fractionation on serum amylase activity. *Acta Oncologica* 26: 139-142.

3. Tomassi, I.; Balzi, M.; Cremonini, D.; Becciolini, A.; Giannardi, G.; and Pelu, G. 1979. Radiation effects on the parotid gland of mammals. Part 3. Behavior of enzyme activity after irradiation. *Strahlentherapie* 155: 570-573.

4. Becciolini, A.; Giannardi, G.; Cionini, L.; Porciani, S.; Fallai, C.; and Pirtoli, L. 1984. Plasma amylase activity as biochemical indicator of radiation injury to salivary glands. *Acta Radiol.* [Oncol.] 23: 9-14.

5. Chen, W.; Kereiakes, J. G.; Silberstein, E. B.; Aron, B. S.; and Saenger, E. L. 1973. Radiation induces changes in serum and urinary amylase levels in man. *Radiat. Res.* 54: 141-151.

6. Van Den Brenk, H. A. S.; Hurley, R. A.; Gomez, C.; and Richter, W. 1969. Serum amylase as a measure of salivary gland radiation damage: Hyperamylasaemia following fractionated exposure to 4 MV x-rays delivered in high pressure oxygen. *Br. J. Radiol.* 42: 688-700.

7. Beccioloni, A.; Balzi, M.; Cremonini, D.; Tomassi, I.; Giannardi, G.; and Pelu, G. 1980. Radiation effects on the parotid gland of mammals. Part 4. Biochemical and morphological changes after local irradiation. *Strahlentherapie* 156: 69-72.

8. Kashima, H. K.; Kirkham, W. R.; and Andrews, R. J. 1965. Postirradiation sialadenitis: A study of the clinical features, histopathologic changes and serum enzyme variations following irradiation of human salivary glands. *Amer. J. Roentgen.* 94: 271-291.

9. Vranovska, J.; Popisil, J.; and Dienstbier, Z. 1977. Changes of the activity of certain lysosomal enzymes in the blood serum of whole-body irradiated rats. *Strahlentherapie* 153: 496-500.

10. Highman, B., and Hanks, A. R. 1970. Serum alkaline phosphatase in rats after 800 R whole-body or regional X-irradiation. *Proc. Soc. Exp. Biol. Med.* 133: 1201-1206.

11. Horvath, M.; Rode, I. L.; Kralovanszky, J.; and Volant, M. 1980. Investigation of a valuable biochemical indicator in radiotherapy. III. Serum lactate dehydrogenase enzyme level on irradiation of cancer patients. *Strahlentherapie* 156: 244-247.

12. Stepan, J.; Havranek, T.; and Jojkova, K. 1977. Serum alkaline phosphatase as indicators of radiation damage in rats. *Radiat. Res.* 70: 406-414.

13. Ely, M. J.; Speicher, J. M.; Catravas, G. N.; and Snyder, S. L. 1985. Radiation effects on diamine oxidase activities in intestine and plasma of the rat. *Radiat. Res.* 103: 158-162.

14. Tanner, N. S. B.; Stamford, I. F.; and Bennett, A. 1981. Plasma prostaglandins in mucositis due to radiotherapy and chemotherapy for head and neck cancer. *Br. J. Cancer* 43: 767-771.

15. Steel, L. K.; Rafferty, M. A.; Wolfe, W. W.; Egan, J. E.; Kennedy, D. A.; Catravas, G. N.; Jackson, W. E., III; and Dooley, M. A. 1986. Urinary excretion of cyclic nucleotides, creatinine, prostaglandin E_2, and thromboxane B_2 from mice exposed to whole-body irradiation from an enhanced neutron field. *Int. J. Radiat. Biol.* 50: 695-715.

16. Abe, M.; Takahashi, M.; Takeuchi, K.; and Fukuda, M. 1968. Studies on the significance of taurine in radiation injury. *Radiat. Res.* 33: 563-573.

17. Donlon, M. A.; Helgeson, E. A.; Lambright, K. T.; and Catravas, G. N. 1981. Increased urinary excretion of histamine by rats following gamma radiation. *Fed. Proc.* 42: 1124.

18. Gerber, G. B.; Gertler, P.; Altman, K. I.; and Hemplemann, L. H. 1961. Dose dependency of radiation-induced creatine excretion in rat urine. *Radiat. Res.* 15: 307-313.

19. Gerber, G. B.; Gerber, G.; Kurohara, S.; Altman, K. I.; and Hemplemann, L. H. 1961. Urinary excretion of several metabolites in persons accidentally exposed to ionizing radiation. *Radiat. Res.* 15: 314-318.

20. Lasser, E. C., and Stenstrom, K. W. 1954. Elevation of circulating blood histamine in patients undergoing deep roentgen therapy. *Amer. J. Roentgen.* 72: 985-988.

21. Young, R. W. 1987. Acute radiation syndrome. In *Military Radiobiology,* edited by J. J. Conklin and R. I. Walker, 165-190. Orlando, FL: Academic Press.

22. Hunt, W.A. Effects of ionizing radiation on behavior and the brain. In reference 21, 321-330.

23. Conklin, J. J., and Walker, R. I. Diagnosis, triage, and treatment of casualties. In reference 21, 231-240.

24. Messerschmidt, O. 1979. *Medical procedures in a nuclear disaster.* Munich: Verlag Karl Thiemig.

25. Nuclear Regulatory Commission. 1985. *Health effects model for nuclear power plant accident consequences analysis* [NUREG/CR-4214, Sandia No. SAND85-7185). Washington, DC: U.S. Government Printing Office.

26. Clifton, D. K., and Bremner, W. J. 1983. The effect of testicular X-irradiation on spermatogenesis in man. *J. Androl.* 4: 387-392.

27. Lushbaugh, C. C.; Hubner, K. F.; and Fry, S. A. 1982. The impact of estimates of human radiation tolerance upon radiation emergency management. In *The Control of Exposure of the Public to Ionizing Radiation in the Event of Accident or Attack.* Proceedings of Symposium, April 1981, 46-57. Washington, DC: National Council on Radiation Protection and Measurements.

28. Altman, K. I. 1971. Criteria for the evaluation and selection of radiation-induced metabolic changes as biochemical indicators of radiation damage. In *Biochemical Indicators of Radiation Injury in Man,* edited by K. I. Altman, 1-9. Vienna: International Atomic Energy Agency.

29. Walden, T. L., Jr.; Draganac, P. S.; and Farkas, W. R. 1984. The elevation of blood levels of zinc protoporphyrin in mice following whole body irradiation. *Blood* 63: 1159-1167.

30. United Nations Scientific Committee on the Effects of Atomic Radiation. 1982. *Ionizing radiation: Sources and biological effects* [1982 Report to the General Assembly]. New York: United Nations.

31. National Council on Radiation Protection and Measurements. 1974. *Radiological factors affecting decision-making in a nuclear attack* [NCRP Report 42]. Washington, DC: National Council on Radiation Protection and Measurements.

32. Gale, R. P. 1987. Immediate medical consequences of nuclear accidents. Lessons from Chernobyl. *JAMA* 258: 625-628.

33. Department of Defense. 1962. Characteristics of acute whole body radiation injury. In *The Effects of Nuclear Weapons,* edited by S. Glasstone, 592-597. Washington, DC: U.S. Atomic Energy Commission.

34. Luk, G. D.; Vaughan, W. P.; Burke, P. J.; and Baylin, S. B. 1981. Diamine oxidase as a plasma marker of rat intestinal mucosal injury and regeneration after administration of 1-B-D-arabinofuranosylcytosine. *Cancer Res.* 41: 2334-2337.

35. Rode, I.; Horvath, M.; Petranyi, J.; and Kiss, B. 1979. Investigation of a valuable biochemical indicator in radiotherapy. I. Immunological tests and reticulocyte number. *Strahlentherapie* 155: 387-391.

36. Horvath, M.; Geszti, O.; Benedek, E.; Farkas, J.; and Reischi, G. 1979. Investigation of a valuable biochemical indicator in radiotherapy. II. Plasma free hemoglobin and haptoglobin level changes. *Strahlentherapie* 155: 579-583.

37. Woo, J.; Treuting, J. J.; and Cannon, D. C. 1979. Metabolic intermediates and inorganic ions. In vol. 1, *Clinical Diagnosis and Management,* edited by J. B. Henry, 262-264. Philadelphia: W. B. Saunders Co.

38. Katz, E. J., and Hasterlik, R. J. 1955. Aminoaciduria following total-body irradiation in the human. *JNCI* 15: 1085-1105.

39. Abe, M.; Takahashi, M.; Takeuchi, K.; and Fukuda, M. 1968. Studies on the significance of taurine in radiation injury. *Radiat. Res.* 33: 563-573.

40. Bender, M. A., and Gooch, P. C. 1962. Types and rates of X-ray-induced chromosome aberrations in human blood irradiated *in vitro. Proc. Natl. Acad. Sci. USA* 48: 522-532.

41. Popescu, H. L.; Pilat, L.; Hilt, M.; and Lancranjan, I. 1972. Evolution of biological changes noticed in three cases of accidental mild gamma irradiation. *J. Occup. Med.* 14: 317-320.

42. El-Alfi, O. S.; Ragab, A. S.; and Eassa, E.-H. M. 1967. Detection of radiation damage in exposed personnel by chromosome study. *Br. J. Radiol.* 40: 760-764.

43. Dolphin, G. W.; Bolton, D.; Humphreys, D. L. O.; Speight, D. L.; and Stradling, G. N. 1970. Biological dosimetry and physical dosimetry after a radiation accident. *Nature* 227: 165.

44. Brandom, W. F.; Saccomanno, G.; Archer, V. E.; Archer, P. G.; and Bloom, A. D. 1978. Chromosome aberrations as a biological dose-response indicator of radiation exposure in uranium miners. *Radiat. Res.* 76: 159-171.

45. Randolph, M. L., and Brewen, J. G. 1980. Estimation of whole-body doses by means of chromosome aberrations observed in survivors of the Hiroshima A-bomb. *Radiat. Res.* 82: 393-407.

46. Schmid, E.; Bauchinger, M.; Bunde, E.; Ferbert, H. F.; and v. Lieven, H. 1974. Comparison of the chromosome damage and its dose response after medical whole-body exposure to Co-60 gamma-rays and irradiation of blood *in vitro*. *Int. J. Radiat. Biol.* 26: 31-37.

47. Liniecki, J.; Bajerska, A.; and Wyszynska, K. 1983. Dose-response relationships for chromosome aberrations in peripheral blood lymphocytes after whole- and partial-body irradiations. II. Decline of aberration-carrying cells in blood with time post exposure. *Mutat. Res.* 110: 103-110.

48. Pantelias, G. E., and Maillie, H. D. 1985. Direct analysis of radiation-induced chromosome fragments and rings in unstimulated human blood lymphocytes by means of the premature chromosome condensation technique. *Mutat. Res.* 149: 67-72.

49. Cornforth, M. N., and Bedford, J. S. 1983. X-ray-induced breakage and rejoining of human interphase chromosomes. *Science* 222: 1141-1143.

50. Waldren, C. A., and Johnson, R. T. 1974. Analysis of interphase chromosome damage by means of premature chromosome condensation after X- and ultraviolet-irradiation. *Proc. Natl. Acad. Sci. USA* 71: 1137-1141.

51. Reddy, M. M.; Goh, K. O.; and Hemplemann, L. H. 1980. Induction of micronuclei in PHA-stimulated human lymphocyte cultures by therapeutic radiation. *Experientia* 36: 343-344.

52. Jessen, D., and Ramel, C. 1978. Factors affecting the induction of micronuclei at low doses of X-rays, MMS, and dimethylnitrosamine in mouse erythroblasts. *Mutat. Res.* 58: 51-65.

53. Schmid, W. 1975. The micronuclei test. *Mutat. Res.* 31: 9-15.

54. Garriott, M. L., and Grahn, D. 1982. Neutron and gamma-ray effects measured by the micronucleus test. *Mutat. Res.* 105: 157-162.

55. Moorhead, P. S.; Nowell, P. C.; Mellman, W. J.; Battips, D. M.; and Hungerford, D. A. 1960. Chromosome preparations of leukocytes cultured from human peripheral blood. *Exp. Cell Res.* 20: 613-616.

56. Bianchi, M.; Bianchi, N. O.; Brewen, J. G.; Buckton, K. E.; Fabry, L.; Fischer, P.; Gooch, P. C.; Kucerova, M.; Leonard, A.; Mukherjee, R. N.; Mukherjee, U.; Nakai, S.; Natarajan, A. T.; Obe, G.; Palitti, F.; Pohl-Ruling, J.; Schwarzacher, H. G.; Scott, D.; Sharma, T.; Takahashi, E.; Tanzarella, C.; and van Buul, P. P. W. 1982. Evaluation of radiation-induced chromosomal aberrations in human peripheral blood lymphocytes *in vitro*. *Mutat. Res.* 96: 233-242.

57. Vulpis, N.; Tognacci, L.; and Scarpa, G. 1978. Chromosome aberrations as a dosimetric technique for fission neutrons over the dose-range 0.2-50 rad. *Int. J. Radiat. Biol.* 33: 301-306.

58. Dolphin, G. W., and Lloyd, D. C. 1974. The significance of radiation-induced chromosome abnormalities in radiological protection. *J. Med. Genet.* 11: 181-189.

59. Hacker, U.; Schumann, J.; and Gohde, W. 1982. Mammalian spermatogenesis as a new system for biologic dosimetry of ionizing irradiation. *Acta Radiol.* [Oncol.] 21: 349-351.

60. Takahashi, E.; Hirai, M.; Tobari, I.; Utsugi, T.; and Nakai, S. 1982. Radiation-induced chromosome aberrations in lymphocytes from man and crab-eating monkey. *Mutat. Res.* 94: 115-123.

61. Das, B. C., and Sharma, T. 1983. Blood lymphocyte culture system: Quantitative analysis of X-ray-induced chromosome aberrations in man, muntjac, and cattle. *Mutat. Res.* 110: 111-139.

62. Maillie, H. D.; Baker, J. V.; Quinn, B. R.; and Fugo, E. D. 1986. Measuring damage to human lymphocytes *in vitro* after low-level radiation exposure using prematurely condensed chromosomes. *Health Phys.* 51: 672-676.

63. Pantelias, G. E., and Maillie, H. D. 1984. The use of peripheral blood mononuclear cell prematurely condensed chromosomes for biological dosimetry. *Radiat. Res.* 99: 140-150.

64. Bloom, A. D. 1972. Induced chromosomal aberrations in man. In vol. 3, *Advances in Human Genetics,* edited by H. Harris and K. Hirschhorn, 99-173. New York: Plenum Press.

65. Van Buul, P. P. W., and Natarajan, A. T. 1980. Chromosomal radiosensitivity of human leukocytes in relation to sampling time. *Mutat. Res.* 70: 61-69.

66. Bille, J.; Scharfenberg, H.; and Manner, R. 1983. Biological dosimetry by chromosome aberration scoring with parallel image processing with the Heidelberg POLYP polyprocessor system. *Comput. Biol. Med.* 13: 49-79.

67. Barkan, S., and Safronova, V. G. 1979. Investigation of intensity of ultraviolet fluorescence of leukocytes and bone marrow cells during chronic exposure to radiation. *Radiobiologiia* 14: 275-278.

68. Baraboi, V. A.; Orel, V. Z.; Sribnaia, A. F.; and Tatsii, I. A. 1978. Mechanism of early postirradiation changes in intensity of spontaneous chemoluminescence of blood serum. *Radiobiologiia* 18: 305-309.

69. Serkiz, Y. I.; Ryabova, E. Z.; and Chebotarev, E. E. 1975. Spontaneous and induced luminescence of blood serum as an index of the degree of radiation damage to animals. *Radiobiologiia* 15: 716-721.

70. Serkiz, Y. A.; Kovtun, T. V.; Ryabova, E. Z.; and Chebotarev, E. E. 1977. Chemoluminescence of alpha- and beta-lipoproteins of blood plasma of rats exposed to fast neutrons. *Radiobiologiia* 17: 803-806.

71. Grunder, F. I., and Moffitt, A. E., Jr. 1979. Evaluation of zinc protoporphyrin in an occupational environment. *Am. Ind. Hyg. Assoc. J.* 40: 686-694.

72. Lamola, A. A., and Yamane, T. 1974. Zinc protoporphyrin in the erythrocytes of patients with lead intoxication and iron-deficiency anemia. *Science* 186: 936-938.

73. Edwards, M. 1987. Chernobyl: One year after. *Natl. Geographic* 171: 633-653.

74. Langlois, R. G.; Bigbee, W. L.; Kyoizumi, S.; Nakamura, N.; Bean, M. A.; Akiyama, M.; and Jensen, R. H. 1987. Evidence for increased somatic cell mutations at the glycophorin A locus in atomic bomb survivors. *Science* 236: 445-448.

75. Mole, R. H. 1984. Sodium in man and the assessment of radiation dose after criticality accidents. *Phys. Med. Biol.* 29: 1307-1327.

76. Conklin, J. J.; MacVittie, T. J.; and Walker, R. I. 1985. Pathophysiology of combined injury and trauma: An overview. In *The Pathophysiology of Combined Injury and Trauma,* edited by R. I. Walker, D. F. Gruber, T. J. MacVittie, and J. J. Conklin, 3-10. Baltimore: University Park Press.

77. Anderson, R. E., and Warner, N. L. 1976. Ionizing radiation and the immune response. *Adv. Immunol.* 24: 215-335.

Chapter 7

BEHAVIORAL AND NEUROPHYSIOLOGICAL CHANGES WITH EXPOSURE TO IONIZING RADIATION

G. ANDREW MICKLEY, Ph.D.,* VICTOR BOGO, M.A.,** and BRUCE R. WEST, M.S.***

*Lieutenant Colonel, United States Air Force; Armed Forces Radiobiology Research Institute, Bethesda, Maryland 20814-5145

**Armed Forces Radiobiology Research Institute, Bethesda, Maryland 20814-5145

***Major, United States Army; Human Response Officer, Radiation Policy Division, Defense Nuclear Agency, 6801 Telegraph Road, Alexandria, Virginia 22310-3398

INTRODUCTION

The use of nuclear weapons in military conflicts will significantly challenge the ability of the armed forces to function. The thermal and overpressure stresses of conventional weapons will be significantly intensified during a nuclear battle. In addition, military personnel will have to contend with the hazards of exposure to ionizing radiation, which will be the main producer of casualties for nuclear weapons of 50 kt or less. Present projections of nuclear combat operations suggest that between one-half and three-quarters of the infantry personnel targeted by a tactical nuclear weapon would receive an initial radiation dose of 1.5–30.0 Gy.[1] This acute dose of ionizing radiation could dramatically affect a soldier's ability to complete combat tasks successfully. This, in turn, may ultimately affect the outcome of the armed conflict.

Information about the consequences of ionizing radiation may be derived from the following: *(a)* the nuclear detonations over Hiroshima and Nagasaki, *(b)* clinical irradiations, *(c)* nuclear accidents, and *(d)* laboratory animal research. Each of these sources has certain constraints. The Hiroshima and Nagasaki data are of limited value since there was no scientific assessment of behavior, and the reports were anecdotal, often conflicting, and not easily tied to specific radiation doses. Clinical irradiations are also of questionable value because precise measures of behavior are not usually recorded, and patients are behaviorally compromised by their illnesses or the chemical therapy being used. Nuclear accidents have been few, and little behavioral information has been obtained from those that have occurred. Although information on human radiation exposure is normally preferred, the paucity of data forces us to rely on animal research.

However, animal research brings with it problems of extrapolation. While the relevance of animal models to human behavior has been frequently shown in the study of toxic effects of ionizing radiation,[2,3] different species (even strains within species) may have different responses or sensitivities to radiation exposure.[4] It is important to understand the specific radiosensitivity of the animal model so that the radiation dose required to produce a similar effect in humans can be reasonably estimated. For example, in humans the lethal dose for 50% of cases after 30 days ($LD_{50/30}$) is 4.5 Gy, whereas in monkeys the $LD_{50/30}$ is 6.0 Gy. Similarly, the monkey is more radiosensitive than the rat ($LD_{50/30}$ = 7.5 Gy) or the mouse ($LD_{50/30}$ = 9.0 Gy).[5,6] Clearly, these classic $LD_{50/30}$ values are estimates, because they will vary with the animal strain, housing conditions, and other factors. However, the values do give a sense of the relative radiosensitivity of the animal models most often used in radiation research, and will help to put into context the radiation doses cited in this chapter.

Variations in radiosensitivity must also be considered when measuring animal behavior. For instance, at specific doses or dose rates, most animal models show a rapid, transient decrease in performance; however, this is not true for some dog or mouse strains.[7-9] Differences in CNS sensitivity to radiation have also been shown. The primate brain may be more sensitive to radiation damage than the rat brain.[10] Although differing sensitivities of animal strains can be enigmatic, they can be meaningful research tools that reveal physiological substrates of natural radioresistance.[9]

BEHAVIORAL CHANGES IN IRRADIATED ANIMALS

Radiation has significant effects on a variety of behavioral factors, including *learning, performance,* and *naturalistic and social behaviors.* However, this list is not a complete taxonomy of behavior. For example, performance can be somewhat arbitrarily separated into tasks having a strong cognitive component and tasks having a strong motor component. Also, an important distinction can sometimes be made between learning and performance. In its simplest form, learning is reflected by a linkage of a stimulus and a response. However, performance also depends on the organism's capacity to make a response. Thus, postirradiation changes in behavior may reflect deficits in either performance or learning (or both). Psychologists consider these concepts to be distinct, but in some cases it is difficult to separate them, especially in animal studies. Whether the mechanism of radiogenic behavioral change is based on deficits in learning, attention, retrieval, capacity to perform, or group disturbance, any of these disruptions can potentially determine an organism's ability to function in a nuclear environment.

Learning and Memory

Pavlovian conditioning paradigms are especially useful in distinguishing between learning and performance in animals. Studies suggest that learning can be altered by exposure to ionizing radiation. For example, rabbits were conditioned to associate a light-and-tone stimulus with the respiratory reflex of apnea that is produced by the inhalation of ammonia vapor.[11] Exposure to 15 Gy of cobalt-60 gamma radiation resulted in the absence or considerable reduction of conditioned apnea. In contrast, the unconditioned apnea (normal response to ammonia inhalation) was enhanced after irradiation, suggesting that the animal's performance capacity was still intact. These classical conditioning data suggest that (at least under the stated circumstances) radiation exposure can alter memory, and that this function is separate from the animal's performance.

Experiments using operant techniques may also be designed to allow some distinction between learning and performance. If a task can be selected in which a learning deficit is represented in a more rapid or vigorous response, then it may be possible to rule out lethargy or reduced physical capacity as the primary mediator of a behavioral change. For example, rats were trained to stay in a lighted area in order to avoid footshock in the adjacent dark area, which they normally preferred.[12] The latency of the subject's movement from the safe, lighted area to the electrified dark side was an indicator of learning. Thus, a rapid move into the hazardous chamber suggested that the subject had a learning deficit. This kind of learning appears to be extremely sensitive to disruption by radiation exposure, since an electron dose of only 0.001–0.1 Gy can produce significant *retrograde amnesia*. Retrograde amnesia is a short-term memory loss, or an inability to recall recent events, following trauma or a novel event. In this case, the forgotten event (footshock) occurred only seconds before the novel event (irradiation). The amnesia lasted for 4 seconds, was dependent on dose rate, and was produced by either electron or X irradiation.[13] The mechanism of radiogenic amnesia is still in question. However, sensory disruption, primarily of the visual system, may explain the memory loss.[12,14,15] These data support the idea that radiation affects some component of learning or memory, and the data agree with others suggesting that radiogenic disruptions in behavior may not merely reflect nonassociative factors.[16]

Human memory may also be impaired by radiation exposure. For instance, a few cases of acute retrograde amnesia were reported by persons who survived the bombing of Hiroshima.[17] Five years after the attack, deficits in memory and intellectual capacity were noted in persons experiencing radiation sickness.[18] These data seem consistent with the Soviet studies reporting memory deficits in patients who had undergone therapeutic irradiations.[19] However, although the human data corroborate the animal studies, they suggest that memory impairments may have been strongly influenced by the other stressors of war or illness.

Improved or unaltered learning capacity or performance after exposure to radiation has been reported. For instance, although radiation caused a dose-dependent decrease in monkey activity and appetite, animals showed no loss of ability to solve "even the most complex learning problems" at doses of 2–10 Gy of X radiation.[20] Task performance was actually enhanced in some studies after 6.5 or 10 Gy of X rays.[21] This enhancement may have been due to decreased general activity and lowered distractibility.[22-25] In fact, performance and learning may have been better in the irradiated animals because the radiation exposure acted as a mild sedative, thus reducing anxiety and distractions.[26] After exposure to several types of radiation, some animals showed superior learning when a premium was placed on paying attention to the site of a food reward, although their performance was worse on tasks requiring attention to peripheral stimuli.[23] In a series of difficult discrimination-learning problems, the performance of monkeys exposed to 3.5 Gy of mixed neutron-gamma radiation was superior to that of control monkeys.[22] Finally, another series of studies with monkeys indicated that radiation does not disrupt performance on memory tasks.[27]

Rodent studies yielded similar findings. For example, adult rats given 2–3 Gy of whole-body radiation did not differ from control animals in learning or remembering a water maze.[28] The rat's ability to maintain a temporal discrimination was not altered following 3 Gy of X rays.[29] Other maze-learning studies were done with rats using either food or water rewards or escapes from aversive water or shock.[30] In these experiments, either no change in the rate of acquisition or improved acquisition (faster running times and improved retention) was found in rats exposed to 1–30 Gy of radiation.[24,28,31,32] Similarly, mice exposed to 8–72 Gy showed no reduction in their ability to acquire an avoidance response.[33,34] When mice were conditioned to shuttle back and forth between adjacent chambers while being exposed to 0.001 Gy/hour (total dose of 10 Gy),[35] no differences were found.

Although some of the behavioral radiobiology literature suggests that learning and performance are rather radioresistant, most studies have reported postirradiation deficits. For instance, maze-learning behavior was reduced after X-ray exposure up to 10 Gy.[36] After it was suggested that more challenging tasks would be more radiosensitive than easy ones, rats were found to have a temporary reduction in their ability to reorganize previously learned material after exposure to 4 Gy of gamma radiation.[37]

Cognitive Performance Tasks

The behavioral tasks in this category generally require discrete physical movements and functional cognitive processes, such as timing, decision making, or concept formation. The tasks that require learning in the laboratory are usually difficult to teach to the animals, and significant time is required to establish stable performance before testing for radiation effects.

Generally, radiation-induced cognitive effects have been reported in primates only after intermediate or high levels of radiation, and often these decrements were still found if the animals were tested months or years later. For instance, a deficit in delayed response was noted in monkeys for a few days after an 80-Gy irradiation.[38] Cynomolgous monkeys tested 2.0–3.5 months after a 20-Gy head-only exposure to X or gamma rays showed a deficit on a discrimination problem series.[39] Their response was similar to that of chimpanzees tested 2–5 years after exposure to 4 Gy of whole-body gamma radiation. In this case, the chimpanzees performed an oddity-discrimination task in which an odd object was selected from a group of similar objects. In other models, delayed (2-week) deficits in performance accuracy occurred in dogs after 3 Gy of X rays,[40] while deficits were found in rats only after prolonged cumulative exposure.[41] Thus, some cognitive deficits occurred only following high radiation exposures, and the deficits were often delayed or chronic.[42]

A recent lever-pressing study examined dose-effect relationships, time-course effects, reversibility of behavioral decrements, and behavioral specificity.[43] In this experiment, rats were maintained under restricted feeding conditions and trained to press a lever under either a fixed-ratio (FR) 50 schedule or a fixed-interval 2-minute schedule of milk reinforcement. In the fixed-ratio task, animals made 50 lever presses for one reward; in the fixed-interval task, the first lever press after 2 minutes was rewarded. Acute doses of 0.5–9.0 Gy of gamma radiation were given at a dose rate of 2.5 Gy/minute. These studies indicated scheduled-controlled performance changes that were dose-dependent, reversible, and behavior-dependent (that is, ratio responses were more affected than interval responses). More important, even at marginally lethal levels using positive reinforcement, radiation disrupted the more physically demanding fixed-ratio performance. These findings suggest that tasks with cognitive components may be radiosensitive if the requirements are sufficiently complex or demanding.[37,44]

Experiments with monkeys have simulated pilot missions after a nuclear confrontation in order to assess crew and aircraft vulnerability and survivability. They involved moderate doses (11 Gy or less) of either neutron or gamma radiation delivered in dose rates simulating either combat (rapid doses) or fallout (protracted doses). The first of this series was a fallout study in which a dose of 3 Gy was delivered over 12 hours to monkeys performing a discrete response task, which required pressing a lever after a light came on. The task was performed for either food reward or shock avoidance.[45,46] A loss of efficiency occurred in two of eight negatively reinforced monkeys and in two of seven food-reinforced monkeys. Delayed reaction time was noted in three monkeys in each group. In addition, four food-reinforced monkeys and one avoidance monkey showed emesis.

In another pilot simulation study, monkeys were required to maintain their chairs in a horizontal position by compensating for pitch and roll to avoid shock.[47,48] Three Gy of gamma radiation were delivered over 72 hours at dose rates from 0.014 Gy/minute to 0.01 Gy/hour. Monkey performance was relatively unimpaired, but all subjects demonstrated classic prodromal symptoms, including productive emesis. Given the common finding that behavioral effects from low dose rates are usually less than those observed from high dose rates, it is not surprising that the pilot simulation study revealed lesser radiation effects than the discrete response task did.

Other flight-simulation research was conducted with monkeys trained to perform a multiple avoidance task and exposed to pulsed doses of 5.0–6.8 Gy of neutron-gamma radiation (5.5:1 ratio).[49] The task required monkeys to respond on an appropriate lever below three randomly illuminated lights. On the exposure day, five subjects exhibited decreased efficiency, seven had increased reaction time, and six experienced productive emesis within 3.5 hours after exposure. Follow-up measurements indicated that as postirradiation time increased, the performance of the subjects gradually decreased. Again, although the behavioral degradation was not severe, it was greater than in the low-dose, low-dose-rate studies. Further research used even higher doses, exposing monkeys to 11 Gy of neutron-gamma radiation.[45] On the exposure day, all eight subjects had significantly degraded response accuracy, seven had increased reaction time, and seven experienced productive emesis. While the onset of degradation produced by 11 Gy was not particularly rapid in the animals, either the emesis alone or similar direct behavioral effects in humans may be sufficient to prevent pilots from flying military missions.

Motor Performance Tasks

Many motor tasks require not only extensive training but also physical conditioning in order to establish baselines of behavior. In general, these are tasks that require physical exertion associated with the movement of large striated muscles.

Several studies revealed chronic deterioration of motor performance after doses of radiation at or below the LD_{50}. For example, long-term (42-week) progressive deterioration of forced wheel-running behavior occurred in mice exposed to an LD_{50} dose of neutron radiation.[50] There was a significant reduction in the motor capacity of rats that daily swam to exhaustion before and after exposure to 3–10 Gy of X rays.[4] In this study, reduced swim times occurred 2 weeks after exposure, with maximum performance deterioration by 4 weeks; the effects were dose related. However, when dogs exercised daily on a treadmill for 30 days after exposure to 1–3 Gy of X rays, long-term deterioration was not confirmed.[51] Performance deteriorated only as dogs neared death after exposure to 3.0 Gy of radiation. The literature on behavioral radiobiology contains frequent examples of experiments in which postirradiation dog performance does not confirm the behavioral decrements seen in the rat, the monkey, or even the human; thus, the dog may not be a valid model for the study of these effects.

These early studies may be contrasted with more recent work identifying the transient changes in motor performance after supralethal doses of ionizing radiation. Significant deficits have been noted in a variety of animal species performing different physically demanding tasks. Miniature pigs that were required to shuttle between adjacent compartments in order to avoid shock experienced transient behavioral deficits after exposure to 15–150 Gy of gamma or mixed neutron-gamma radiation.[52-54] Transient behavioral incapacitations were reported in rats trained to move up to a safe shelf or stay on an accelerating rotating rod in order to avoid shock.[7,55-58] Rhesus monkeys showed a transient reduction in performance in a running wheel task after exposure to 13–49 Gy of mixed neutron-gamma radiation.[59]

Performance of a physically demanding task can alter survival after irradiation. A rat's swimming to exhaustion before and after irradiation will significantly reduce performance and lower the LD_{50} by about 2 Gy.[60] The increased mortality was proportional to the number of exercise trials during the initial 3 weeks after radiation exposure[61] and also to the dose received.[4] Some recent data support this general finding. Rats performing a strenuous, shock-motivated motor task after irradiation had a lower LD_{50} than animals not required to perform this task (Figure 7-1).[62] However, the finding of performance-stimulated mortality is not universal. No mortality changes were noted in dogs and mice that ran in a motorized activity wheel and a motorized treadmill, respectively.[63,64]

The rat-swimming model also revealed a radioresistant benefit when the level of preirradiation physical activity was adjusted. Rats that swam to just short of exhaustion before irradiation showed increased radioresistance and a higher LD_{50}.[65] In a follow-up study, rats recovered from radiation effects sooner if they swam to just short of exhaustion before the radiation exposure.[66] A positive correlation has been found between the initial preirradiation level of spontaneous activity and survival after X irradiation.[67] It was speculated that the beneficial effects for rats of swimming to pre-exhaustion came from radioprotective anoxia. Apparently, animals that reach exhaustion before or after irradiation will show increased radiation effects, in contrast to rats who became more radioresistant if their preirradiation exercise was stopped before exhaustion. The timing and stress of the physical exercise may explain the differing results reported here.

Sensitive measures of the strength and endurance of monkeys reveal that the force of pulling is not reliably impaired after a 4-Gy radiation exposure.[68] Similarly, the postirradiation force of motor response in rats is quite stable for days after a dose of 4.5 or 9.0 Gy.[69] A significant reduction in these measures of strength is seen only when death is imminent.

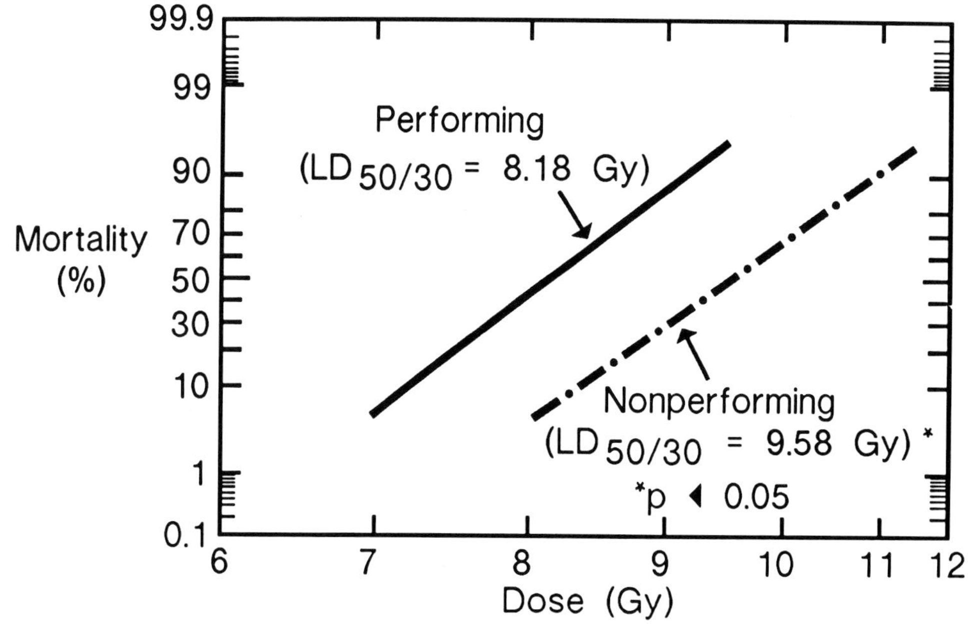

Fig. 7-1. $LD_{50/30}$ profiles after exposure to gamma radiation. Rats either rested or performed a motor task (accelerated rod).

Naturalistic Behaviors

Naturalistic behaviors are a normal part of an animal's response repertoire, and their performance requires no laboratory training. Naturalistic behaviors often evaluated in the study of radiation effects are spontaneous locomotion, social interaction (such as sexual and aggressive behaviors), consumption behaviors (eating and drinking), taste aversions and emesis.

Locomotion. Spontaneous locomotion is a naturalistic behavior that is convenient to measure and provides a relatively powerful tool for studying performance. Activity is of interest because radiation is known to produce malaise, along with other prodromal symptoms of general weakness, fatigue, headache, nausea, anorexia, vomiting, hemorrhage, and drowsiness or insomnia.[70]

An acute whole-body dose of 2–7 Gy of X radiation produced immediate depression in the rat's volitional activity-wheel performance.[71] These data were confirmed by others using guinea pigs, hamsters, rats, and primates.[36,38,72,73] Locomotion was even depressed in rats that were deprived of food for 6 weeks after irradiation and tested daily.[74] (These data are significant because food deprivation normally increases activity.) This locomotor depression lasted a few days, and was followed by partial recovery.[71] At doses above 4 Gy, a second decrease in activity occurred after 1 week, suggesting that more than one response mechanism may be involved. This biphasic response[75] is similar to clinical symptoms in humans.[67]

In a recent study of the effects of sublethal doses of gamma rays on locomotion, mice were monitored for 30 days after exposure to 0.5–7.0 Gy of cobalt-60 radiation.[76] Locomotion after the 7-Gy exposure gradually dropped until it reached a significant low 15 days later. Recovery of locomotion occurred by day 19. Thus, alterations in locomotion were detected at less than the $LD_{50/30}$ (7.6 Gy).

Curiosity and Investigative Behaviors. Curiosity and investigation are other naturalistic behaviors that have been measured. Chimpanzees given 4 Gy of gamma radiation made fewer attempts to solve a variety of puzzles.[25] This deficit seemed to be independent of changes in capacity, because measures of dexterity and strength were unchanged in the same animals. After monkeys were exposed to 4 Gy of X rays, their manipulation of objects in the home cage and their rapid expenditure of energy decreased; sitting time lengthened; and chewing, scratching, grooming, and number of cage movements decreased.[68] A systematic study of home-cage behavior was made with pairs of monkeys after 4 Gy of whole-body exposure of both animals in each pair.[10] Ten-minute structured observations were made twice daily. To control for debilitation, the instances of each category of behavior were divided by the number of times that the identifiable behavior occurred in that time period. The irradiated animals showed reliable deficits in curiosity, more inner-cage-directed movements to well-known stimuli, and fewer instances of outer-directed movements or attention to things outside the cage. Similarly, reduced curiosity or reduced visual exploration (looking around) has been observed in rats after receiving 50 Gy of X rays.[72] Since some of the procedures with the monkeys tried to factor out general malaise, these findings suggest a specific change in curiosity and attention that developed after irradiation.[77]

Social Behavior. Because military units are social structures, the effect of radiation exposure on social behavior is a military concern. The most commonly studied social behaviors are aggression and fighting. Primate studies showed that aggression in monkeys[10, 30, 78, 79] and the social interactions of chimpanzees[39] significantly decreased following irradiation. Fighting among male mice (a very common group home-cage activity) decreased with an increasing dose of X radiation, but all signs of fighting were not totally suppressed until shortly before death.[80] An intruder mouse introduced into the home cage of another mouse continued to be attacked for several days after the resident mouse had received 10 Gy of gamma radiation.[81] These behaviors persisted until the resident mouse showed radiogenic moribund behavior.

An extreme variant of aggression is muricide (mouse killing), which some rats exhibit spontaneously. Muricide was frequently suppressed after radiation exposure.[82] Footshock can be used to induce aggression, however, and 7 Gy of gamma radiation can stimulate this response.[83] The increase in this unnatural type of aggression may be related to radiation-induced increased irritability.[5] This hypothesis is consistent with the report that head-irradiated male rats were more "emotional" than were the sham-irradiated controls during the first 30 days after exposure.[72]

Changes in aggressiveness may reflect a more general social phenomenon. Several investigators reported that mortality following irradiation will increase if rats are kept in high-density housing.[30,84-86] Presumably, the combined stresses of maintaining territory and being exposed to radiation increased the rat's mortality from the radiation. The mechanism of this aggregate toxicity is being studied.[87] The effects of emotionality or dominance following irradiation have been studied, but neither factor seemed to alter postirradiation mortality.[85] Finally, frequent sexual activity during the 30 days after exposure was found to increase the mortality rate of male mice.[88]

Consumption Behaviors. Exposure to ionizing radiation is known to reduce food and water consumption and to produce nausea and vomiting.[30,67] Intake will be decreased, at least initially, depending on the radiation dose and dose rate.[29,72] Instances of radiation-induced anorexia and adipsia have been noted.[75,89] Subjects will not perform for food after 10 Gy of radiation, but will continue to work to avoid electric shock, suggesting that consumption behaviors are relatively radiosensitive.[90]

Changes in food preferences have also occurred after irradiation. Monkeys chose apples and carrots more frequently and peanuts less often after exposure to 4 Gy of whole-body X radiation.[91,92] The changed preferences lasted 4 weeks and were dose dependent. Because the mouth, throat, and stomach are highly sensitive to abrasion after irradiation, the newly preferred foods may have been easier for the monkeys to swallow.[10]

Taste Aversions and Emesis. Animals readily learn to associate gastrointestinal upset and malaise with a novel taste and smell, and will avoid the new substance when later exposed to it.[93] Results indicate that a *conditioned taste aversion* (CTA) can occur at doses as low as 0.25 Gy and can be reliably achieved at 0.5 Gy. Because this may be the most reliable and radiosensitive form of behavioral conditioning, CTA has been extensively used as a model of radiation-induced gastrointestinal distress and emesis.[94]

The relationship of emesis and performance decrement is complex. When gamma radiation is used, the ED_{90} (effective dose for 90% of cases) for monkey emesis is 8 Gy.[95] Emesis is more likely to be produced after irradiation with neutrons than after gamma-ray exposure.[96] Up to 10 Gy, increasing doses of radiation in the monkey correspond with the enhanced likelihood of emesis.[97] However, above 10 Gy, the number of monkeys that vomit decreases with increasing dose. The reason for this high-dose inhibition of emesis is largely unknown, but it may be that doses above 10 Gy interfere with the transmission or reception of afferent vagal impulses from injured organs, which normally play a part in this response. The report that no emesis occurs during early behavioral incapacitations is fairly common. No relationship was found between emesis and early performance deficits in monkeys exposed to up to 50 Gy of mixed neutron-gamma radiation and performing in a physical-activity wheel.[59] Similar visual-discrimination performance results were seen in monkeys pulsed with 22 Gy of radiation.[44,98] Animals not incapacitated but receiving the same dose as incapacitated animals will vomit as expected.[94] Although the data are revealing, the relationship between radiation-induced emesis and behavioral deficits must be clarified.

Despite some ambiguity in the animal data, emesis will almost certainly interfere with the performance of some critical military tasks, such as those that require the wearing of artificial breathing devices.

COMBINED INJURIES

Nuclear war will produce few "pure" radiation injuries. It is more likely that victims will experience burns, wounds, and perhaps trauma from chemical agents and environmental stresses combined with the damage from ionizing radiation. The physiological effects and treatment of these combined injuries have received significant attention.[99,100] Less clear are the behavioral consequences from combined traumas that include irradiation.

Mice were exposed to 3 Gy of neutron-gamma radiation and some of them were then exposed to the further trauma of a wound or burn.[101] The radiation exposure alone caused significantly depressed measures of locomotion. In addition, the wound injury increased the harmful effects of radiation, while the burn injury did not.

In a study of the combined effects of radiation (7 Gy) and an anticholinesterase agent (physostigmine, 0.1 mg/kg), rats were evaluated on a behavioral test battery that included measuring their balance on a rotating rod and recording several components of their locomotor activity.[102,103] At 45 minutes after irradiation, a radiation-only group had a 30% deficit in performance, while a physostigmine-only group had a 40% deficit. A combined-treatment group showed a 60% performance deficit on the rotating rod task. In fact, all measures of performance indicated that the effect of combined ionizing radiation and physostigmine was much greater than the effect of either insult alone. In a follow-up dose-response study, rats were required to balance on a rotating rod.[104] As in the above experiment, physostigmine and radiation each produced a dose-dependent behavioral decrement when presented alone. A synergistic behavioral effect was observed after combined treatment with the chemical and radiation.

Environmental and combat stresses may also combine with radiation injuries to increase behavioral decrements. For example, a study in monkeys to test for synergy between radiation and motion effects reported an emesis ED_{50} of 4.5 Gy for radiation alone and 2.6 Gy for radiation plus motion.[78] Radiation may reduce the tolerance of animals to the stress of G forces (acceleration) as measured by lethality and pathomorphological and cardiovascular end points.[105-107] But other experiments report that an animal's resistance to critical acceleration increases for several days after irradiation (7–8.5 Gy).[107,108] The variables of timing and direction of acceleration combine with radiation dose factors to complicate the issue. However, to the best of our knowledge, only one behavioral experiment has studied the combined effects of radiation and G forces. Rats were exposed to 9.5 Gy of X rays over a 24-hour period, followed 5–7 days later by 4 minutes of positive 10 G of acceleration stress.[109] Compared to animals that were only irradiated, the authors reported that rats that received both stresses exhibited a significant (about 25%) but transient decrease in the ability to learn new mazes. However, no change in the number of errors in an already-learned maze was observed in rats after combined treatment with positive G forces and radiation.

Other environmental stresses can alter the effectiveness of radiation on behavior or lethality. For instance, daily exhaustive exercise, continuous exposure to cold (6°C), or continuous exposure to high altitude (15,000 feet) considerably reduced the time to death and the incidence of death after irradiation.[30] Taken together, these data suggest that the behavioral effects of radiation may summate or act synergistically with other stresses. Therefore, any estimates of battlefield performance decrements that do not include these factors will probably be lower in number and degree than the behavioral decrements actually observed in a military conflict.

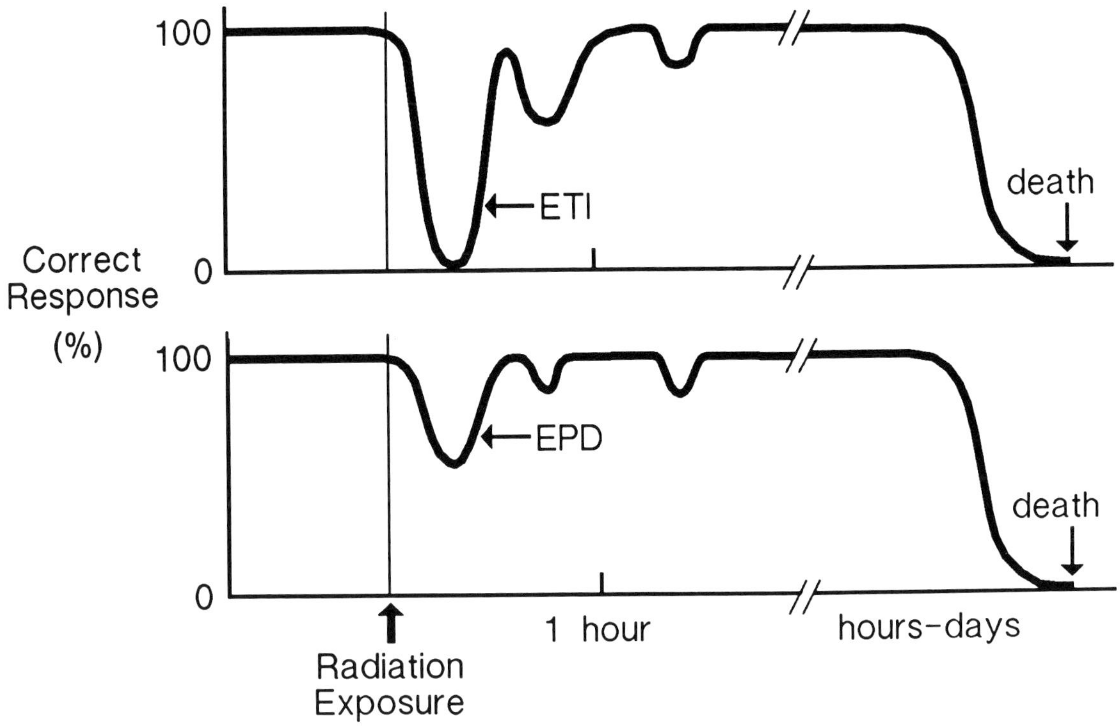

Fig. 7-2. Idealized performance time-course profiles for acute radiation-induced behavioral decrement. Soon after a sufficiently large dose of radiation, several animal species exhibit ETI (upper panel) or EPD (lower panel). Smaller transient deficits may occur around 45 minutes and 4 hours later.

EARLY TRANSIENT INCAPACITATION AND OTHER EARLY PERFORMANCE DEFICITS

For the military, an abrupt inability to perform—aptly termed early transient incapacitation (ETI)—is a potentially devastating behavioral consequence of radiation exposure.[110] An idealized individual ETI profile is shown in Figure 7-2. Prior to irradiation, performance is at maximum efficiency. But 5–10 minutes after exposure to a large, rapidly delivered dose of ionizing radiation, performance falls rapidly to near zero, followed by partial or total recovery 10–15 minutes later. Delayed ETIs may also occur at about 45 minutes and 4 hours after irradiation. In various animal models, ETI is a strikingly short, intense phenomenon. A less severe variant of ETI is *early performance decrement* (EPD), in which performance is significantly degraded rather than totally suppressed (Figure 7-2). Until recently, it was presumed that ETI and EPD would occur only at supralethal radiation doses and that, after behavioral recovery, death would occur in hours or days. However, more recent data reveal that high doses may not be necessary to produce these effects.[44,111]

Transient EPDs occur in monkeys, rats, and pigs performing a variety of tasks, and the deficits are believed to occur in humans. However, this finding is not universal in animals, since EPD does not occur in some strains of mice[9,112] and dogs.[8,113,114]

Task Complexity

When ETI was first observed in monkeys in the early 1950s, the dose levels reported to produce it were quite high, perhaps because the behaviors tested were relatively undemanding and were therefore radioresistant to disruption (Table 7-1).[110,115,116] These early measurements involved either the simple observation of untrained monkeys or their performance of a relatively easy continuous-avoidance task (pressing a lever to avoid shock when a light came on in the operant chamber). In the context of these minimal requirements, the effective

TABLE 7-1

RADIATION-INDUCED EARLY TRANSIENT INCAPACITATION (ETI) AS A FUNCTION OF TASK COMPLEXITY OR TASK DIFFICULTY

Rank Order of Task Difficulty*	Task or Behavioral Criterion	Dose to Produce ETI (Gy)	Reference
1	Observation	50–300	110,115
2	Continuous avoidance**	50–100	116
3	Visual-discrimination task***	22	117,118
4	Speed-stress visual-discrimination task†	9††	44

*Ranked from least to most difficult or complex

**Presentation of light required monkey to press a lever every 20 seconds to avoid shock

***Circle and square randomly presented every 10 seconds on two backlit press-plates. Subject had 5 seconds to touch the square to avoid shock.

†Subject had 0.7 seconds to avoid shock

††Calculated ED_{50}= median effective dose. Other numbers in this column were empirically observed instances of ETI and were not derived from curve fitting.

ETI-producing radiation doses were found to be 50 Gy or more. When a more complex shock-avoidance visual-discrimination task was later used, the median effective dose to produce ETI was reduced to approximately 22 Gy (Table 7-1).[117,118] On this visual-discrimination task, monkeys were required to discriminate (within 5 seconds) between a circle and a square (the square was always the correct choice) randomly presented on backlit press-plates every 10 seconds. Monkeys were trained later on a variant of this visual-discrimination task, in which the temporal response criterion (set at 0.7 seconds) approached the reaction time of the animal.[44] Under these conditions (speed-stress visual discrimination), the median effective dose to produce ETI was approximately 9 Gy (Figure 7-3). Thus, the dose of radiation required to disrupt behavior is directly related to the complexity of the task that the animal is required to perform; that is, complex or demanding tasks are more radiosensitive than easy tasks.

Another reason that the radiation dose required to disrupt performance was presumed to be high is that ETI is an all-or-none, relatively insensitive end point. When the ETI data are analyzed with a more sensitive behavioral end point (that which measures a significant change from a baseline response rather than only a total cessation of response), the disruptive dose is even lower (Table 7-2), approaching the LD_{50} for the monkey.[44] Furthermore, the ED_{50} for transient behavioral deficits in monkeys may be as low as 3 Gy if the animals are performing a more difficult task requiring both visual discrimination and memory.[111] If these data can be generalized to the human, they suggest that under certain circum-

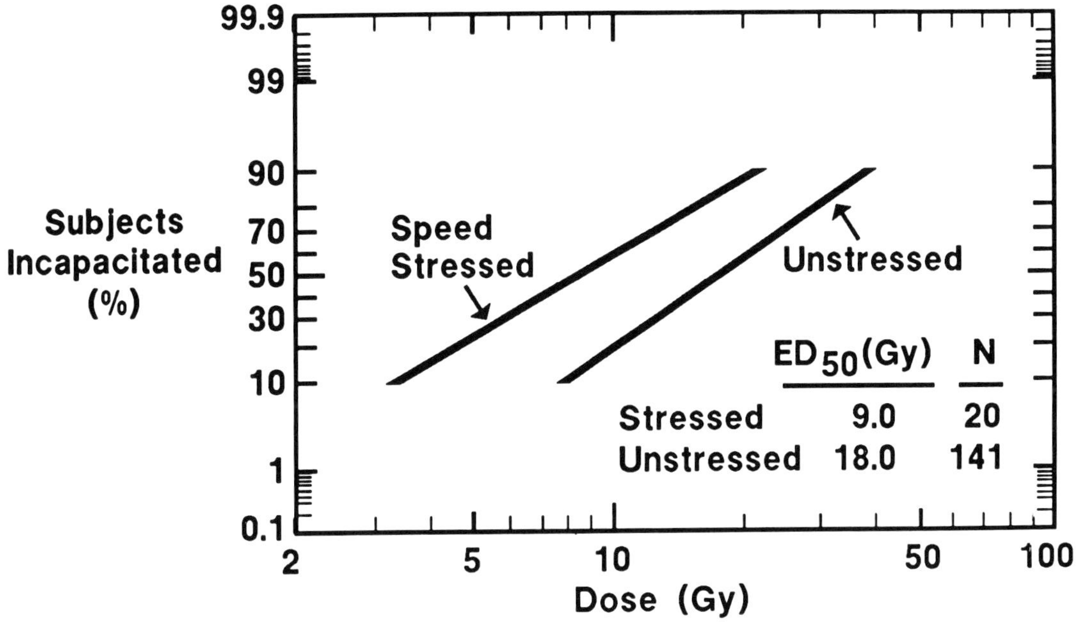

Fig. 7-3. ETI as a function of radiation dose for monkeys performing a visual-discrimination task in which criterion of minimum response time was either 5 seconds (unstressed) or 0.7 seconds (stressed). Incapacitation is defined as at least 1 minute of nonresponding.

stances, relatively low doses of radiation may cause rapid, transient disruptions in performance.

The issues of task demands and task complexity influencing the effective radiation level are common in the investigation of ETI. For instance, the dose of radiation required to disrupt performance was compared for three tasks: the visual-discrimination task (described above, with a 5-second response time), a physical activity task, and an equilibrium-maintenance task. In the physical activity task, monkeys ran at 1–5 mph in a nonmotorized, circular cage.[59] In the equilibrium task, monkeys maintained horizontal alignment by compensating for the pitch and roll of a platform on which they were seated.[119] Performance on all three tasks was assessed in monkeys exposed to a 25-Gy pulse of neutron-gamma radiation. Visual-discrimination performance with a 5-second response time was disrupted the least, with performance returning to about 80% of baseline by 20 minutes after irradiation (Figure 7-4). Wheel-running performance was disrupted the most, and performance returned to only about 50% of baseline at 60 minutes after irradiation. The above data suggest a hierarchy of behavioral effectiveness, with obvious implications for military missions.[44,86]

Radiation Dose

A variety of radiation parameters, including dose, can significantly influence EPD. Low doses of radiation can sometimes produce behavioral changes, such as locomotor activation,[120] that are in contrast to the locomotor depression observed after high doses.[121] Beyond a certain threshold, more radiation tends to produce increasingly depressed measures of performance.[7,44,59] For example, in a recent study, 7.2 Gy was the ED_{50} for the speed-stress visual-discrimination task.[44] However, all monkeys

TABLE 7-2

MEDIAN EFFECTIVE DOSES REQUIRED TO ACHIEVE DIFFERENT BEHAVIORAL END POINTS IN IRRADIATED MONKEYS

Task	End Point	ED_{50} (Gy)	Reference
Speed-stress visual-discrimination task*	Early transient incapacitation (ETI)**	9	44
Speed-stress visual-discrimination task	Early performance decrement (EPD)***	7	44
Delayed match-to-sample task	EPD+	3–5	111

*Response time 0.7 seconds or less

**Defined as six consecutive ommissions or 1 minute of nonperformance

***EPD defined as 2 z-scores below baseline performance levels

exposed to 14.1 Gy of mixed neutron-gamma radiation showed transient EPD, while only one of five subjects showed this deficit at 6.8 Gy. Thus, at 7.3 Gy (Figure 7-3), the incidence of performance suppression ranged from 10% to 90%. These radiation dose-response curves for measures of behavior in some ways parallel the curves observed for a number of end points, such as emesis and lethality.[122]

Radiation Dose Rate

Another radiation factor that can influence behavior is exposure dose rate. Monkeys trained to perform a delayed matching-to-sample task, involving visual discrimination and short-term memory, were exposed to 10 Gy of gamma radiation at dose rates of 0.3–1.8 Gy/minute (Figure 7-5).[111] Only 7% of the subjects demonstrated transient EPD after a dose rate of 0.3 Gy/minute, while 81% showed behavioral decrement after 1.8 Gy/minute. This increase of 1.5 Gy/minute raised the incidence of early EPDs by 73%.

Fractionated (or split) doses have less impact on behavior. For instance, monkeys performing a visual-discrimination task were exposed to a total dose of 50 Gy of gamma-neutron radiation delivered in a reactor pulse.[123,124] One group of monkeys received the radiation treatment in one 50-Gy dose; the other groups received 25 Gy at two intervals separated by zero time and intervals of 20, 30, and 40 minutes and 1, 3, 4.5, and 6 hours (Figure 7-6). Performance was more severely disrupted for subjects who received the whole dose at once than for subjects in the split-dose conditions. In a recent study with rats, a single acute exposure to 7.5 Gy of gamma radiation disrupted performance by reducing the rate of lever-pressing under an FR 20 schedule (thus, 20 lever presses would be required to terminate electric foot-shock).[125] Behavioral disruption was characterized by decreased response rates over the 40-day period after exposure. However, when a different group of rats received a total dose of 7.5 Gy delivered at 1.5 Gy/day over 5 days, disruption in FR performance was significantly less.[125] Although other behavioral dose-rate effects have been reported,[126-131] this finding is not universal and may depend on the behavior being measured.[89]

threshold that lasted 2–5 weeks did occur in dogs after as little as 0.39 Gy of X rays.[29] At larger doses of 10–70 Gy, cochlear microphonics decreased in guinea pigs.[136]

The physiological substrate of hearing deficits has also been explored. Changes in the mouse ear following 20–30 Gy of whole-body X rays included cellular necrosis in the organ of Corti and in the epithelial cells of the ear canals.[30] Rats exposed to a whole-body dose of 1–30 Gy of gamma or X radiation demonstrated damage in the cochlea but not in the cristae of the vestibular inner ear or the middle ear. Human patients who received 40–50 Gy of therapeutic gamma radiation developed inflammation of the middle ear but only a temporary loss of auditory sensitivity and temporary tinnitus.[141] After being exposed to 20–80 Gy of X radiation, the hearing organs of guinea pigs were generally resistant to radiation.[142]

Vestibular function may be more radiosensitive than audition. Depressed vestibular function was reported in dogs after exposure to 3.5–5.0 Gy of proton radiation or 2 Gy of gamma radiation.[143] In another study, 5 Gy of gamma radiation depressed the electromyogram of vestibular-tonic reflexes of rear extremity muscles in the guinea pig.[144] At higher doses of 4–22 Gy, loss of the pinna reflex (ear twitch) was noted in the mouse, and disturbances in equilibrium and other vestibular functions were noted in the burro and hamster.[131] Thus, depression in vestibular function may exist at doses close to the LD_{50}, and symptoms of vestibular disruption may last longer at higher than at lower doses.

Other Senses. Although the literature is sparse, olfactory and gustatory changes have been reported in patients exposed to therapeutic radiation.[145] Altered taste perceptions were also found in patients exposed to 36 Gy of X rays, with a metallic taste being the most common report. Transient changes in taste and olfactory sensitivity were also reported in radiotherapy patients and in the rat.[30]

The effects of radiation on the skin senses have also not been fully assessed. In the work that does exist, it is difficult to separate the direct receptor changes from the secondary changes arising from effects on the vascular system.[70] However, radiation-induced changes in pain perception have been addressed empirically. Gamma photons produced a dose-dependent analgesia in mice,[146] but data suggest that X or gamma rays did not alter the analgesic effects of morphine or the anesthetic effects of halothane in rats except under certain conditions.[147,148]

In summary, whole-body radiation doses below the LD_{50} do not appear to produce permanent sensory changes; however, transient alterations were reported at doses of 1–5 Gy. High levels of radiation can cause longer-lasting sensory impairments. Furthermore, high radiation doses that affect CNS morphology will also impair perceptual function.

Radiation-Induced Changes in the Nervous System

Although it is true that other organ systems may contribute to radiogenic lethargy and reduced responsiveness, the nervous system's central role in behavior makes it the presumed primary mediator of radiation-induced performance deficits. This presumption is supported by the fact that electrical or chemical stimulation of the brain can overcome some radiation-induced behavioral deficits.[121,149] In addition, experiments with partial-body shielding revealed the effectiveness of head-only irradiations in producing behavioral changes.[30] In this regard, severe long-term changes on a conditioned avoidance task (jumping a low barrier) and color visual-discrimination learning were reported in monkeys whose heads were irradiated with 20 Gy.[39] These data suggested functional derangement in the posterior association areas. Also, monkeys whose heads received X radiation (frontal and posterior association areas) 2 years earlier showed retarded learning on a problem-solving task.[38] Studies with rats, in which 50 Gy was delivered directly to the frontal cerebrum[16] or 25 Gy to the whole cerebrum, revealed a decreased ability to learn an alteration running pattern motivated by delayed reward.[150] Decreased learning was observed in rats whose heads were exposed to up to 8 Gy of X radiation and who then were required to learn a 14-unit maze.[151] Although the importance of the brain in radiation-induced behavioral change is well established, the question still remains: What specific changes in the CNS mediate the performance deficits observed after exposure to ionizing radiation? The answer is complex.

One hypothesis is that a sufficiently large radiation dose causes permanent brain lesions, demyelination, and necrosis, which in turn produce chronic behavioral deficits. In addition, short-lived behavioral phenomena may be mediated by transient vascular changes that induce edema or ischemia in the CNS. A second hypothesis is that performance changes are mediated by significant alterations in brain function due to changes in neurochemistry and neurophysiology. As is often the case, there is some truth in both hypotheses.

Radiogenic Pathology of the Nervous System

Radiogenic damage to brain morphology may occur after an exposure of less than 15 Gy and is a well-accepted finding at higher doses. However, these two conclusions have not always been reported. A review of many standard radiobiology textbooks reveals the common belief that the adult nervous system is relatively resistant to damage from ionizing radiation exposure.[152] This conclusion has been derived, in part, from early clinical reports suggesting that radiation exposures, given to produce some degree of tumor control, produced no immediate morphological effects on the nervous system.[153] However, this view was eroded when it was later shown that the latency period for the appearance of radiation damage in the nervous system is simply longer than it is in other organ systems.[154] Subsequent interest in the pathogenesis of delayed radiation necrosis in clinical medicine has produced a significant body of literature. Recent studies of radiation-induced brain damage in human patients have used the technology of computed axial tomography (CAT) to confirm CNS abnormalities that are not associated with the tumor under treatment but occur because of the radiotherapy.[155]

General (although not universal) agreement exists that there is a threshold dose below which no late radiation-induced morphological sequelae in the CNS occur. In laboratory animals, single doses of radiation up to 10 Gy produced no late morphological changes in the brain or spinal cord.[156,157] Necrotic lesions were seen in the forebrain white matter from doses of 15 Gy but not 10 Gy.[158,159] In humans, the "safe" dose has been a topic of considerable debate. Depending on the radiation field size, the threshold for CNS damage was estimated to be 30–40 Gy if the radiation is given in fractions,[160] although spinal cord damage may occur with fractionated doses as low as 25 Gy.[161] The difference between a safe and a pathogenic radiation dose to the brain may be as small as 4.3 Gy.[162]

It is clear that the technique used to assess neuropathology can profoundly influence its detection. In a recent preliminary inspection of neutron-irradiated brain tissue stained with silver to detect degenerating neural elements, punctate brain lesions were found within 3 days after a 2.57-Gy neutron exposure.[163] This effect was transient, and no degeneration was observed 30 days after irradiation. The lesions were not detectable using standard H and E stains. These effects are similar to a multi-infarction syndrome in which the effects of small infarctions accumulate and may become symptomatic. Since this pathology was observed at a dose of radiation previously believed to be completely safe, confirmation of these new data may profoundly influence our view of the radiosensitivity of brain tissue.

In an organ like the brain, different topographical regions may have varying susceptibility to ionizing radiation. The most sensitive area is the brain stem.[164] The brain cortex may be less sensitive than the subcortical structures,[157] such as the hypothalamus,[165] the optic chiasm, and the dorsal medulla.[166] Although radiation lesions tend to occur more frequently in brain white matter,[167-169] the radiosensitivity of white matter also appears to vary from region to region.[157]

In this regard, researchers have produced measures of the functional sensitivity of some brain areas and the insensitivity of others.[121,170] The activation of behaviors through electrical stimulation of the lateral hypothalamus (but not the septal nucleus or substantia nigra) is still possible after 100 Gy.[121,171] However, years after clinical irradiations, dysfunctions of the hypothalamus are prominent even without evidence of hypothalamic necrosis.[172] Local subcortical changes may exist in the reticular formation and account for radiation-induced convulsability of the brain.[173,174] Similarly, postirradiation spike discharges are more likely to be seen in the hippocampal electroencephalograph (EEG) than in the cortical EEG.[175] This idea of selective neurosensitivity is further supported by experiments in which electrical recordings were made from individual nerve fibers after irradiation.[176] These data reveal a hierarchy of radiosensitivity in which gamma nerve fibers are more sensitive than beta fibers, and alpha nerve fibers are the least sensitive.

The functional radiosensitivity of specific brain nuclei may in part explain the ability of a particular dose of ionizing radiation to disrupt one type of behavior but not another. For example, monkeys will continue to perform a visual-discrimination task but not a more physically demanding task (wheel running) after a similar dose of ionizing radiation.[59] These data agree with the suggestion that classically conditioned reflexes are more radioresistant than motor coordination, and that this selective disruption of particular behaviors "indicate[s] that ionizing radiation mainly affects the functions of the subcortico-[brain]stem formations of the brain."[170]

The phenomenon of latent CNS radiation damage with doses above threshold has been well documented.[152,177,178] The long latent period has led to considerable speculation on the likely pathogenesis of late radiation lesions: *(a)* radiation may act primarily on the vascular system, with necrosis secondary to edema and ischemia, and *(b)* radiation may have a primary effect on cells of the neural parenchyma, with vascular lesions exerting a minor influence.[153]

The first evidence in support of a vascular hypothesis was obtained when human brains that had been exposed to X rays were examined.[154] It was suggested that delayed damage of capillary endothelial cells may occur, leading to a breakdown of the blood-brain barrier. This would result in vasogenic edema, the elevated pressure-impaired circulation of cerebral spinal fluid, and eventually neuronal and myelin degeneration.[159,179] The finding that hypertension accelerates the appearance of vascular lesions in the brain after irradiation with 10–30 Gy also supports a hypothesis of vascular pathogenesis.[180] The occlusive effects of radiation on arterial walls may cause a transient cerebral ischemia.[181] Sequential monkey-brain CAT scans revealed brain edema and hydrocephalis that accompanied hypoactivity and the animal's loss of alertness following 20 Gy of radiation.[182] The exposure of forty-five rabbit heads to 4, 6, or 8 Gy of X radiation produced a disturbance of the permeability of the blood-brain barrier that returned to normal only after 6 days.[183] The transient nature of the vascular phenomena may partially explain some of the behavioral deficits observed after exposure to intermediate or large doses of ionizing radiation.[184,185]

Evidence for the direct action of radiation on the parenchymal cells of the nervous system, rather than the indirect effect through the vascular bed, was first provided when brain tissue in irradiated human patients was examined.[186] None of the brain lesions could be attributed to vascular damage because they were *(a)* predominantly in white matter and not codistributed with blood vessels, *(b)* not morphologically typical of ischemic necrosis, and *(c)* often found in the absence of any vascular effects.[187-191] Thus, it appears that direct neuronal or glial mechanisms caused at least some of the observed radiogenic brain lesions.

In the brain, hypertension accelerates the onset of radiogenic vascular damage but not white matter lesions.[180] These data help to separate vascular damage from the pathogenesis of white-matter lesions, making it difficult to support the view that ischemia and edema are important in white-matter pathogenesis. It may be that selective necrosis of white matter is due to the slow reproductive loss of glia or their precursors. The radiosensitivity of certain types of glial cells (beta astrocyte) is well recognized.[192,193] The earliest sign of their damage is widening of the nodes of Ranvier and segmental demyelination as early as 2 weeks after a dose of 5–60 Gy.[194] Clinical evidence also suggests that radiogenic demyelination may occur. Several patients experienced sensations like electric shock (referenced to sensory levels below the neck) after radiotherapy for head and neck cancers.[195] The symptoms gradually abated and disappeared after 2–36 weeks. Similarly, this transient radiation myelopathy could be a result of temporary demyelination of sensory neurons. In addition, mitotic activity in the subependymal plate (important in glia production) did not recover after radiation doses producing necrosis, but did recover after doses not producing necrosis. This supports the hypothesis that glia are a primary target for radiogenic brain damage.[196]

Both vascular and glial changes may be important in the development of late radiation damage to the CNS.[153] The preponderance of one type of cell damage over another depends on the radiation dose used. "Vascular effects occur at lower dose levels but after a longer latent period than effects mediated through damage to the neuroglia."[153] Perhaps the most important points for the present chapter are that *(a)* radiogenic brain damage is a well-accepted finding after high doses (greater than 15 Gy), and *(b)* it may occur after doses of less than 15 Gy under certain circumstances. The mechanisms of this damage are still debatable.

In addition to axonal demyelination, other direct neuronal damage may occur in the irradiated adult animal. Although mitotic neurons of the prenatal or neonatal CNS are known to be extremely sensitive to radiation, the neurons of more mature animals are thought to be quite resistant and less likely to result in cell death.[30,145,197] However, as early as 1962, neurogenesis was thought to take place in the cerebral cortex of adult rats.[198] Adult and juvenile neurogenesis was found to be especially prominent in the granule cell populations of the hippocampus and the olfactory bulb. These newly formed cells had the ultrastructural characteristics of neurons,[199] and the number of granule cells in the hippocampus increased in the adult rat.[200,201] Although these findings have not been confirmed in primates (thus reducing their ability to be generalized to the human), they suggest that certain neuron populations in the adult brain are radiosensitive due to their mitotic state.[202] Neurogenesis was reported in the hippocampal subgranular cell layer of the adult rabbit, and these cells were quite radiosensitive (4.0–4.5 Gy).[203,204] Therefore, it may be that certain populations of proliferating neurons in the adult can be damaged or destroyed by relatively low doses of ionizing radiation.

Radiogenic changes in brain morphology are not limited to necrotic lesions or cell death. Subtle dendritic alterations following X irradiation, including decreased dendritic intersections, branchings, and length, as well as reduced packing density of neuronal elements in the irradiated cerebral cortex of the monkey, were reported.[205]

Alterations in Nervous System Function

Given the above data, we can say that (except for the possibility of mitotic neurons in the CNS) the adult brain is indeed relatively resistant to radiation when the end point measured is cell death or change in neuronal morphology. However, the point is that the CNS is quite sensitive to functional changes brought on by alterations in neurophysiology and neurochemistry. It is likely that these functional changes, brought about by low or intermediate doses (less than 15 Gy) of ionizing radiation, account for many of the behavioral changes observed.

Supporting this view, changes in brain metabolism were reported after very low (0.11–0.24 Gy) doses of ionizing radiation.[206] In a more detailed analysis with the ^{14}C-2-deoxyglucose method of measuring local cerebral glucose utilization, a dose of 15 Gy of X radiation was administered to the rat brain.[207] Significantly lower rates of glucose use were found in sixteen different rat brain structures at 4 days after irradiation and in twenty-five structures at 4 weeks. Although large radiogenic changes exist in the metabolism of some brain nuclei, a weighted average rate for the irradiated brains, as a whole, was approximately 15% below that for the controls.

Electrophysiology. Measures of electrophysiology have been used to illustrate changes in brain function after exposure to ionizing radiation. Several studies were reviewed in which cortical EEG changes were observed in humans and in animals following doses of less than 0.05 Gy.[208] Typically, an initial temporary increase in bioelectric amplitude was followed, within minutes, by a depression. Other investigations have frequently needed higher doses of radiation in order to observe changes in EEG. For example, changes were not seen in EEGs after 0.03–0.04 Gy, but significant alterations were observed after 2 Gy.[209] At a higher dose (15 Gy), monkey cortical EEG abnormalities consisted of the slowing of activity, with an increase in amplitude.[166] Spiking and patterns of grand mal seizure also occurred. A rapid onset of high-amplitude slow waves (delta waves) seemed to relate to periods of behavioral incapacitation.[210] Exposures to 4–6 Gy of gamma radiation seem to stimulate spontaneous activity in the neocortex, whereas exposures of higher than 9 Gy inhibit all brain activities.[211]

The hippocampus shows significant changes in physiological activities after gamma irradiation with even less than half of the 18-Gy threshold dose needed to produce changes in cortical activities.[164,212] One of the most striking effects was hippocampal spike discharges, first identified in cats[175] and later confirmed in rabbits.[212] This spiking developed soon after irradiation (2–4 Gy) when no other clinical signs of neurological damage or radiation sickness were present. The apparent radiosensitivity of the hippocampus and its importance in critical functions like learning, memory, and motor performance have recently led others to investigate the electrophysiology of this brain area. The firing of hippocampal neurons was found to be altered by exposure to 4 Gy of gamma radiation.[213] In addition, *in vitro* experiments suggest that spontaneous discharges of hippocampal pacemaker-like neurons are induced by X and gamma rays at a dose of 0.08 Gy.[214] If confirmed, these data suggest that hippocampal electrophysiology may be the most sensitive measure of functional brain changes after irradiation.

Alterations in the thresholds and patterns for audiogenic and electroconvulsive seizures have been produced by exposing animals to ionizing radiations. Such effects are generally interpreted as reflecting gross changes in CNS reactivity. Early work with dogs showed that spontaneous seizures sometimes occurred following very large doses of radiation.[154] Later experiments confirmed that seizures can be induced by whole-body or head-only exposures to 30–250 Gy in a variety of species. For example, rats were exposed to 5 Gy of X radiation and the electroconvulsive shock (ECS) threshold was determined for 180 days after irradiation.[173] ECS thresholds were reduced in irradiated rats over the entire test period. In later studies,[174] it was reported that considerably lower doses (perhaps less than 0.01 Gy) also reduced the thresholds for ECS seizures and audiogenic seizures.[215,216]

Unlike the CNS, peripheral nerves are quite resistant to the functional alterations produced by ionizing radiation. Most data indicate that peripheral nerves do not show any changes in electrophysiology with X-ray exposures below 100 Gy.[217] After higher doses, the action-potential amplitude and the conduction velocity temporarily increase but then gradually decrease.[217-221] Also, alpha and beta particles are more destructive to peripheral nerves than are gamma or X rays, and usually cause a monophasic depression of function without the initial enhancement of activity.[222-224] Perhaps the lowest dose of ionizing radiation ever found to produce an alteration in the function of peripheral nerves was reported in a study in which T-shaped preparations of isolated frog sciatic nerves were produced when the nerves were partially divided longitudinally.[225] Electrical stimulation was applied to the intact stem of the T, and electrical recordings were made from the ends of the two branches. A small segment of one of the branches was irradiated with 0.04–0.06 Gy of alpha particles, producing a definite decrease in action-potential amplitude and an increase in chronaxie. These results are remarkable, given the much higher doses that have been required to affect these peripheral nerve functions in most other studies.

Relatively little radiobiology research has been done using single isolated nerve fibers. However, the results that do exist agree with those from experiments with nerve trunks. In single fibers isolated from a frog sciatic nerve, effects on peripheral nerve functions included the induction of an injury current in the irradiated segment and, with increased exposure, a sequence consisting of increased threshold, reduced action potential, and finally a conduction block.[224]

It has been known for some time that paralysis of the hind limbs of animals can result from localized irradiation of the spinal cord. Rabbits developed this paralysis at 4–33 weeks after exposure of the upper thoracic region to 30–110 Gy of X radiation at 2.5 Gy/day.[226] The minimum single exposure found to produce paralysis at 5 months was 20 Gy.[227] As in other model systems, the time interval between irradiation and the appearance of neurological symptoms decreases as dose increases. For example, 50 Gy of X rays to the monkey midthoracic spinal cord produced immediate paraplegia, whereas 40 Gy was effective only after a latent period of about 5.5 months.[228]

Radiation effects on the electrophysiology of the synapse were first studied using the cat spinal reflex.[229-233] These studies showed that excitatory synaptic transmission is significantly increased by X-ray exposures of 4–6 Gy. Synaptic transmission at the upper cervical ganglion of the cat is also facilitated 15–20 minutes after exposure to 8 Gy of X rays.[234] Both mono- and polysynaptic spinal reflexes are significantly augmented immediately after exposure to 5 Gy of X radiation. It is of interest that significant augmentation of monosynaptic excitatory postsynaptic potentials (EPSP) was found immediately after exposure to 6–12 Gy of X rays, whereas inhibitory postsynaptic potentials (IPSP) recorded from the same cell were not significantly affected by a 12-Gy exposure.[232,233] Similarly, polysynaptic EPSPs were significantly augmented as the dose increased, whereas the polysynaptic IPSPs were little influenced by even an exposure of 158 Gy. At higher doses (50–200 Gy), ionizing radiation may damage both synaptic and postsynaptic functioning, probably through different molecular mechanisms.[235] These radiogenic changes in synaptic transmission may be important factors underlying the complicated functional changes that occur in the CNS following radiation exposures.

Neurochemistry. One of the most important mechanisms of postirradiation nervous transmission to be studied has been the ion flow across the neuronal semipermeable membrane. In particular, the flow of sodium ions is believed to be involved in the control of neuronal excitability[236] and apparently can be disrupted after either a very high or very low dose of radiation. A study using the radioactive isotope sodium-24 compared the sodium intake across the membrane of the squid giant axon before and after exposure to X rays.[237] A significant increase in sodium intake was found to occur during the initial hyperactive period induced by a dose of 500 Gy. These observations were confirmed in a study of frog sciatic nerves that had been irradiated with 1,500–2,000 Gy of alpha particles, although a simultaneous decrease in the rate of sodium extrusion also occurred.[222] Peripheral nerves may be less radiosensitive than CNS neurons and perhaps differ in their radiation response. In a study that used a different technique, the artificially stimulated uptake of sodium into brain synaptosomes was significantly reduced by an ionizing radiation exposure (high-energy electrons) of 0.1–1,000.0 Gy.[238] This CNS effect was later confirmed for 1–100 Gy of gamma radiation.[239]

The brain has been described as a radiosensitive biochemical system,[206] and in fact, many significant changes in brain neurochemistry have been observed after irradiation. An early study revealed that 1–2 days after an exposure to 3 Gy of X radiation, neurosecretory granules in the hypophysial-hypothalamic system showed a transient increase in number over the controls.[240] A leaking of brain monoamines from the neuronal terminals of rats irradiated with 40 Gy of X rays has also been observed.[241] These changes in neuronal structure may correlate with radiogenic alterations of neurotransmitter systems.

Normal catecholamine functioning appears to be damaged following exposure to intermediate or high doses of ionizing radiation. After 100 Gy, a transient disruption in dopamine functioning (similar in some ways to dopamine-receptor blockade) was demonstrated.[242] This idea is further supported by the finding that a 30-Gy radiation exposure increases the ability of haloperidol (a dopamine-receptor-blocking drug) to produce cataleptic behavior.[243] Radiation-induced effects on dopamine have been correlated in time with ETI, suggesting that changes in this neurotransmitter system may play a role in behavioral disruptions. However, other neuromodulators (such as prostaglandins) also seem to influence dopaminergic systems to help produce some radiation-induced behavioral changes.[243] A transient reduction in the norepinephrine content of a monkey hypothalamus was also observed on the day of exposure to 6.6 Gy of gamma radiation. Levels of this neurotransmitter returned to normal 3 days later.[244] Similar effects have been reported,[245] but another study found no change in noradrenaline after 8.5 Gy of X rays.[246] Monoamine oxidase (MAO), an enzyme which breaks down catecholamines, was significantly reduced by a supralethal 200-Gy dose of mixed neutron-gamma radiation. This enzymatic change occurred within 4 minutes of exposure and lasted for at least 3 hours. In contrast, a very marked increase in MAO activity was observed when animals received the same dose of radiation rich in gamma rays.[247]

Contradiction exists in the literature concerning radiation's effects on 5-hydroxytryptamine (5-HT). Some investigators reported a radiogenic stimulation of 5-HT release at approximately 10 Gy, while others observed a decrease or no change in the levels of this neurotransmitter.[246] Although the physiological mediators of transient functional deficits may not be the mediators of radiation-induced mortality, it is interesting that dopamine and 5-HT have been suggested as radioprotectants for prolonging the survival of X-irradiated rats or mice.[248,249]

A variety of functions involving the neurotransmitter acetylcholine (ACH) is significantly altered by exposure to ionizing radiation. ACH synthesis rapidly increases in the hypothalamus of the rat after less than 0.02 Gy of beta radiation, but is inhibited at only slightly higher radiation doses.[206] A dose of 4 Gy of cobalt-60 gamma radiation produced a long-term increase in the rate of ACH synthesis in dogs.[250] Also, high-affinity choline uptake (a correlate of ACH turnover and release) slowly increased to 24% above control levels 15 minutes after irradiation with 100 Gy.[242] Choline uptake was back to normal by 30 minutes after exposure. Massive doses of gamma or X rays (up to 600 Gy) are required to alter brain acetylcholinesterase activity,[251] whereas much smaller doses depress plasma acetylcholinesterase by 30%.[252]

Cyclic nucleotides, such as cyclic AMP (adenosine-3',5'-cyclic monophosphate), act as second messengers in synaptic transmission. It is interesting that after irradiation (50 Gy), concentrations of cyclic AMP are reduced in rats[253] and monkeys.[254] The transient nature of these changes also suggests their possible role in EPDs.

Exposure to large doses of ionizing radiation results in postirradiation hypotension in monkeys,[111,255,256] with arterial blood pressure decreasing to less than 50% of normal.[257] Postirradiation hypotension also produces a decrease in cerebral blood flow immediately after a single dose of either 25 or 100 Gy of cobalt-60 gamma radiation.[127,258,259] This hypotension may be responsible for the ETI observed after a supralethal dose of ionizing radiation.[111,260,261] In support of this hypothesis, the antihistamine chlorpheniramine maleate was effective in reducing the monkeys' performance decrements and at the same time reducing postirradiation hypotension.[257] A study with untrained monkeys, whose postirradiation blood pressures were maintained by norepinephrine or other pressor drugs, showed that as long as arterial pressure remained above a critical level, the monkeys appeared to remain attentive and alert.[262] However, in a follow-up study on monkeys trained to perform a task, norepinephrine maintained blood pressure but did not consistently improve their performance during the first 30 minutes after irradiation.[263] Other authors have not seen a close association between blood pressure and behavioral changes.[210] Further contrary evidence was obtained from experiments with the spontaneously hypertensive rat (SHR), in which exposure to ionizing radiation reduced the blood pressure of most of them to near-normal levels. However, these irradiated SHRs still showed a significant behavioral deficit after exposure to 100 Gy of high-energy electrons.[264] Finally, a significant association was found between the degree of hypotension and the frequency of EPDs.[111] Still, half the monkeys with a 50% drop in blood pressure did not show behavioral decrements. Thus, even though the relationship between decreased blood pressure and impaired performance is intriguing, simple changes in blood pressure may not be sufficient to explain EPDs.

The massive release of histamine that is observed after exposure to a large dose of ionizing radiation has been proposed as a mediator of radiogenic hypotension and EPDs.[265] Histamine is a very active biogenic amine and putative neurotransmitter located in neurons and mast cells throughout the body, especially around blood vessels.[266] Attempts to alter the development of behavioral deficits by treating animals with antihistamines before exposure have been encouraging.[257,267] Monkeys pretreated with chlorpheniramine (H_1-receptor blocker) performed better and survived longer after irradiation than did controls.[267] Similar benefits were observed in irradiated rats.[268] Further, the use of diphenhydramine (a histamine H_1-receptor antagonist) inhibited radiation-induced cardiovascular dysfunction.[269] Since these antagonists produced only partial relief from radiation effects, it appears that the histamine hypothesis explains only a portion of the behavioral and physiological deficits observed after radiation exposure.[270]

When most animal species are exposed to a sufficiently large dose of ionizing radiation, they exhibit lethargy, hypokinesia, and deficits in performance.[30,54,121] Because these behaviors seem similar to those observed after a large dose of morphine, a role for endogenous opioids (endorphins) has been proposed in the production of radiation-induced behavioral changes.[271,272] Endogenous morphine-like substances may be released as a reaction to some[273-275] but not all[276] stressful situations. Like a sufficiently large injection of morphine itself, endogenous opioids can produce lethargy, somnolence, and reduction in behavioral responsiveness.[276,277]

Cross-tolerance between endorphins and morphine has been demonstrated for a variety of behavioral and physiological measures.[278,279] Given the similarity of radiation- and opiate-induced symptoms, it is not surprising that endorphins appear to be involved in some aspects of radiogenic behavioral change. Ionizing radiation can produce dose-dependent analgesia in mice, and this radiogenic analgesia can be reversed by the opiate antagonist naloxone.[146] In another experiment, morphine-induced analgesia of the rat was significantly enhanced 24 hours after neutron (but not gamma) irradiation, suggesting some combined delayed effects of endogenous and exogenous analgesics that may be radiation-specific.[148] Ionizing radiation exposure can also attenuate the naloxone-precipitated abstinence syndrome in morphine-dependent rats.[280]

Further supporting the hypothesis that endorphins are involved in radiation-induced behavioral change, C57Bl/6J mice exhibited a stereotypic locomotor hyperactivity similar to that observed after morphine injection, after receiving 10–15 Gy of cobalt-60 gamma radiation.[9] This radiogenic behavior was reversed by administering naloxone or by preexposing the mice to chronically stressful situations (a procedure that produces endorphin tolerance).[281] Further, opiate-experienced C57Bl/6J mice reduced the self-administration of morphine after irradiation, suggesting that the internal production of an endorphin reduced the requirement for an exogenous opioid compound.[282] Biochemical assays also revealed changes in mouse brain beta-endorphin after exposure to ionizing radiation.[283] Rats and monkeys had enhanced blood levels of beta-endorphin after irradiation,[284,285] and morphine-tolerant rats showed less performance decrement after irradiation than nontolerant subjects.[286] In addition, naloxone (1 mg/kg) given immediately before exposure to 100 Gy of high-energy electrons significantly attenuated the ETI observed in rats.[284] Conversely, rats either underwent no change[62] or were made more sensitive to radiation effects after chronic treatment with naloxone on a schedule that increased the number of endorphin receptors.[287] However, the manipulation of opioid systems did not produce total control over postirradiation performance deficits. Thus, these data do not suggest an exclusive role for endorphins in radiogenic behavioral change.

THE HUMAN EXPERIENCE WITH RADIATION

Humans have been exposed to radiation from environmental and industrial sources, clinical therapy, accidents, wartime detonations at Hiroshima and Nagasaki, and even experiments. Many of these exposures contribute little information about the behavioral effects of ionizing radiation. In most of the cases, behavioral data were not collected. Many of the data that were gathered are difficult to evaluate because there is no information about the radiation dose received, the level of baseline performance, or other circumstances. But the data are interesting, at least in a qualitative context, because they partially validate some work with animal models and also suggest new hypotheses for testing.

Two radiation accidents are particularly instructive. Both exposures occurred in the early days of the production of fissionable radiation material for nuclear weapons and involved radiation doses large enough to produce an ETI. In spite of safety precautions to ensure that the plutonium-rich holding tanks did not contain enough fissionable material to permit the occurrence of a critical reaction, an accidental critical event took place in 1958 at the Los Alamos Scientific Laboratory.[288] Mr. K. received an average (and fatal) total body dose of 45 Gy and an upper abdominal dose estimated at 120 Gy of mixed neutron-gamma radiation. During the event, Mr. K. either fell or was knocked to the floor. For a short period, he was apparently dazed and turned his plutonium-mixing apparatus off and on again. He was able to run to another room but soon became ataxic and disoriented. Because he kept repeating, "I'm burning up, I'm burning up," his co-workers helped him to a shower, but by this time he could not stand unaided. He was incapacitated and drifted in and out of consciousness for over a half hour before he was rushed to a local hospital. Before his death at 35 hours after irradiation, Mr. K. regained consciousness and a degree of coherence. From approximately 2 to 30 hours after the accident, he showed significant behavioral recovery and at some points actually experienced euphoria, although his clinical signs were grave. The last few hours before Mr. K.'s death were characterized by irritability, uncooperativeness, mania, and eventually coma.[288]

The 1964 case of Mr. P., an employee of a uranium-235 recovery plant, closely parallels that of Mr. K. This accident took place in Providence, Rhode Island, when Mr. P. was trying to extract fissionable material from uranium scraps. A criticality occurred, and Mr. P. was thrown backward and stunned for a period of time. He received a head dose of 140 Gy and an average body dose of 120 Gy. Unlike Mr. K., however, Mr. P. did not lose consciousness. After a period of disorientation and confusion, he stood up and ran from the building to an emergency shack, a distance of over 200 yards. Mr. P.'s awareness of his surroundings during this early period has been questioned because he ran into a 4-inch-wide sapling even though it was quite visible. Unfortunately, Mr. P. rode in an ambulance for almost 2 hours, during which time behavioral observations were not made. When he arrived at Rhode Island Hospital, he had transient difficulty enunciating words. Significant behavioral recovery occurred from 8 to 10 hours after the accident. During this period, Mr. P. was alert, cooperative, and talked of future activities in a euphoric manner, inconsistent with his terminal diagnosis. In the hours before his death at 49 hours after the accident, Mr. P.'s condition deteriorated significantly, and he exhibited restlessness, anxiety, extreme fatigue, and disorientation.[289]

These cases of radiation accidents involving humans are consistent with the animal literature suggesting that a supralethal radiation dose can produce EPDs. Both of the accident victims experienced behavioral deficits to some degree soon after exposure. These deficits were transient and were most prominent in Mr. K. The data agree with general conclusions reached in a review of several radiation accidents, in which a remission of early symptoms occurred before the onset of the manifest illness phase was recorded.[290] In comparison with these high-dose accidents, lower radiation doses or partial-body exposures may produce milder but more persistent behavioral changes characterized by weakness and fatigability. An accident victim exposed to ionizing radiation from an unshielded klystron tube received as much as 10 Gy to portions of his upper torso and experienced fatigability that lasted for more than 210 days after exposure.[291]

The 1986 Chernobyl nuclear reactor accident also produced behavioral deficits in persons attempting to perform their duties in high-radiation environments. A Soviet fireman who fought the blaze of the burning reactor core suffered performance deficits and eventually had to withdraw because of his exposure to radiation.[292] Similarly, a Soviet physician who had received significant radiation exposures while treating patients could not perform his duties.[293] Both persons eventually recovered from their behaviorally depressed states and are (at this writing) still alive. These recent accident data add to the growing literature suggesting that sublethal doses of radiation can induce human performance decrements.

A few attempts have been made to assess human performance after clinical irradiations. The Halsted test battery for frontal-lobe functional deficits was used in four patients exposed to 0.12–1.90 Gy of mixed neutron-gamma radiations.[294] Test scores at days 1–4 and 1 year after exposure were within the normal range. Patients with advanced neoplastic disease were whole-body irradiated with 0.15–2.0 Gy given as a single dose or in 2–5 fractions separated by intervals of up to 1 hour.[42] The subjects were pretrained and served as their own controls in performing tests designed to assess hand-eye coordination. Tests were performed immediately after exposure and at later intervals, but at no time did a performance decrement exist that could be ascribed to these relatively low radiation doses. However, because the behavioral design of these experiments was secondary to medical treatment, the results are inconclusive. The paucity of radiobiological data on human behavior and the need to predict military performance after ionizing radiation exposure have led to an extensive Defense Nuclear Agency program on the estimation of human radiation effects.[295]

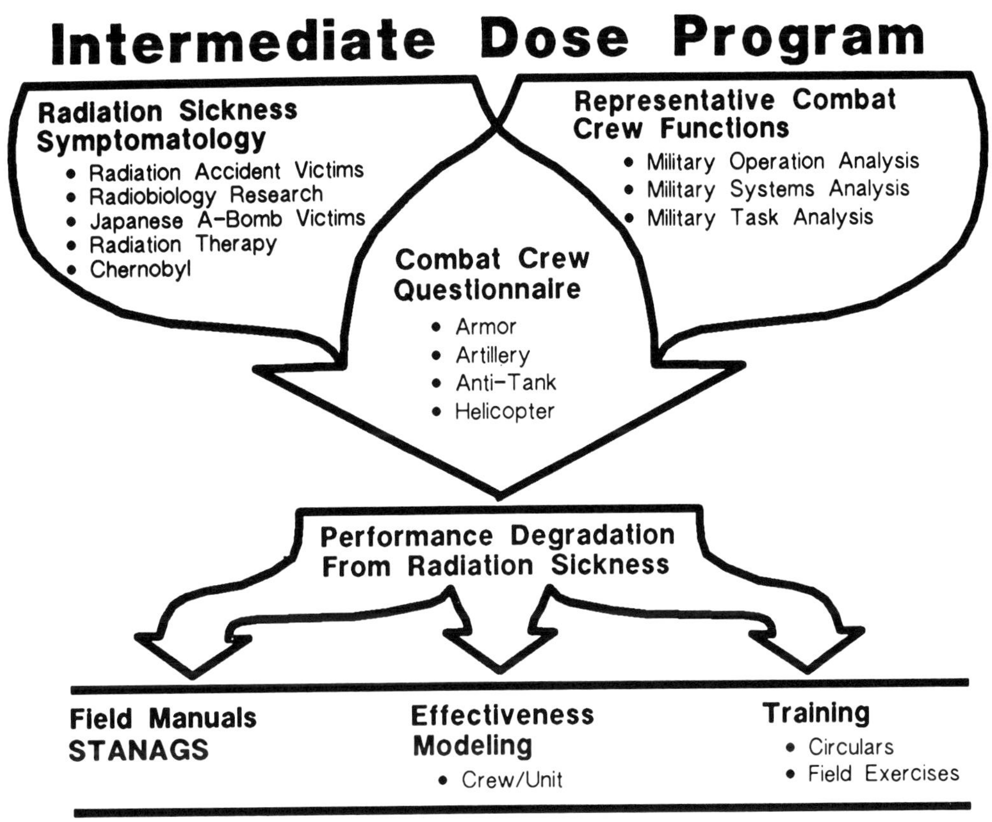

Fig. 7-8. Outline of empirical approach used by Defense Nuclear Agency to estimate performance deficits after an intermediate dose (0.75–45 Gy) of ionizing radiation

RADIATION-INDUCED CHANGES IN MILITARY PERFORMANCE

The U.S. Army has predicted certain distributions of effect for combat personnel exposed to ionizing radiation. For every soldier who receives a radiation dose of greater than 30 Gy (a supralethal and behaviorally incapacitating dose), another will receive a lethal (4.5 Gy) dose that may alter behavior. Two more soldiers will receive doses that are sublethal but greater than the present maximum (0.5 Gy) allowed for troop safety.[296] Given this wide range of expected doses and the ambiguity of the expected outcomes for human behavior, the Defense Nuclear Agency established methods for estimating the behavioral effects of acute radiation doses (0.75–45.0 Gy) on combat troops.

To predict human radiation-induced performance deficits, the Defense Nuclear Agency used a survey method of first identifying the physical symptoms expected after various radiation doses and then determining the soldiers' estimates of their own changes in performance while experiencing these symptoms (Figure 7-8). Briefly, this involved *(a)* an extensive review of the literature on human radiation (including radiation-therapy patients, Japanese atomic-bomb victims, and radiation-accident victims) to identify the symptoms to be expected after the radiation doses of interest; *(b)* the

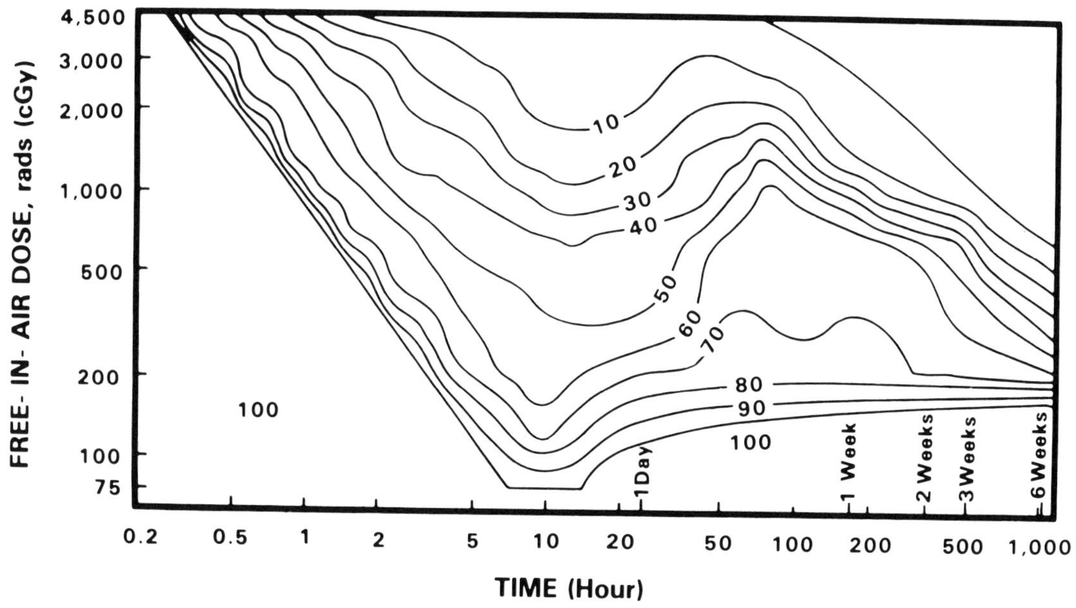

Fig. 7-9. Expected changes in performance at various times after a gun-crew chief is exposed to a single radiation dose, as specified. Contours represent a person's average performance in increments of capability (such as performing at 10% of normal capacity).
Source: Data are derived from the Human Response Program of the Defense Nuclear Agency

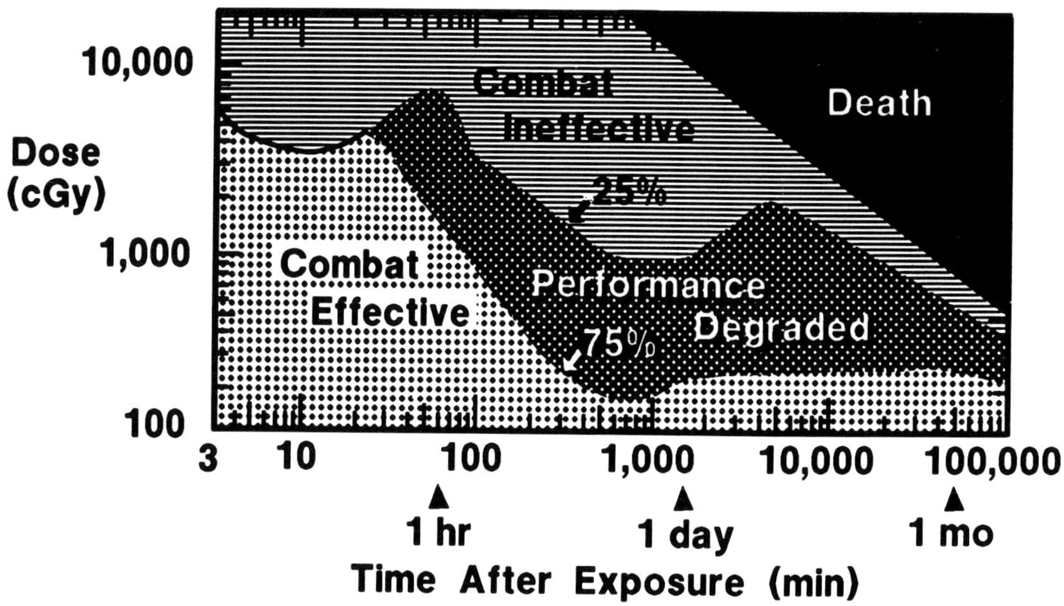

Fig. 7-10. Expected behavioral response to radiation exposure for persons performing a physically demanding task. Combat effective: 75%–100% normal capacity. Degraded: 25%–75%. Combat ineffective: 0–25%. (1 cGy = 1 rad)
Source: Data are derived from the Human Response Program of the Defense Nuclear Agency

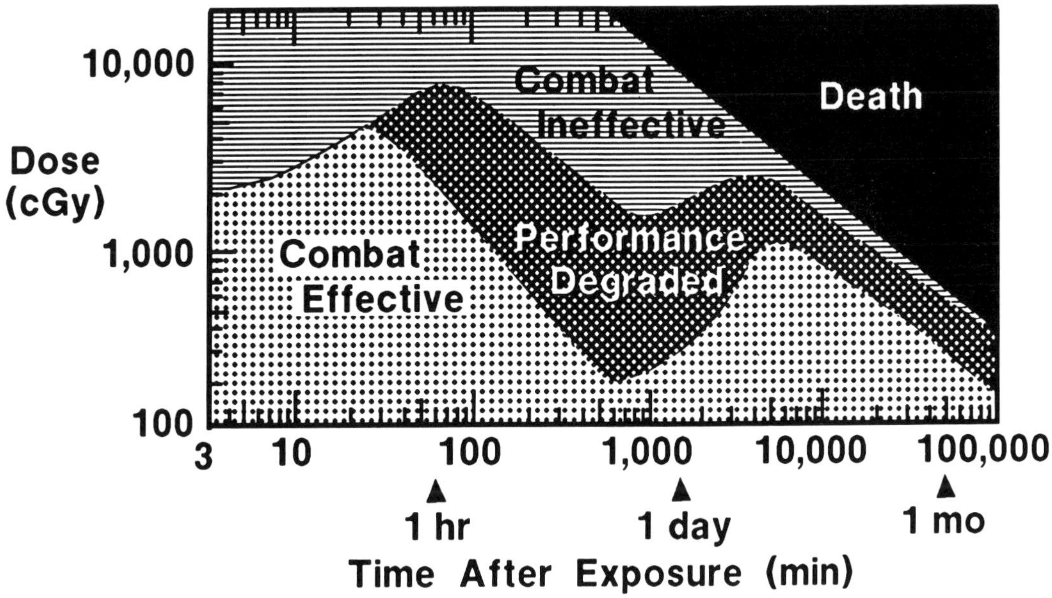

Fig. 7-11. Expected behavioral response to radiation exposure for persons performing a physically undemanding task. Combat effective: 75%-100% normal capacity. Degraded: 25%-75%. Combat ineffective: 0-25%.
Source: Data are derived from the Human Response Program of the Defense Nuclear Agency

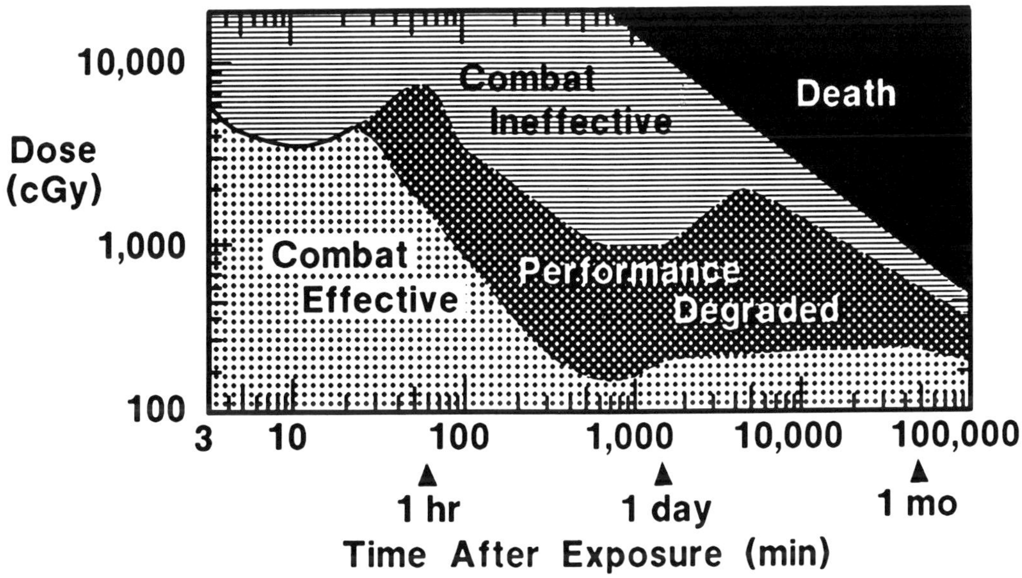

Fig. 7-12. Expected behavioral response to radiation exposure for persons performing tasks required of a CH-47 helicopter crew. Combat effective: 75%-100% normal capacity. Degraded: 25%-75%. Combat ineffective: 0-25%.
Source: Data are derived from the Human Response Program of the Defense Nuclear Agency

compilation of symptom complexes that reflect various combinations of the expected radiogenic symptoms, including gastrointestinal distress, fatigability, weakness, hypotension, infection, bleeding, fever, fluid loss, and electrolyte imbalance;[297] *(c)* the development of accurate descriptions of the severity of each symptom category at each postirradiation time of interest; *(d)* an analysis of tasks performed by five different crews, including a field artillery gun (155-mm SP Howitzer) crew, a manual-operations field artillery fire-direction crew, a tank (M60A3) crew, a CH-47 (Chinook helicopter) crew, and an anti-tank guided missile crew in a TOW vehicle; *(e)* the development of questionnaires that require experienced crewmembers (NCOs or warrant officers) to predict task degradation (slowing of performance) during particular symptom complexes; and *(f)* the evaluation of monkey performance data from a visual-discrimination (physically undemanding) task or a wheel-running (physically demanding) task.[298] This analysis of animal data was performed, in the absence of sufficient human data, in order to estimate the rapid behavioral decrements that follow large (10–45 Gy) radiation doses.

For each crew position, sophisticated statistical techniques made possible the construction of minute-by-minute performance estimates and also smoothed the summary curves as a function of radiation dose and time (Figure 7-9). The analysis involved grouping the results from individual crew members into two categories: physically demanding tasks and physically undemanding tasks (Figures 7-10 and 7-11). A separate analysis of helicopter tasks was also made (Figure 7-12). The degree of performance deficit for each of the five crew positions was described in terms of the following categories: *(a)* performance capability 75%–100% of normal is *combat effective, (b)* performance capability 25%–75% of normal is *degraded,* and *(c)* performance capability 0–25% of normal is *combat ineffective.*

This scheme was then used to summarize the expected changes in the performance of combatants after various doses of radiation exposure.[295] In general, the data indicate that the capabilities of crew members performing tasks of similar demand are degraded similarly. The capabilities of crew members performing physically demanding tasks are degraded more than the capabilities of members performing physically undemanding tasks. This latter observation agrees with the data from animal studies on physical effort after irradiation (Figure 7-4). Figures 7-10, 7-11, and 7-12 illustrate the behavioral changes that might be expected during a one-month period after various doses of ionizing radiation. For example, if crew members performing a physically demanding task are exposed to 10 Gy (Figure 7-10), they will be combat effective for only a little over 1 hour. This period will be followed by an extended time (roughly 1 month) of degraded performance before they become combat ineffective before death. The outlook for performance (but not ultimate prognosis) is a little better for a person performing a physically undemanding task after a 10-Gy irradiation (Figure 7-11). This soldier would remain combat effective for 1.7 hours after exposure. Following this initial period of coping, a transient performance degradation of 2.8 days would ensue before a short recovery and then a gradual decline, ending in death at 1 month after irradiation.

In order to obtain an independent check of the performance degradations predicted for radiation sickness by this study, results were compared (where possible) to actual performance decrements measured in members of the U.S. Coast Guard. The decrements occurred during motion-sickness episodes with symptoms similar to those of radiation sickness. This comparison revealed that the estimates of radiogenic performance decrements made by responders to the questionnaire were similar to the actual declines in short-term task performance that were measured during motion sickness.

Although these are the best estimates of human radiation-induced behavioral deficits that are currently available, their limitations are recognized. These predictions apply to the physiological effects of prompt whole-body irradiation. The data do not predict the behavioral effects of protracted radiation exposures that would occur with fallout, nor do they attempt to account for degradation from the psychological effects that are unique to nuclear combat.

RADIOPROTECTION AND BEHAVIOR

Relatively few studies have addressed the problem of normalizing the behavioral changes that are seen immediately (and up to 24 hours) after irradiation. Research suggests that antihistamines and opiate antagonists (such as naloxone) may offer behavioral radioprotection under certain circumstances.

Some data suggest that estrogens (known to reduce lethal effects of ionizing radiation)[299,300] can reduce the intensity and duration of radiation-induced early transient behavioral deficits in castrated rats trained to perform an avoidance task.[56] Amphetamines can continue to produce locomotor hyperactivity in rats after irradiation with 100 Gy of electrons at a time when the animals would normally be hypoactive. Experiments have also been performed to evaluate the behavioral toxicity of radioprotectants that have the ability to *(a)* reduce the lethal effects of radiation or *(b)* challenge the emesis that sometimes accompanies intermediate doses of ionizing radiation.[62]

Radioprotectants that Reduce Mortality

Traditionally, the development of radioprotectants has meant searching for compounds to protect from the lethal effects of ionizing radiation.[301] More recently, radioprotective compounds have been evaluated for their ability not only to decrease mortality but also to preserve behavioral capacities after irradiation.[62,302] Two early studies administered n-decylaminoethanethiosulfuric acid (WR-1607) (10 mg/kg, intravenous) to monkeys and reported some behavioral benefits.[90,303] In the first study, monkeys trained to perform a continuous-avoidance task were exposed to 100–400 Gy of pulsed neutron-gamma radiation.[90] Protection from ETI was observed up to 4 hours after irradiation, and WR-1607 extended the lives of the subjects for almost 5 hours beyond that observed in control animals. In the second study, monkeys trained to perform a visual-discrimination task were exposed to 25 or 40 Gy of mixed neutron-gamma radiation.[303] ETI was blocked during the first hour, but performance started to fall 2 hours after exposure. Although these behavioral results were promising, WR-1607 produced severe emesis. This side effect may explain the current shift of interest to another promising drug, WR-2721 (ethiofos).[302]

Many experiments have assessed the behavioral toxicity of drugs that are known to offer protection from radiation mortality. Researchers have been studying ethiofos extensively, hoping that it has fewer side effects than WR-1607.[301] Troops who are incapacitated on the battlefield from a radioprotectant are as great a loss as troops incapacitated by ionizing radiation. Ethiofos has been tested in mice, rats, and monkeys for its behavioral toxicity and its potential ability to block radiogenic performance decrements, using spontaneous locomotor activities as well as accelerating-rod and visual-discrimination performance tests.[62,75,98,101,302,304-306] In all of the species and tasks analyzed, ethiofos was behaviorally toxic when given alone (it disrupted trained behavior or it reduced locomotor activity), and it increased rather than decreased the radiation-induced performance decrements. Thus, although ethiofos protects from the lethal effects of radiation, it has limited use when the recipient must remain functional. This concept of a behaviorally tolerated drug dose is very important in evaluating the radio-protectant candidates for military use.

Efficacy of Antiemetics

Although considerable research on antiemetics exists, its focus has been mainly limited to drugs that are effective in radiation therapy.[96,307,308] In this regard, various anti-inflammatory drugs (such as dexamethasone and steroids) have been useful in managing the emesis of patients.[309,310] However, therapy makes few task demands on the recipients; in the military, antiemetics that are effective against radiation-induced vomiting must also not disrupt performance capabilities. These requirements significantly reduce the field of potentially useful antiemetics. For example, metoclopramide, dazopride, and zacopride (5-HT3-receptor blockers) were tested for antiemetic effects in monkeys exposed to 8 Gy of gamma radiation.[308] All three drugs were found to be effective antiemetics. However, only zacopride had no readily observable behavioral effects; metoclopramide disrupted motor performance, and dazopride produced drowsiness.[95] Additional work assessed the behavioral toxicity of zacopride in monkeys performing the speed-stress visual-discrimination task [311] and in rats performing the accelerating-rod task.[312] No behavioral toxicity was observed in either performance model. In the future, these more refined behavioral measures will be used to assess the military usefulness of these and other putative antiemetics after radiation exposure.

Shielding

In addition to pharmacological radioprotection, the immediate effects of radiation may be mitigated by shielding (placing material between the radiation source and the subject). Studies have focused on either head shielding (body exposed) or body shielding (head exposed). In one study of ETI, pigs were trained to traverse a shuttle-box on cue and then were either body-exposed or head-exposed to 60–130 Gy of mixed neutron-gamma radiation.[313] The investigators reported that head shielding offered significant protection from ETI. Other short-term shielding experiments were conducted with monkeys trained to perform a visual-discrimination task.[118,314] The monkeys were exposed to mixed neutron-gamma radiation at doses of 25, 45, or 100 Gy. In the 25- and 100-Gy-dose groups, ETI was about equally severe for all shielding conditions. However, the incidence of ETI in the 45-Gy-dose group was lowest in the head-shielded condition. The results from several other shielding studies with monkeys do not clearly indicate that head or body shielding offers any differing protection from ETI.[127,258,260,315,316] These equivocal results also raise questions about the exclusive role of the CNS in the production of radiation-induced performance deficits. As with radiation-induced taste aversion, postirradiation behaviors may be influenced by peripheral mechanisms that have not been fully explored.[94]

Bone-Marrow Factors

Bone-marrow transplants have been used to challenge radiation-induced damage to the blood-forming systems. It is interesting that this manipulation seems also to provide some subchronic behavioral benefits.[317] Measures of activity and lethality were recorded in rats that were irradiated with 6.5 Gy of X rays. Twenty percent of the nontreated rats died, whereas 86% of the marrow-treated group survived. It is more important here that the initial decreases in spontaneous locomotor activity were less severe in the marrow-treated rats. Instead of showing a second drop in activity 10 days after irradiation, the treated rats showed near-normal activity for the entire 35 days of testing.[71] A similar outcome for behavior was observed in rats exposed to 7.5 Gy of whole-body X rays except for shielded marrow-containing bones.[317]

Bone-marrow transplantation may be impractical in military situations. However, shielding may enable stem cells to survive so that certain immunomodulators of growth factors may promote regeneration and thereby enhance performance.

Radiation in Space

The behavioral scientist who is interested in these issues is constantly challenged by a variety of military-relevant tasks that require empirical analysis. As military operations move to outer space, new radiation hazards will challenge the human's abilities to carry out missions.[86,318] The behavioral effects of ionizing radiations (such as protons and high-Z particles) in space are beginning to be explored.[319,320] Preliminary indications are that radiations in space may be significantly more disruptive to behavior than are the radiations in the earth's environments.

SUMMARY

The success or failure of military operations can be measured in terms of missions completed or tasks performed. Under many circumstances, exposure to ionizing radiation can significantly impede performance. In the case of low-to-intermediate doses of radiation (up to 10 Gy), performance deficits may be slow to develop, may be relatively long lasting, and will usually abate before the onset of chronic radiation effects, such as cancers. After large doses, the behavioral effects are often rapid (within minutes), and they usually abate before the onset of the debilitating chronic radiation sickness. These rapid effects can also occur after intermediate doses. But all tasks are not equally radiosensitive; tasks with complex, demanding requirements are more easily disrupted than simple tasks. The exceptions may be certain naturalistic behaviors which are also quite radiosensitive. Radiation parameters such as dose, dose rate, fractionation, and quality can all influence the observed degree of performance decrements. Electron radiation is more able to produce behavioral deficits than are other radiations, such as neutron radiation. In addition, combined injuries will probably be prevalent in any future nuclear conflicts; present data suggest that trauma can act synergistically with radiation exposure to greatly increase the behavioral deficits.

Possible sensory and neurophysiological mediators of radiation-induced behavioral deficits have been identified. Long-term changes in performance may be mediated in part by radiogenic brain damage from ischemia, edema, or direct damage to the parenchymal tissues themselves (such as dendrites and glia). More transient cerebrovascular changes after radiation exposure may also produce short-lived behavioral deficits. Postirradiation alterations in brain metabolism and the disruption of the normal electrophysiology of the axon and synapse may have important roles in certain performance deficits. In addition, a wide range of radiogenic neurochemical alterations have been characterized. These include the reduced ability of synaptic sodium channels to respond to stimulation. The nervous system's radiosensitivity is revealed by the fact that alterations in the basic substrate of neural excitation have been observed at doses of less than 1 Gy. Various levels of neurotransmitters (such as acetylcholine and dopamine), putative neurotransmitters (such as endorphins), and other neurochemicals and biogenic amines (such as histamine) undergo significant changes after radiation exposure. Like the modifications of morphology and electrophysiology, many of these neurochemical changes may also be capable of mediating the performance decrements observed after ionizing radiation exposure.

The literature on performance deficits in animals is quite extensive compared to that for humans. Human data are derived from radiation accidents or therapeutic studies, and many confirm the information from animal studies. Based on all data now available, the Human Response Program of the Defense Nuclear Agency has estimated the expected performance changes in irradiated soldiers. These projections depend on such factors as radiation dose, time after exposure, and task difficulty. Although the topics are complex, the human and laboratory animal data should permit the description, prediction, and (eventually) amelioration of the behavioral effects of ionizing radiation exposure. Thus far, however, many of the pharmacological compounds that protect animals from the lethality of ionizing radiation have been found to have severe behavioral toxicity. We must further explore the potential for using behaviorally compatible antiemetics and selective physical shielding to help maintain performance after radiation exposure.

REFERENCES

This chapter addresses most of the significant issues on behavioral and neurophysiological changes after ionizing radiation exposure, but is not exhaustive. For more detail and less military orientation, consult references 10, 20, 30, 67, 145, and 196. A number of U.S. and NATO military publications (including U.S. Army Field Circular 50-10, NATO STANAG 2083, and NATO STANAG 2866) concern troop performance in a variety of combat situations.

1. Young, R. W., and Auton, D. L. 1984. The Defense Nuclear Agency Intermediate Dose Program: An overview. In *Proceedings of the Psychology in the Department of Defense, Ninth Symposium* [Technical Report TR-84-2; NTIS AD-A141-043-0], edited by G. E. Lee and T. E. Ulrich, 85-89. Colorado Springs: U.S. Air Force Academy.

2. Mickley, G. A. 1987. Psychological phenomena associated with nuclear warfare: Potential animal models. In *Proceedings of the DNA Symposium/Workshop on the Psychological Effects of Tactical Nuclear Warfare* [Technical Report TR-87-209; NTIS AD-A194-754-8-XAB], edited by R. W. Young, 7.1-7.35. Washington, DC: Defense Nuclear Agency.

3. Bogo, V. 1988. Early behavioral toxicity produced by acute ionizing radiation. *Comments on Toxicology* 2: 265-276.

4. Kimeldorf, D. J.; Jones, D. C.; and Castanera, T. J. 1953. Effect of X-irradiation upon the performance of daily exhaustive exercise by the rat. *Am. J. Physiol.* 174: 331-335.

5. Casarett, A. P. 1968. *Radiation biology.* Englewood Cliffs, NJ: Prentice-Hall, Inc.

6. Hall, E. J. 1973. *Radiobiology for the radiologist.* Hagerstown, MD: Harper and Row.

7. Bogo, V. 1984. Effects of bremsstrahlung and electron radiation on rat motor performance. *Radiat. Res.* 100: 313-320.

8. Casarett, A. P. 1973. Swim-tank measurement of radiation-induced behavioral incapacitation. *Psychol. Rep.* 33: 731-736.

9. Mickley, G. A.; Stevens, K. E.; White, G. A.; and Gibbs, G. L. 1983. Endogenous opiates mediate radiogenic behavioral change. *Science* 220: 1185-1187.

10. Davis, R. T. 1965. The radiation syndrome. In *Behavior of Nonhuman Primates,* edited by A. M. Schrier, H. F. Harlow, and F. Stollnitz, 495-524. New York: Academic Press.

11. Meyerson, F. G. 1958. Effect of damaging doses of gamma-radiation on unconditioned and conditioned respiratory reflexes. In *Works of the Institute of Higher Nervous Activity.* Vol. 4 of the Pathophysiological Series [Israel Program Sci. Transl. OTS:61-31,021, 1962], 25-41. Moscow, USSR: Izd. Akad. Nauk.

12. Wheeler, T. G., and Hardy, K. A. 1985. Retrograde amnesia produced by electron beam exposure: Causal parameters and duration of memory loss. *Radiat. Res.* 101: 74-80.

13. Wheeler, T. G., and Tilton, B. M. 1983. *Duration of memory loss due to electron beam exposure* [Technical Report TR-83-33; NTIS AD-A132-941-6]. Brooks Air Force Base, TX: School of Aerospace Medicine.

14. Page, K. R., and Wheeler, T. G. 1985. *Potency of photoflash-produced retrograde amnesia in rats* [Technical Paper TP-85-1; NTIS AD-A159-149-4-XAB]. Brooks Air Force Base, TX: School of Aerospace Medicine.

15. Wheeler, T. G. 1982. *Amnesia production by visual stimulation* [Technical Report TR-82-45; NTIS AD-A124-822-8]. Brooks Air Force Base, TX: School of Aerospace Medicine.

16. Burt, D. H., and Ingersoll, E. H. 1965. Behavioral and neuropathological changes in the rat following X-irradiation of the frontal brain. *J. Comp. Physiol. Psychol.* 59: 90-93.

17. Janis, I. L. 1951. *Air war and emotional stress.* New York: McGraw-Hill.

18. Committee for the Compilation of Materials on Damage Caused by the Atomic Bombs in Hiroshima and Nagasaki. 1981. Psychological trends among A-bomb victims. In *Hiroshima and Nagasaki: Physical, Mental and Social Effects of the Atomic Bombings,* translated by E. Ishikawa, E. and D. Swain, 485-500. New York: Basic Books.

19. Jammet, H.; Mathe, G.; Pendic, B.; Duplan, J. F.; Maupin, B.; Laterjet, R.; Kalic, D.; Schwarzenberg, L.; Djukic, Z.; and Vigne, J. 1959. Study of six cases of accidental whole-body irradiation. *Rev. Franc. Etud. Chim. Biol.* 4: 210-225.

20. Van Cleave, C. D. 1963. *Irradiation and the nervous system.* New York: Rowman and Littlefield, Inc.

21. Harlow, H. F., and Moon, L. E. 1956. The effects of repeated doses of total-body X-irradiation on motivation and learning in rhesus monkeys. *J. Comp. Physiol. Psychol.* 49: 60-65.

22. Riopelle, A. J.; Gradsky, M. A.; and Ades, H. W. 1956. Learned performance of monkeys after single and repeated X-irradiations. *J. Comp. Physiol. Psychol.* 49: 521-524.

23. McDowell, A. A. 1958. Comparisons of distractibility in irradiated and nonirradiated monkeys. *J. Genet. Psychol.* 93: 63-72.

24. Blair, W. C., and Arnold, W. J. 1956. The effects of cranial X-irradiation on retention of maze learning in rats. *J. Comp. Physiol. Psychol.* 49: 525-528.

25. Brown, W. L., and McDowell, A. A. 1962. Some effects of radiation on psychologic processes in rhesus monkeys. In *Response of the Nervous System to Ionizing Radiation,* edited by T. J. Haley and R. S. Snider, 729-746. New York: Academic Press, Inc.

26. McDowell, A. A., and Brown, W. L. 1958. Facilitative effects of irradiation on performance of monkeys on discrimination problems with reduced stimulus cues. *J. Genet. Psychol.* 93: 73.

27. Kaplan, S. J., and Gentry, G. 1954. *Some effects of a lethal dose of X-radiation upon memory. A case study* [Report NP-5321]. Randolph Air Force Base, TX: School of Aviation Medicine.

28. Furchtgott, E. 1951. Effects of total body X-irradiation on learning: An exploratory study. *J. Comp. Physiol. Psychol.* 44: 197-203.

29. Jarrard, L. E. 1963. Effects of X-irradiation on operant behavior in the rat. *J. Comp. Physiol. Psychol.* 56: 608-611.

30. Kimeldorf, D. J., and Hunt, E. L. 1965. *Ionizing radiation: Neural function and behavior.* New York and London: Academic Press.

31. Blair, W. C. 1958. The effects of cranial X-irradiation on maze acquisition in rats. *J. Comp. Physiol. Psychol.* 51: 175-177.

32. Scarborough, B. B.; Martin, J.; and McLaurin, W. A. 1966. Ionizing radiation: Effects of repeated low dose exposure. *Physiol. Behav.* 1: 147-150.

33. Ordy, J. M.; Barnes, H. W.; Samorajski, T.; Curtis, H. J.; Wolin, L.; and Zeman, W. 1964. Pathologic and behavioral studies in mice after deuteron irradiation of the central nervous system. *Radiat. Res.* 18: 31-45.

34. Ordy, J. M.; Samorajski, T.; Zeman, W.; Collins, R. L.; and Curtis, H. J. 1963. Long-term pathologic and behavioral changes in mice after local deuteron irradiation of the brain. *Radiat. Res.* 20: 30-42.

35. Meier, G. W. 1962. Irradiation, genetics, and aging: Behavioral implications. In *Effects of Ionizing Radiation on the Nervous System; Proceedings*, 187-196. Vienna: International Atomic Energy Agency.

36. Fields, P. E. 1957. The effect of whole-body X-radiation upon activity drum, straightaway, and maze performances of white rats. *J. Comp. Physiol. Psychol.* 50: 386-391.

37. Urmer, A. H., and Brown, W. L. 1960. The effect of gamma radiation on the reorganization of a complex maze habit. *J. Genet. Psychol.* 97: 67-76.

38. McDowell, A. A., and Brown, W. L. 1960. Visual acuity performance of normal and chronic focal-head irradiated monkeys. *J. Genet. Psychol.* 93: 139-144.

39. Riopelle, A. J. Some behavioral effects of ionizing radiation on primates. In reference 25, 719-728.

40. Dimascio, A.; Fuller, J. F.; Azrin, N. H.; and Jetter, W. 1956. The effect of total-body X-irradiation on delayed-response performance of dogs. *J. Comp. Physiol. Psychol.* 49: 600-604.

41. Brown, W. L.; Overall, J. E.; Logie, L. C.; and Wicker, J. E. 1960. Lever-pressing behavior of albino rats during prolonged exposures to X-irradiation. *Radiat. Res.* 13: 617-631.

42. Payne, R. B. 1959. Effects of ionizing radiation exposure on human psychomotor skills. *U.S. Armed Forces Med. J.* 10: 1009-1021.

43. Mele, P. C.; Franz, C. G.; and Harrison, J. R. 1988. Effects of sublethal ionizing radiation on schedule-controlled performance in rats. *Pharmacol. Biochem. Behav.* 30: 1007-1014.

44. Bogo, V.; Franz, C. F.; and Young, R. W. 1987. Effects of radiation on monkey discrimination performance. In *Proceedings of the Eighth International Congress of Radiation Research* (Abstract), edited by E. M. Fielden, J. F. Fowler, J. H. Hendry, and D. Scott, 259. Edinburgh, Scotland: International Congress of Radiation Research.

45. Brown, G. C. 1984. *Behavioral and pathological changes following a 1100-rad radiation exposure.* Ann Arbor, MI: University Microfilms International.

46. Yochmowitz, M. G., and Brown, G. C. 1977. Performance in a 12-hour, 300-rad profile. *Aviat. Space Environ. Med.* 48: 241-247.

47. Barnes, D. J.; Patrick, R. P.; Yochmowitz, M. G.; Yaeger, R. J.; Lof, N. E.; Hardy, K. A.; and Bastien, R. W. 1977. *Protracted low-dose ionizing radiation effects upon primate performance* [Technical Report TR-77-30; NTIS AD-A054-958-4]. Brooks Air Force Base, TX: School of Aerospace Medicine.

48. Yochmowitz, M.; Patrick, R.; Jaeger, R.; and Barnes, D. 1977. Protracted radiation-stressed primate performance. *Aviat. Space Environ. Med.* 48: 598-606.

49. Yochmowitz, M. G.; Brown, G. C.; and Hardy, K. A. 1985. Performance following a 500-675 rad neutron pulse. *Aviat. Space Environ. Med.* 56: 525-533.

50. Stapleton, G. E., and Curtis, H. J. 1946. *The effects of fast neutrons on the ability of mice to take forced exercise* [U.S. Atomic Energy Commission Report MDDC-696]. Oak Ridge, TN: Oak Ridge National Laboratory.

51. Jetter, W. W.; Lindsley, O. R.; and Wohlwill, F. J. 1953. *The effects of X-irradiation on physical exercise and behavior in the dog; related hematological and pathological control studies* [U.S. Atomic Energy Commission Report NYO-4548]. New York: Atomic Energy Commission.

52. George, R. E.; Chaput, R. L.; Verrelli, D. M.; and Barron, E. L. 1971. The relative effectiveness of fission neutrons for miniature pig performance decrement. *Radiat. Res.* 48: 332-345.

53. Chaput, R. L., and Barron, E. L. 1973. Postradiation performance of miniature pigs modified by tasks. *Radiat. Res.* 53: 392-401.

54. Chaput, R. L., and Wise, D. 1970. Miniature pig incapacitation and performance decrement after mixed gamma-neutron irradiation. *Aerospace Med.* 41: 290-293.

55. Casarett, A. P., and Comar, C. L. 1973. Incapacitation and performance decrement in rats following split dose of fission spectrum radiation. *Radiat. Res.* 53: 455-461.

56. Mickley, G. A. 1980. Behavioral and physiological changes produced by a supralethal dose of ionizing radiation: Evidence for hormone-influenced sex differences in the rat. *Radiat. Res.* 81: 48-75.

57. Bogo, V. Comparative effects of bremsstrahlung, gamma, and electron radiation on rat motor performance. In reference 1, 68-72.

58. Wheeler, T. G.; Hardy, K. A.; Anderson, L. B.; and Richards, S. 1984. *Motor performance in irradiated rats as a function of radiation source, dose, and time since exposure* [Technical Report TR-84-8; NTIS AD-A141-209-7]. Brooks Air Force Base, TX: School of Aerospace Medicine.

59. Franz, C. G. 1985. Effects of mixed neutron-gamma total body irradiation on physical activity performance of rhesus monkeys. *Radiat. Res.* 101: 434-441.

60. Kimeldorf, D. J., and Jones, D. C. 1951. The relationship of radiation dose to lethality among exercised animals exposed to roentgen rays. *Am. J. Physiol.* 167: 626-632.

61. Jones, D. C.; Kimeldorf, D. J.; Rubadeau, D. O.; and Castanera, T. J. 1953. Relationships between volitional activity and age in the male rat. *Am. J. Physiol.* 172: 109-114.

62. Bogo, V. 1988. Behavioral radioprotection. *Pharmacol. Ther.* 39: 73-78.

63. Martin, B. A., and Michaelson, S. M. 1966. Exercise performance of upper-body x-irradiated dogs. *Am. J. Physiol.* 211: 457-461.

64. Smith, F., and Smith, W. W. 1951. Exercise effects on tolerance to radiation. *Am. J. Physiol.* 165: 662-666.

65. Brown, W. L., and White, R. K. 1958. Preirradiation fatigue as a factor in the prevention of irradiation deaths in rats. *J. Genet. Psychol.* 93: 287-290.

66. Brown, W. L., and White, R. K. 1960. A study of fatigue and mortality in irradiated rats. *Radiat. Res.* 13: 610-616.

67. Furchtgott, E. 1975. Ionizing radiations and the nervous system. In vol. 3, *Biology of Brain Dysfunction,* edited by G. E. Galli, 343-379. New York: Plenum Press.

68. Leary, R. W., and Ruch, T. C. 1955. Activity, manipulation drive, and strength in monkeys subjected to low-level irradiation. *J. Comp. Physiol. Psychol.* 48: 336-342.

69. Alderks, C. E.; Mickley, G. A.; and Harris, A. H. 1987. Effects of ionizing irradiation on time and force measures during a shock avoidance task. Paper presented at 13th Convention of the Association for Behavior Analyses, Nashville, Tennessee.

70. Furchtgott, E. 1971. Behavioral effects of ionizing radiations. In *Pharmacology and Biophysical Agents and Behavior,* edited by E. Furchtgott, 1-64. New York: Academic Press.

71. Jones, D. C.; Kimeldorf, D. J.; Rubadeau, D. O.; Osborn, G. K.; and Castanera, T. J. 1954. Effects of X-irradiation on performance of volitional activity by the adult male rat. *Am. J. Physiol.* 177: 243-250.

72. Arnold, W. J. Behavioral effects of cranial irradiation of rats. In reference 25, 669-682.

73. Castanera, T. J.; Jones, D. C.; and Kimeldorf, D. J. 1959. The effects of X irradiation on the diffuse activity performance of rats, guinea pigs and hamsters. *Br. J. Radiol.* 32: 386-389.

74. McDowell, A. A., and Brown, W. L. 1960. Comparisons of running wheel activity of normal and chronic radiated rats under varying conditions of food deprivation. *J. Genet. Psychol.* 96: 79-83.

75. Landauer, M. R.; Davis, H. D.; Dominitz, J. A.; and Weiss, J. F. 1988. Long-term effects of the radioprotector WR-2721 on locomotor activity and body weight of mice following ionizing radiation. *Toxicology* 49: 315-323.

76. Landauer, M. R.; Davis, H. D.; Dominitz, J. A.; and Pierce, S. J. 1987. Effects of acute gamma radiation exposure on locomotor activity in Swiss-Webster mice. *The Toxicologist* 7: 253.

77. McDowell, A. A.; Davis, R. T.; and Steele, J. P. 1956. Application of systematic direct observational methods to analysis of the radiation syndrome in monkeys. *Percept. Mot. Skills* (Monograph Suppl. 3), 6: 117-130.

78. Mattsson, J. L., and Yochmowitz, M. G. 1980. Radiation-induced emesis in monkeys. *Radiat. Res.* 82: 191-199.

79. McDowell, A. A. 1954. The immediate effects of single dose of whole body X radiation upon the social behavior and self-care of caged rhesus monkeys. *Am. Psychol.* 9: 423.

80. Vogel, H., Jr. 1950. The effect of X irradiation on fighting behavior in male mice. *Anat. Rec.* 108: 547.

81. Maier, D. M., and Landauer, M. R. 1987. Effects of gamma radiation on aggressive behavior in male swiss webster mice. *Soc. Neurosci. Abstr.* 13(2): 933.

82. O'Boyle, M. 1976. Suppresssion of mouse-killing in rats following irradiation. *Percept. Mot. Skills* 42: 511-514.

83. Burke, R. D.; Mattsson, J. L.; and Fischer, J. R. 1981. *Effect of ionizing radiation on shock-elicited aggression of male rats* [Technical Report TR-81-18; NTIS AD-A103-329-9]. Brooks Air Force Base, TX: School of Aerospace Medicine.

84. Ader, R., and Hahn, E. W. 1963. Effects of social environment on mortality to whole body x-irradiation in the rat. *Psychol. Rep.* 13: 211-215.

85. Ader, R. and Hahn, E. W. 1963. Dominance and emotionality in the rat and their effects on mortality after whole-body x-irradiation. *Psychol. Rep.* 13: 617-618.

86. Mickley, G. A.; Bogo, V.; Landauer, M. R.; and Mele, P. C. 1988. Current trends in behavioral radiobiology. In *Terrestrial Space Radiation and Its Biological Effects,* edited by C. E. Swenberg, 517-536. New York: Plenum Press.

87. Maier, D. M. Personal communication, 1987.

88. Rugh, R., and Grupp, E. 1960. X-irradiation lethality aggravated by sexual activity of male mice. *Am. J. Physiol.* 198: 1352-1354.

89. Morse, D. G., and Mickley, G. A. 1988. Dose-rate and sex effects on the suppression of appetitive behavior following exposure to gamma-spectrum radiation. In *Abstracts of 36th Annual Meeting of Radiation Research Society,* 163. Philadelphia: Radiation Research Society.

90. Sharp, J. C.; Kelly, D. D.; and Brady, J. V. 1968. The radio-attenuating effects of n-decylaminoethanethiosulfuric acid in the rhesus monkey. In *Use of Nonhuman Primates in Drug Evaluation,* edited by H. Vagtborg, 338-346. San Antonio, TX: Southwest Foundation for Research and Education.

91. Leary, R. W. 1955. Food-preference changes of monkeys subjected to low-level irradiation. *J. Comp. Physiol. Psychol.* 48: 343-346.

92. Davis, R. T. 1958. Latent changes in the food preferences of irradiated monkeys. *J. Genet. Psychol.* 92: 53-59.

93. Garcia, J.; Kimeldorf, D. J.; and Koelling, R. A. 1955. A conditioned aversion towards saccharin resulting from exposure to gamma radiation. *Science* 122: 157-158.

94. Rabin, B. M., and Hunt, W. A. 1986. Mechanisms of radiation-induced conditioned taste aversion learning. *Neurosci. Biobehav. Rev.* 10: 55-65.

95. Dubois, A.; Fiala, N.; and Bogo, V. 1987. Treatment of radiation induced vomiting and gastric emptying suppression with zacopride. Part 2. *Gastroenterology* 92(5): 1376.

96. Young, R. W. 1986. Mechanisms and treatment of radiation-induced nausea and vomiting. In *Nausea and Vomiting: Mechanisms and Treatment,* edited by C. J. Davis, G. V. Lake-Bakaar, and G. V. Grahame-Smith, 94-109. New York: Springer-Verlag.

97. Middleton, G. R., and Young, R. W. 1975. Emesis in monkeys following exposure to ionizing radiation. *Aviat. Space Environ. Med.* 46: 170-172.

98. Bogo, V.; Franz, C. G.; Jacobs, A. F.; Weiss, J. F.; and Young, R. W. 1988. WR-2721, radiation, and visual discrimination performance. *Pharmacol. Ther.* 39: 93-95.

99. Walker, R. I.; Gruber, D. F.; MacVittie, T. J.; and Conklin, J. J., eds. 1985. *The pathophysiology of combined injury and trauma: Radiation, burn, and trauma.* Baltimore: University Park Press.

100. Gruber, D.; Walker, R. I.; MacVittie, T. J.; and Conklin, J. J., eds. 1987. *The pathophysiology of combined injury and trauma: Management of infectious complications in mass casualty situations.* Orlando, FL: Academic Press.

101. Landauer, M. R.; Ledney, G. D.; and Davis, H. D. 1987. Locomotor behavior in mice following exposure to fission-neutron irradiation and trauma. *Aviat. Space Environ. Med.* 58: 1205-1210.

102. Wheeler, T. G., and Cordts, R. E. 1983. *Combined effects of ionizing radiation and anticholinesterase exposure on rodent motor performance* [Technical Report TR-83-30; NTIS AD-A131-847-6]. Brooks Air Force Base, TX: School of Aerospace Medicine.

103. Bogo, V.; Hill, T. A.; and Young, R. W. 1981. Comparison of accelerod and rotarod sensitivity in detecting ethanol- and acrylamide-induced performance decrement in rats: Review of experimental considerations of rotating rod systems. *Neurotoxicology* 2: 765-787.

104. Wheeler, T. G., and Cordts, R. E. 1984. *Nonlinear performance interaction upon exposure to anticholinesterase and ionizing radiation* [Technical Report TR-84-5; NTIS AD-A139-909-6]. Brooks Air Force Base, TX: School of Aerospace Medicine.

105. Casey, H. W., Cordy, D. R., Goldman, M., and Smith, A. H. 1967. Influence of chronic acceleration on the effects of whole-body irradiation in rats. *Aerospace Med.* 38: 451-457.

106. Mattsson, J. L.; Cordts, R. E.; and Deyak, R. R. 1981. Radiation and G tolerance in rats. *Aviat. Space Environ. Med.* 52: 404-407.

107. Antipov, V. V.; Davyov, B. I.; Verigo, V. V.; and Svirezhev, Y. M. 1975. Combined effect of flight factors. In *Ecological and Physiological Bases of Space Biology and Medicine,* Vol. 2, Book 2 of *Foundations of Space Biology and Medicine,* edited by M. Calvin and O. G. Gazenko, 639-667. Washington, DC: National Aeronautics and Space Administration.

108. Zellmer, R. W.; Womack, G. W.; McNee, R. C.; and Allen, R. G. 1963. Significance of combined stresses of G-forces and irradiation. *Aerospace Med.* 34: 626-629.

109. Livshits, N. N.; Apanasenko, Z. I.; Kuznetsova, M. A.; Meizerov, E. S.; and Zakirova, R. M. 1975. Effects of acceleration on the higher nervous activity of previously irradiated rats. *Radiobiologiia* 15: 92-99.

110. Seigneur, L. J., and Brennan, J. T. 1966. *Incapacitation in the monkey (Macaca mulatta) following exposure to a pulse of reactor radiation* [Scientific Report SR66-2]. Bethesda, MD: Armed Forces Radiobiology Research Institute.

111. Bruner, A. 1977. Immediate dose-rate effects of ^{60}Co on performance and blood pressure in monkeys. *Radiat. Res.* 70: 378-390.

112. Blondal, H. 1958. Initial irradiation reaction in mice. *Nature* 182: 1026-1027.

113. Pitchford, T. L. 1968. *Beagle incapacitation and survival time after pulsed mixed gamma-neutron irradiation* [Scientific Report SR68-24]. Bethesda, MD: Armed Forces Radiobiology Research Institute.

114. Thorp, J. W. 1970. *Beagle and miniature pig response to partial body irradiation: Dose relationships* [Technical Note TN70-5; NTIS AD-717-591]. Bethesda, MD: Armed Forces Radiobiology Research Institute.

115. Langham, W. R.; Kaplan, S. J.; Pickering, J. E.; Lushbaugh, C. C.; Haymaker, W.; Storer, J. B.; and Harris, P. S. 1952. *The effects of rapid, massive doses of gamma radiation on the behavior of sub-human primates* [Technical Report LA-1558; OCLC 13613209]. Los Alamos, NM: Los Alamos National Laboratory.

116. Sharp, J. C., and Keller, B. K. 1965. *A comparison between the effects of exposure to a mixed fission spectrum delivered in a single "pulse" and X-rays delivered at a slower rate upon conditioned avoidance behavior of the primate* [Technical Report TR4]. Washington, DC: Walter Reed Army Institute of Research.

117. Curran, C. R.; Conrad, D. W.; and Young, R. W. 1971. *The effects of 2000 rads of pulsed gamma-neutron radiation upon the performance of unfettered monkeys* [Scientific Report SR71-3; NTIS AD-724-653]. Bethesda, MD: Armed Forces Radiobiology Research Institute.

118. Thorp, J. W., and Young, R. W. 1971. Monkey performance after partial body irradiation. *Aerospace Med.* 42: 503-507.

119. Barnes, D. J. 1966. *An initial investigation of the effects of pulsed ionizing radiation on the primate equilibrium function* [Technical Report TR-66-106; OCLC 1768649]. Brooks Air Force Base, TX: School of Aerospace Medicine.

120. Hunt, E. L., and Kimeldorf, D. J. 1964. Behavioral arousal and neural activation as radiosensitive reactors. *Radiat. Res.* 21: 91-110.

121. Mickley, G. A., and Teitelbaum, H. 1978. Persistence of lateral hypothalamic-mediated behaviors after a supralethal dose of ionizing radiation. *Aviat. Space Environ. Med.* 49: 863-873.

122. Young, R. W. 1979. *Prediction of the relative toxicity of environmental toxins as a function of behavioral and non-behavioral end points* [OCLC 5897233]. Washington, DC: The Catholic University of America.

123. Young, R. W., and McFarland, W. L. 1972. *Performance of the monkey (Macaca mulatta) after two 2500-rad pulses of mixed gamma-neutron radiation* [Scientific Report SR72-19; NTIS AD-759-017]. Bethesda, MD: Armed Forces Radiobiology Research Institute.

124. Germas, J. E., and Shelton, Q. H. 1969. *Performance of the monkey following multiple supralethal pulses of radiation* [Scientific Report SR69-21; NTIS AD-698-481]. Bethesda, MD: Armed Forces Radiobiology Research Institute.

125. Mele, P. C.; Franz, C. G.; and Harrison, J. R. 1987. Effects of ionizing radiation on fix-ratio escape performance in rats. *Soc. Neurosci. Abstr.* 13(2): 998.

126. Davis, R. T., and Steele, J. P. 1963. Performance selections through radiation death in rhesus monkeys. *J. Psychol.* 56: 119.

127. Chapman, P. H., and Young, R. J. 1968. Effect of cobalt-60 gamma irradiation on blood pressure and cerebral blood flow in the *Macaca mulatta*. *Radiat. Res.* 35: 78-85.

128. Hunt, W. A. 1983. Comparative effects of exposure to high-energy electrons and gamma radiation on active avoidance behaviour. *Int. J. Radiat. Biol.* 44: 257-260.

129. Chaput, R. L.; Berardo, P. A.; and Barron, E. L. 1973. *Increased brain radioresistance after supralethal irradiation* [Scientific Report SR73-7; NTIS AD-764-885-0]. Bethesda, MD: Armed Forces Radiobiology Research Institute.

130. Barnes, D. J.; Brown, G. C.; and Fractor, Z. M. 1971. *Differential effects of multiple and single irradiations upon the primate equilibrium function* [Technical Report TR-71-7; NTIS AD 722-058]. Brooks Air Force Base, TX: School of Aerospace Medicine.

131. George, R. E.; Chaput, R. L.; and Barron, E. L. 1972. *The dependence of miniature pig performance decrement upon gamma ray dose rate* [Scientific Report SR72-20; NTIS AD-757-039]. Bethesda, MD: Armed Forces Radiobiology Research Institute.

132. Bogo, V.; Zeman, G. H.; and Dooley, M. A. 1989. Radiation quality and rat motor performance. *Radiat. Res.* 118: 341-352.

133. Gleitman, H. 1983. *Basic psychology.* New York: W. W. Norton and Co.

134. Graham, E. S.; Farrer, D. N.; Carsten, A. L.; and Roizin, L. 1971. Decrements in the visual acuity of rhesus monkeys as a delayed effect of occipital irradiation. *Radiat. Res.* 45: 373-383.

135. Caveness, W. F.; Tanaka, A.; Hess, K. H.; Kemper, T. L.; Tso, M. O.; and Zimmerman, L. E. 1974. Delayed brain swelling and functional derangement after X-irradiation of the right visual cortex in the *Macaca mulatta. Radiat. Res.* 57: 104-120.

136. Minamisawa, T.; Sugiyama, H.; Tsuchiya, T.; and Ito, H. 1970. Effects of X-irradiation on evoked potentials from visual systems in rabbits. *J. Radiat. Res.* 11: 127-133.

137. Minamisawa, T.; Tsuchiya, T.; and Ito, H. 1972. Changes in the averaged evoked potentials of the rabbit during and after fractionated X-irradiation. *Electroencephalogr. Clin. Neurophysiol.* 33: 591-601.

138. Kekcheyev, K. 1941. Changes in the threshold of achromatic vision of man by the action of ultrashort, ultraviolet, and X-rays waves. *Probl. Fiziol. Opt.* 1: 77-79.

139. Lenoir, A. 1944. Adaptation und roentgenbesstrahlung. *Radio. Clin.* 13: 264-276.

140. Murphy, J. E., and Harris, J. D. 1961. Negligible effects of X-irradiation of the head upon hearing in the rat. *J. Aud. Res.* 1: 117-132.

141. Borsanyi, S. 1962. The effects of radiation therapy on the ear: With particular reference to radiation otitis media. *South. Med. J.* 55: 740-743.

142. Tokimoto, T., and Kanagawa, K. 1985. Effects of X-ray irradiation on hearing in guinea pigs. *Acta Otolaryngol.* (Stockh.) 100: 266-272.

143. Moskovskaya, N. V. 1959. Effect of ionizing radiations on the functions of the vestibular analyzer. *Vestn. Otorinolaringol.* 21: 59-62.

144. Apanasenko, Z. I. 1967. *Combined effect of double exposure to vibration and chronic irradiation on the functional state of vestibular apparatus* [Technical Translation F-413], 212-228. Washington, DC: National Aeronautics and Space Administration.

145. Furchtgott, E. 1963. Behavioral effects of ionizing radiation: 1955-61. *Psychol. Bull.* 60: 157-199.

146. Teskey, G. C., and Kavaliers, M. 1984. Ionizing radiation induces opioid-mediated analgesia in male mice. *Life Sci.* 35: 1547-1552.

147. Doull, J. 1967. Pharmacological responses in irradiated animals. *Radiat. Res.* 30: 333-341.

148. Burghardt, W. F., and Hunt, W. A. The interactive effects of morphine and ionizing radiation on the latency of tail withdrawal from warm water in the rat. In reference 1, 73-76.

149. Mickley, G. A., and Stevens, K. E. 1986. Stimulation of brain muscarinic acetylcholine receptors acutely reverses radiogenic hypodipsia. *Aviat. Space Environ. Med.* 57: 250-255.

150. Ingersoll, E. H.; Carsten, A. L.; and Brownson, R. H. 1967. Behavioral and structural changes following X-irradiations of the forebrain in the rat. *Proc. Soc. Exp. Biol. Med.* 125: 382-385.

151. Arnold, W. J. 1952. Maze learning and retention after X-irradiation of the head. *J. Comp. Physiol. Psychol.* 45: 358-361.

152. Cassaret, G. W. 1980. *Radiation histopathology.* Vol. II. Boca Raton, FL: CRC Press.

153. Hopewell, J. W. 1979. Late radiation damage to the central nervous system: A radiobiological interpretation. *Neuropathol. Appli. Neurobiol.* 5: 329-343.

154. Lyman, R. S., Kupalov, R. S., and Scholz, W. 1933. Effects of roentgen rays on the central nervous system. Results of large doses on the brains of adult dogs. *AMA Arch. Neurol. Psychiat.* 29: 56-87.

155. Hohwieler, M. L.; Lo, T. C.; Silverman, M. L.; and Freiberg, S. R. 1986. Brain necrosis after radiotherapy for primary intracerebral tumor. *Neurosurgery* 18: 67-74.

156. Haymaker, W. Morphological changes in the nervous system following exposure to ionizing radiation. In reference 35, 309-358.

157. Lindgren, M. 1958. On tolerance of brain tissue and sensitivity of brain tumors to irradiation. *Acta Radiol.* [Suppl.] 170: 5-75.

158. Kemper, T. L.; O'Neill, R.; and Caveness, W. F. 1977. Effects of single dose supervoltage whole brain radiation in *Macaca mulatta. J. Neuropathol. Exp. Neurol.* 36: 916-940.

159. Caveness, W. F. 1977. Pathology of radiation damage to the normal brain of the monkey. *Natl. Cancer Inst. Monogr.* 46: 57-76.

160. Pallis, C. A.; Louis, S.; and Morgan, R. L. 1961. Brain myelopathy. *Brain* 84: 460-479.

161. Dynes, J. B., and Smedal, M. J. 1960. Radiation myelitis. *Am. J. Roentgenol. Rad. Ther. Nuc. Med.* 83: 78-87.

162. Marks, J. E., and Wong, J. 1985. The risk of cerebral radionecrosis in relation to dose, time and fractionation. *Prog. Exp. Tumor Res.* 29: 210-218.

163. Switzer, R. C. Personal communication, 1988.

164. Arnold, A.; Bailey, P.; and Harvey, R. A. 1954. Intolerance of primate brain stem and hypothalamus to conventional high energy radiations. *Neurology* 4: 575-585.

165. Yoshii, Y.; Maki, Y.; Tsunemoto, H.; Koike, S.; and Kasuga, T. 1981. The effect of total-head irradiation on C3H/He mice. *Radiat. Res.* 86: 152-170.

166. Ross, J. A. T.; Levitt, S. R.; Holst, E. A.; and Clemente, C. D. 1954. Neurological and electroencephalographic effects of X irradiation of the head in monkeys. *AMA Arch. Neurol. Psychiat.* 71: 238-249.

167. Roizin, L.; Akai, K.; Carsten, A.; Liu, J. C.; and Eisenberg-Gelber, B. 1976. Post-X-ray myelinopathy (pathogenic mechanisms). In *International Symposium on the Aetiology and Pathogenesis of Demyelinating Diseases* [OCLC 8943192], edited by T. Yonawa, 29-57. Neiho-Sha: Japan Press Co.

168. Ibrahim, M. Z. M.; Haymaker, W.; Miquel, J.; and Riopelle, A. J. 1967. Effects of radiation on the hypothalamus in monkeys. *Archiv. fur Psychiatrie und Zeitschrift f.d. ges. Neurologie* 210: 1-15.

169. van der Kogel, A. J. 1986. Radiation-induced damage in the central nervous system: An interpretation of target cell responses. *Br. J. Cancer* (Suppl. VII) 53: 207-217.

170. Abdullin, G. Z. 1962. *Study of comparative radiosensitivity of different parts of brain in terms of altered function* [Atomic Energy Commission TR-5141]. Washington, DC: OTS/Department of Commerce.

171. Christensen, H. D.; Flesher, A. M.; and Haley, T. J. 1969. Changes in brain self-stimulation rates after exposure to X-irradiation. *J. Pharm. Sci.* 58: 128-129.

172. Mechanick, J. I.; Hochberg, F. H.; and LaRocque, A. 1986. Hypothalamic dysfunction following whole brain irradiation. *J. Neurosurg.* 65: 490-494.

173. Rosenthal, F., and Timiras, P. S. 1961. Changes in brain excitability after whole-body X-irradiation in the rat. *Radiat. Res.* 18: 648-657.

174. Rosenthal, F., and Timiras, P. S. 1961. Threshold and pattern of electroshock seizures after 250 R whole-body X-irradiation in rats. *Proc. Soc. Exp. Biol. Med.* 108: 267-270.

175. Gangloff, H. Acute effects of X-irradiation on brain electrical activity in cats and rabbits. In reference 35, 123-138.

176. Gerstner, H. B. 1956. Effect of high-intensity X-irradiation on the A group fibers of the frog sciatic nerve. *Am. J. Physiol.* 184: 333-337.

177. Russel, D. S.; Wilson, C. W.; and Tansley, K. 1949. Experimental radionecrosis in the brains of rabbits. *J. Neurol. Neurosurg. Psychiat.* 12: 187-195.

178. Berg, N. O., and Lindgren, M. 1958. Time dose relationship and morphology of delayed radiation lesions of the brain of the rabbit. *Acta Radiol.* [Suppl.] 167: 1-118.

179. Caveness, W. F. 1980. Experimental observations: Delayed necrosis in normal monkey brain. In *Radiation Damage to the Nervous System,* edited by H. A. Gilbert and A. R. Kagen, 1-38. New York: Raven Press.

180. Hopewell, J. W., and Wright, E. A. 1970. The nature of latent cerebral irradiation damage and its modification by hypertension. *Br. J. Radiol.* 43: 161-167.

181. Hirata, Y.; Matsukado, Y.; Mihara, Y.; and Kochi, M. 1985. Occlusion of the internal carotid artery after radiation therapy for the chiasmal lesion. *Acta Neurochem.* 74: 141-147.

182. Halpern, J.; Kishel, S. P.; Park, J.; Tsukada, Y.; Johnson, R. J. R.; and Ambrus, J. L. 1984. Radiation-induced brain edema in primates, studied with sequential brain CAT scanning and histopathology. *Res. Commun. Chem. Pathol. Pharmacol.* 45: 463-470.

183. Winkler, H. 1957. Untersuchungen uber die Wirkung von Roentgensstrahlen auf die Bluthirnschranke mit hilfe von P32. Zbl. allg. *Pathol. Anat.* 97: 301-307.

184. McMahon, T., and Vahora, S. 1986. Radiation damage to the brain. *Neuropsychiatric Aspects* 8: 437-441.

185. Sheline, G. E.; Wara, W. M.; and Smith, V. 1980. Therapeutic irradiation and brain injury. *Int. J. Radiat. Oncol. Biol. Phys.* 6: 1215-1228.

186. O'Connel, J. F. A., and Brunschwig, A. 1937. Observations on the roentgen treatment of intracranial gliomata with special reference to the effects of irradiation upon the surrounding brain. *Brain* 60: 230-258.

187. Crompton, M. R., and Layton, D. D. 1961. Delayed radionecrosis of the brain following therapeutic x-irradiation of the pituitary. *Brain* 84: 85-101.

188. Innes, J. R., and Carsten, A. 1961. Demyelination or malacic myelopathy. *Arch. Neurol.* 4: 190-199.

189. Zeman, W. 1963. Disturbances of nucleic acid metabolism preceeding delayed radionecrosis of nervous tissue. *Proc. Natl. Acad. Sci. USA* 50: 626-630.

190. Hopewell, J. W., and Wright, E. A. 1975. The effects of dose and field size on late radiation damage to the rat spinal cord. *Int. J. Radiat. Biol.* 28: 325-333.

191. Pourquier, H.; Baker, J. R.; Giaux, G.; and Benirschke, K. 1958. Localized roentgen-ray beam irradiation of the hypophysohypothalamic region of the guinea pig with a 2 million volt van de Graaf generator. *Am. J. Roentgenol. Rad. Ther. Nuc. Med.* 80: 840-850.

192. Reyners, H.; Gianfelici de Reyners, E.; and Maisin, J.-R. 1982. The beta-astrocyte: A newly recognized radiosensitive glial cell type in the cerebral cortex. *J. Neurocytol.* 11: 967-983.

193. Reyners, H., Gianfelici de Reyners, E., and Maisin, J.-R. 1986. Early cell regeneration processes after split-dose X-irradiation of the cerebral cortex of the rat. *Br. J. Cancer* (Suppl. VII) 53: 218-220.

194. Mastaglia, F. L.; McDonald, W. I.; Watson, J. V.; and Yogendran, K. 1976. Effects of X-irradiation on the spinal cord: An experimental study of the morphological changes in central nerve fibers. *Brain* 99: 101-122.

195. Jones, A. 1964. Transient radiation myelopathy (with reference to Lhermitte's sign of electrical paresthesia). *Br. J. Radiol.* 37: 727-744.

196. Cavanagh, J. B., and Hopewell, J. W. 1972. Mitotic activity in the subependymal plate of rats and the long-term consequences of X-irradiation. *J. Neurol. Sci.* 15: 471-482.

197. Furchtgott, E. 1956. Behavioral effects of ionizing radiation. *Psychol. Bull.* 53: 321-334.

198. Altman, J. 1962. Are new neurons formed in the brains of adult mammals? *Science* 135: 1127-1129.

199. Kaplan, M. S., and Hinds, J. W. 1977. Neurogenesis in the adult rat: Electron microscopic analysis of light radioautographs. *Science* 197: 1092-1094.

200. Bayer, S. A., and Altman, J. 1975. Radiation-induced interference with postnatal hippocampal cytogenesis in rats and its long-term effects on the acquisition of neurons and glia. *J. Comp. Neurol.* 163: 1-20.

201. Bayer, S. A. 1985. Neuron production in the hippocampus and olfactory bulb of the adult rat brain: Addition or replacement. In *Hope for a New Neurology,* edited by F. Nottebohm, 163-172. New York: N. Y. Acad. Sci.

202. Rakic, P. DNA synthesis and cell division in the adult primate brain. In reference 201, 193-211.

203. Gueneau, G.; Drouet, J.; Privat, A.; and Court, L. 1979. Differential radiosensitivity of neurons and neuroglia of the hippocampus in the adult rabbit. *Acta Neuropathol.* (Berl.) 48: 199-209.

204. Gueneau, G.; Baille, V.; and Court, L. 1986. Protracted postnatal neurogenesis and radiosensitivity in the rabbit's dentate gyrus. In *Radiation Risks to the Developing Nervous System,* edited by H. Kriegel, W. Schmahl, G. B. Gerber, and F.-E. Stieve, 133-140. Stuttgart: Gustav Fischer Verlag.

205. Schade, J. P., and Caveness, W. F. 1968. Alterations in dendritic organization. *Brain Res.* 7: 59-86.

206. Egana, E. 1962. Some effects of ionizing radiations on the metabolism of the central nervous system. *Int. J. Neurol.* 3: 631-647.

207. Ito, M.; Patronas, N. J.; Di Chiro, G.; Mansi, L.; and Kennedy, C. 1986. Effect of moderate level X-radiation to brain on cerebral glucose utilization. *J. Comput. Assist. Tomogr.* 10: 584-588.

208. Lebedinsky, A. V.; Grigoryev, U. G.; and Demirchoglyan, G. G. 1958. On the biological effect of small doses of ionizing radiation. In *Proceedings of Second United Nations International Conference on Peaceful Uses of Atomic Energy.* [OCLC 2216641]. Vol. 22, 17-28. Geneva: United Nations.

209. Haley, T. J. Changes induced in brain activity by low doses of X-irradiation. In reference 35, 171-185.

210. McFarland, W. L, and Levin, S. G. 1974. Electroencephalographic responses to 2500 rads of whole-body gamma-neutron radiation in the monkey *Macaca mulatta. Radiat. Res.* 58: 60-73.

211. Monnier, M., and Krupp, P. Action of gamma radiation on electrical brain activity. In reference 25, 607-617.

212. Gangloff, H., and Haley, T. J. 1960. Effects of E-irradiation on spontaneous and evoked brain electrical activity in cats. *Radiat. Res.* 12: 694-704.

213. Bassant, M. H., and Court, L. 1978. Effects of whole-body gamma irradiation on the activity of rabbit hippocampal neurons. *Radiat. Res.* 75: 593-606.

214. Peimer, S. I.; Dudkin, A. O.; and Swerdlov, A. G. 1986. Response of hippocampal pacemaker-like neurons to low doses of ionizing radiation. *Int. J. Radiat. Biol.* 49: 597-600.

215. Pollack, M., and Timiras, P. S. 1964. X-ray dose and electroconvulsive responses in adult rats. *Radiat. Res.* 21: 111-119.

216. Miller, D. S. Effects of low level radiation on audiogenic convulsive seizures in mice. In reference 25, 513-531.

217. Sato, M. 1978. Electrophysiological studies on radiation-induced changes in the adult nervous system. In vol. 7, *Advances in Radiation Biology*, edited by J. T. Lett, and H. Adler, 181-210. New York: Academic Press.

218. Bachofer, C. S. 1957. Enhancement of activity of nerves by X-rays. *Science* 125: 1140-1141.

219. Bachofer, C. S., and Gautereaux, M. E. 1959. X-ray effects on single nerve fibers. *J. Gen. Physiol.* 42: 723-735.

220. Bachofer, C. S., and Gautereaux, M. E. 1960. Bioelectric activity of mammalian nerves during X-irradiation. *Radiat. Res.* 12: 575-586.

221. Bachofer, C. S., and Gautereaux, M. E. 1960. Bioelectric response in situ of mammalian nerves exposed to X-rays. *Am. J. Physiol.* 198: 715-717.

222. Gaffey, C. T. Bioelectric effects of high energy irradiation on nerve. In reference 25, 277-296.

223. Gasteiger, E. L., and Campbell, B. Alteration of mammalian nerve compound action potentials by beta irradiation. In reference 25, 597-605.

224. Yamashita, H., and Miyasaka, T. 1952. Effects of beta rays upon a single nerve fiber. *Proc. Soc. Exp. Biol. Med.* 80: 375-377.

225. Kroebel, W., and Kroem, G. 1959. Die wirkung geringer strahlungsdosen auf die signalerzeugungs und fortleitungs-eigenshaftens-eigenschaften in froschnerven. *Atomkernenergie* 4: 280-286.

226. Scholz, W.; Ducho, E. G.; and Breit, A. 1959. Experimentelle Roentgenspatschaden am ruchenmark des erwachsenen kaninchens. Ein weiterer beitrag zur wirkungsweise ionisierender strahlen auf das zentralnervose gewebe. *Psychiat. Neurol. Japan* 61: 417-442.

227. Scholz, W.; Schlote, W.; and Hirschberger, W. Morphological effect of repeated low dosage and single high dosage of X-irradiation to the central nervous system. In reference 25, 211-232.

228. Davidoff, L. M.; Dyke, C. G.; Elsberg, C. A.; and Tarlov, I. M. 1938. The effect of radiation applied directly to brain and spinal cord. I. Experimental investigations on *Macaca* rhesus monkeys. *Radiology* 31: 451-463.

229. Lott, J. R. Changes in ventral root potentials during X-irradiation of the spinal cord in the cat. In reference 35, 85-92.

230. Sato, M.; Austin, G. M.; and Stahl, W. The effects of ionizing radiation on spinal cord neurons. In reference 25, 561-671.

231. Sato, M.; Austin, G. M.; and Stahl, W. Delayed radiation effects on neuronal activity in the spinal cord of the cat. In reference 35, 93-110.

232. Sato, M.; Stahl, W.; and Austin, G. M. 1963. Acute radiation effects on synaptic activity in the mammalian spinal cord. *Radiat. Res.* 18: 307-320.

233. Sato, M., and Austin, G. 1964. Acute radiation effects on mammalian synaptic activities. In *Response of the Nervous System to Ionizing Radiation,* edited by T. J. Haley and R. S. Snider, 279-289. Boston: Little, Brown and Co.

234. Mtskhvetadze, A. V., and Kucherenko, T. M. 1968. Direct and indirect effect of irradiation on the transmission of the stimulus in the upper neck sympathetic ganglion of cats. *Radiobiologiia* 8: 624-627.

235. Tolliver, J. M., and Pellmar, T. C. 1987. Ionizing radiation alters neuronal excitability in hippocampal slices of the guinea pig. *Radiat. Res.* 112: 555-563.

236. Catterall, W. A. 1984. The molecular basis of neuronal excitability. *Science* 223: 653-661.

237. Rothenberg, M. A. 1950. Studies on permeability in relation to nerve function. II. Ionic movements across axonal membranes. *Biochim. Biophys. Acta* 4: 96-114.

238. Wixon, H. N., and Hunt, W. A. 1983. Ionizing radiation decreases veratridine stimulated uptake of sodium in rat brain synaptosomes. *Science* 220: 1073-1074.

239. Mullin, M. J.; Hunt, W. A.; and Harris, R. A. 1986. Ionizing radiation alters the properties of sodium channels in rat brain synaptosomes. *J. Neurochem.* 47: 489-495.

240. Tanimura, H. 1957. Changes of the neurosecretory granules in hypothalamo-hypophysical system of rats by irradiating their heads with X-rays. *Acta Anat. Nippon.* 32: 529-533.

241. Dahlstrom, A.; Haggendal, J.; and Rosengren, B. 1973. The effect of Roentgen irradiation on monoamine containing neurons of the rat brain. *Acta Radiol. Ther. Phys. Biol.* 12: 191-200.

242. Hunt, W. A.; Dalton, T. K.; and Darden, J. H. 1979. Transient alterations in neurotransmitter activity in the caudate nucleus of rat brain after a high dose of ionizing radiation. *Radiat. Res.* 80: 556-562.

243. Joseph, J. A.; Kandasamy, S. B.; Hunt, W. A.; Dalton, T. K.; and Stevens, S. 1988. Radiation-induced increases in sensitivity of cataleptic behavior to haloperidol: Possible involvements of prostaglandins. *Pharmacol. Biochem. Behav.* 29: 335-341.

244. Kulinski, V. I., and Semenov, L. F. 1965. Content of catecholamines in the tissues of macaques during the early periods after total gamma irradiation. *Radiobiologiia* 5: 494-500.

245. Varagic, V.; Stepanovic, S.; Svecenski, N.; and Hajdukovic, S. 1967. The effect of X-irradiation on the amount of catecholamines in heart atria and hypothalamus of the rabbit and in brain and heart of the rat. *Int. J. Radiat. Biol.* 12: 113-119.

246. Johnsson, J. E.; Owman, C. H.; and Sjoberg, N.-O. 1970. Tissue content of noradrenaline and 5-hydroxytryptamine in the rat after ionizing radiation. *Int. J. Radiat. Biol.* 18: 311-316.

247. Catravas, G. N., and McHale, C. G. 1973. *Activity changes of brain enzymes in rats exposed to different qualities of ionizing radiation* [Scientific Report SR73-19; NTIS AD-777-383-1]. Bethesda, MD: Armed Forces Radiobiology Research Institute.

248. Rixon, R. H., and Baird, K. M. 1968. The therapeutic effect of serotonin on the survival of X-irradiated rats. *Radiat. Res.* 33: 395-402.

249. Prasad, K. N., and Van Woert, M. H. 1967. Dopamine protects mice against whole-body irradiation. *Science* 155: 470-472.

250. Davydov, B. I. 1961. Acetylcholine metabolism on the thalamic region of the brain of dogs after acute radiation sickness. *Radiobiologiia* 1: 550-554.

251. Sabine, J. C. 1956. Inactivation of cholinesterases by gamma radiation. *Am. J. Physiol.* 187: 280-282.

252. Lundin, J.; Clemedson, C. J.; and Nelson, A. 1957. Early effects of whole-body irradiation on cholinesterase activity in guinea pig's blood with special regard to radiation sickness. *Acta Radiol.* 48: 52-64.

253. Hunt, W. A., and Dalton, T. K. 1980. Reduction in cyclic nucleotide levels in the brain after a high dose of ionizing radiation. *Radiat. Res.* 83: 210-215.

254. Catravas, G. N.; Wright, S. J.; Trocha, P. J.; and Takenaga, J. 1981. Radiation effects on cyclic AMP, cyclic GMP, and amino acid levels in the CSF of the primate. *Radiat. Res.* 87: 198-203.

255. Hawkins, R., and Forcino, D. 1988. Postradiation cardiovascular dysfunction. *Comments on Toxicology* 2: 243-252.

256. Cockerham, L. G.; Pautler, E. L.; and Hampton, J. D. 1984. Postradiation blood flow in the visual cortex of primates. *The Toxicologist* 5: 82.

257. Doyle, T. F.; Curran, C. R.; and Turns, J. E. 1974. The prevention of radiation-induced early transient incapacitation of monkeys by an antihistamine. *Proc. Soc. Exp. Biol. Med.* 145: 1018-1024.

258. Chapman, P. H., and Young, R. J. 1968. *Effect of head versus trunk fission-spectrum radiation on learned behavior in the monkey* [Technical Report TR-68-80]. Brooks Air Force Base, TX: School of Aerospace Medicine.

259. Cockerham, L. G.; Doyle, T. F.; Paulter, E. L.; and Hampton, J. D. 1986. Disodium cromoglycate, a mast-cell stabilizer, alters postradiation regional cerebral blood flow in primates. *J. Toxicol. Environ. Health* 18: 91-101.

260. Chapman, P. H., and Young, R. J. 1968. Effect of high energy x-irradiation of the head on cerebral blood flow and blood pressure in the *Macaca mulatta*. *Aerospace Med.* 3: 1316-1321.

261. Turbyfill, C. L.; Roudon, R. M.; and Kieffer, V. A. 1972. Behavior and physiology of the monkey *(Macaca mulatta)* following 2500 rads of pulse mixed gamma-neutron radiation. *Aerospace Med.* 7: 41-45.

262. Miletich, D. J., and Strike, T. A. 1970. *Alteration of postirradiation hypotension and incapacitation in the monkey by administration of vasopressor drugs* [Scientific Report SR70-1; NTIS AD-702-723]. Bethesda, MD: Armed Forces Radiobiology Research Institute.

263. Turns, J. E.; Doyle, T. F.; and Curran, C. R. 1971. *Norepinephrine effects on early post-irradiation performance decrement in the monkey* [Scientific Report SR71-16; NTIS AD-737-213]. Bethesda, MD: Armed Forces Radiobiology Research Institute.

264. Mickley, G. A.; Teitelbaum, H.; Parker, G. A.; Vieras, F.; Dennison, B. A.; and Bonney, C. H. 1982. Radiogenic changes in the behavior and physiology of the spontaneously hypertensive rat: Evidence for a dissociation between acute hypotension and incapacitation. *Aviat. Space Environ. Med.* 53: 633-638.

265. Doyle, T. F., and Strike, T. A. 1977. Radiation-released histamine in the rhesus monkey as modified by mast cell depletion and antihistamine. *Experientia* 33: 1047-1049.

266. Douglas, W. W. 1985. Histamine and 5-hydroxytryptamine (serotonin) and their antagonists. In *Goodman and Gilman's The Pharmacological Basis of Therapeutics.* 7th ed., 605-615. New York: Macmillan Publishing Co.

267. Doyle, T. F., Turns, J. E., and Strike, T. A. 1971. Effect of antihistamine on early transient incapacitation of monkeys subjected to 4000 rads of mixed gamma-neutron radiation. *Aerospace Med.* 42: 400-403.

268. Mickley, G. A. 1981. Antihistamine provides sex-specific radiation protection. *Aviat. Space Environ. Med.* 52: 247-250.

269. Alter, W. A.; Catravas, G. N.; Hawkins, R. N.; and Lake, C. R. 1984. Effect of ionizing radiation on physiological function in the anesthetized rat. *Radiat. Res.* 99: 394-409.

270. Carpenter, D. O. 1979. *Early transient incapacitation: A review with considerations of underlying mechanisms* [Scientific Report SR79-1; NTIS AD-A071-803-1]. Bethesda, MD: Armed Forces Radiobiology Research Institute.

271. Iverson, S. D., and Iverson, L. L. 1981. *Behavioral pharmacology.* New York: Oxford University Press.

272. DeRyck, M.; Schallert, T.; and Teitelbaum, P. 1980. Morphine versus haloperidol catalepsy in the rat: A behavioral analysis of postural support mechanisms. *Brain Res.* 201: 143-172.

273. Grevert, D., and Goldstein, A. 1977. Some effects of naloxone on behavior in the mouse. *Psychopharmacology* 53: 111-113.

274. Herman, B. H., and Panksepp, I. 1978. Effects of morphine and naloxone on separation distress and approach attachment: Evidence for opiate mediation of social effect. *Pharmacol. Biochem. Behav.* 9: 213-220.

275. Akil, H.; Madden, J.; Patrick, R. L., III; and Barchas, J. D. 1976. Stress-induced increase in endogenous opioid peptides: Concurrent analgesia and its reversal by naloxone. In *Opiates and Endogenous Opiate Peptides,* edited by H. W. Kosterlitz, 63. Amsterdam: Elsevier North-Holland.

276. Margules, D. L. 1979. Beta-endorphin and endoloxone: Hormones of the autonomic nervous system for the conservation of expenditure of bodily resources and energy in anticipation of famine or feast. *Neurosci. Biobehav. Rev.* 3: 155-162.

277. Katz, R. J.; Carroll, B. J.; and Baldrighi, G. 1978. Behavioral activation by enkephalins in mice. *Pharmacol. Biochem. Behav.* 8: 493-496.

278. Szekely, J. E., Ronai, A. Z., Dunai-Kovacs, Z., Bajusz, S., and Graf, L. 1977. Cross tolerance between morphine and beta-endorphin *in vivo. Life Sci.* 20: 1259-1264.

279. Brown, R. G., and Segal, D. S. 1980. Alterations in beta-endorphin-induced locomotor hyperactivity in morphine tolerant rats. *Neuropharmacology* 19: 619-621.

280. Dafny, N., and Pellis, N. R. 1986. Evidence that opiate addiction is in part an immune respose: Immune system destruction by irradiation altered opiate withdrawal. *Neuropharmacology* 25: 815-818.

281. Mickley, G. A.; Sessions, G. R.; Bogo, V.; and Chantry, K. H. 1983. Evidence for endorphin-mediated cross-tolerance between chronic stress and the behavioral effects of ionizing radiation. *Life Sci.* 33: 749-754.

282. Mickley, G. A.; Stevens, K. E.; White, G. A.; and Gibbs, G. L. 1983. Changes in morphine self-administration after exposure to ionizing radiation: Evidence for the involvement of endorphins. *Life Sci.* 33: 711-718.

283. Mickley, G. A. 1983. Ionizing radiation alters beta-endorphin-like immunoreactivity in brain but not blood. *Pharmacol. Biochem. Behav.* 19: 979-983.

284. Alter, W.; Mickley, G. A.; Catravas, G.; Mueller, G.; Keiffer, V.; Doyle, T.; and Kovski, A. Role of histamine and beta-endorphin in radiation-induced hypotension and acute performance decrement in the rat. Paper presented at the 1980 Annual Scientific Meeting of Aerospace Medical Association, Los Angeles, 225-226.

285. Danquechin-Dorval, E.; Mueller, G. P.; Eng, R. R.; Durakovic, A.; Conklin, J. J.; and Dubois, A. 1985. Effect of ionizing radiation on gastric secretion and gastric motility in monkeys. *Gastroenterology* 89: 374-380.

286. Mickley, G. A.; Stevens, K. E.; Burrows, J. M.; White, G. A.; and Gibbs, G. L. 1983. Morphine tolerance offers protection from radiogenic performance decrements. *Radiat. Res.* 93: 381-387.

287. Morse, D. E., and Mickley, G. A. 1988. Interaction of the endogenous opioid system and radiation in the suppression of appetite behavior. *Society for Neuroscience Abstracts* 14(2): 1106.

288. Shipman, T. L.; Lushbaugh, C. C.; Peterson, D. F.; Langham, W. H.; Harris, P. S.; and Lawrence, J. N. P. 1961. Acute radiation death resulting from an accidental nuclear critical excursion. *J. Occup. Med.* 3: 146-192.

289. Karas, J. S., and Stanbury, J. B. 1965. Fatal radiation syndrome from an accidental nuclear excursion. *N. Engl. J. Med.* 272: 755-761.

290. Wald, N., and Thoma, G. E. 1961. *Radiation accidents: Medical aspects of neutron and gamma ray exposure* [U.S. Atomic Energy Commission Report ORNL-2748, Part B; OCLC 12779642]. Oak Ridge, TN: Oak Ridge National Laboratory.

291. Howland, J. W.; Ingram, M.; Mermagen, H.; and Hansen, C. L. 1961. The Lockport incident: Accidental exposure of humans to large doses of X-irradiation. In *Diagnosis and Treatment of Acute Radiation Injury*, 11-26. Geneva: World Health Organization.

292. Telyatnikov, L. 1987. The top story of 1987. Paper presented at the Great American Firehouse Exposition and Muster, Baltimore, Maryland, 1987 [OCLC 18595371].

293. Young, R. Personal communication, 1987.

294. Hasterlik, R. J., and Marinelli, L. D. 1956. Physical dosimetry and clinical observations on four human beings involved in an accidental critical assembly excursion. In vol. 11, *Proceedings of the International Conference on Peaceful Uses of Atomic Energy* [OCLC 514057], 25-34. Geneva: International Atomic Energy Commission.

295. Anno, G. H.; Wilson, D. B.; and Dore, M. A. 1985. *Nuclear weapon effect research at PSR—1983: Acute radiation effects on individual crewmember performance* [Technical Report TR-85-52; NTIS AD-A166-282-4-XAB]. Washington, DC: Defense Nuclear Agency.

296. Young, R. W., and Myers, P. H. 1986. The human response to nuclear radiation. *Medical Bulletin* 43, No. 7: 20-23.

297. Baum, S. J.; Anno, G. H.; Young, R. W.; and Withers, H. R. 1985. *Nuclear weapon effect research at PSR—1983.* In vol. 10, *Symptomatology of Acute Radiation Effects in Humans After Exposure to Doses of 75 to 4500 Rads (cGy) Free-in-air* [Technical Report TR-85-50; NTIS AD-A166-280-8-XAB]. Washington, DC: Defense Nuclear Agency.

298. Franz, C. G.; Young, R. W.; and Mitchell, W. E. 1981. *Behavioral studies following ionizing radiation exposures: A data base* [Technical Report TR81-4; NTIS AD-A115-825-2]. Bethesda, MD: Armed Forces Radiobiology Research Institute.

299. Shapiro, N. I.; Nuzhdin, N. I.; and Kuzin, A. M. 1955. The action of estrogens on the radiation reaction in mice. In *Collected Works on Radiobiology*, edited by N. I. Nuzhdin [Atomic Energy Commission TR-3740; OCLC 14622095], 13-29. Moscow: USSR Academy of Science.

300. Thompson, J. S.; Reilly, R. W.; Crawford, M.; and Russe, H. P. 1965. The effect of estradiol and estriol on the survival of sublethally and lethally irradiated mice. *Radiat. Res.* 26: 567-583.

301. Giambarresi, L., and Jacobs, A. J. 1987. Radioprotectants. In *Military Radiobiology*, edited by J. J. Conklin and R. I. Walker, 265-301. Orlando FL: Academic Press, Inc.

302. Bogo, V.; Jacobs, A. J.; and Weiss, J. F. 1985. Behavioral toxicity and efficacy of WR-2721 as a radioprotectant. *Radiat. Res.* 104: 182-190.

303. Turbyfill, C. L; Roudon, R. M.; Young, R. W.; and Kieffer, V. A. 1972. *Alteration of radiation effects by 2-(n-decylamino) ethanethiolsulfuric acid (WR1607) in the monkey* [Scientific Report SR72-3; NTIS AD-745-284]. Bethesda, MD: Armed Forces Radiobiology Research Institute.

304. Williams, C. D.; Weiss, J. F.; and Bogo, V. 1987. Motor performance evaluation of behavioral toxicity in mice: Effect of radiation and radioprotective agents. *Proc. of Society of Armed Forces Medical Laboratory Scientists* 16: 25.

305. Bogo, V., and Weiss, J. F. 1987. Ability of selenium and WR-2721 to mitigate radiation-induced performance decrement in rats. *Proceedings of the 1st International Neurotoxicology Association Meeting* [OCLC 18421514], 148. Lunteren, Netherlands: International Neurotoxicology Association.

306. Landauer, M. R.; Davis, H. D.; Dominitz, J. A.; and Weiss, J. F. 1987. Dose and time relationships of the radioprotector WR-2721 on locomotor activity in mice. *Pharmacol. Biochem. Behav.* 27: 573-576.

307. Young, R. W. Acute radiation syndrome. In reference 301, 165-190.

308. Dubois, A. 1988. Effect of ionizing radiation on the gastrointestinal tract. *Comments on Toxicology* 2: 233-242.

309. Salazer, O. M.; Rubin, P.; Keller, B.; and Scarantino, C. 1978. Systemic (half body) radiation therapy: Response to toxicity. *Int. J. Radiat. Oncol. Biol. Phys.* 4: 937-950.

310. Barrett, A.; Barrett, A. J.; and Powles, R. L. 1979. Total body irradiation and marrow transplantation for acute leukemia. The Royal Marsden Hospital experience. *Pathol. Biol.* 27: 357-359.

311. Bogo, V.; Boward, C.; Fiala, N.; and Dubois, A. 1988. Zacopride: A promising radiation antiemetic. *The Toxicologist* 8(1): 77.

312. Dubois, A.; Fiala, N.; Boward, C. A.; and Bogo, V. 1988. Prevention and treatment of the gastric symptoms of radiation sickness. *Radiat. Res.* 115: 595-604.

313. Thorp, J. W.; Chaput, R. L.; and Kovacic, R. T. 1970. Performance of miniature pigs after partial body irradiation. *Aerospace Med.* 41: 379-382.

314. Thorp, J. W., and Germas, J. E. 1969. *Performance of monkeys after partial body irradiation* [Scientific Report SR69-18; NTIS AD-699-127]. Bethesda, MD: Armed Forces Radiobiology Research Institute.

315. Chapman, P. H. 1968. *Behavioral and circulatory responses to x-irradiation delivered at 200 rads per minute to whole body and trunk only* [Technical Report TR-68-111]. Brooks Air Force Base, TX: School of Aerospace Medicine.

316. Chapman, P. H., and Hurst, C. M. 1968. *The effect of head versus trunk X-irradiation on avoidance behavior in the rhesus monkey* [Technical Report TR-68-37]. Brooks Air Force Base, TX: School of Aerospace Medicine.

317. Jones, D. C.; Kimeldorf, D. J.; Castanera, T. J.; Rubadeau, D. O.; and Osborn, G. K. 1957. Effect of bone marrow therapy on the volitional activity of whole-body X-irradiated rats. *Am. J. Physiol.* 189: 21-23.

318. Bogo, V. 1988. Radiation: Behavioral implications for humans in space. *Toxicology* 49: 299-307.

319. Hunt, W. A.; Rabin, B. M.; Joseph, J. A.; Dalton, T. K.; Murray, W. E.; and Stevens, S. A. 1988. Effects of ion particles on behavior and brain function: Initial studies. In reference 86, 537-551.

320. Philpott, D. E.; Sapp, W.; Miquel, J.; Kato, K.; Corbett, R.; Stevenson, J.; Back, S.; Lindseth, K. O.; and Benton, E. V. 1985. The effect of high energy (HZE) particle radiation (^{40}Ar) on aging parameter of mouse hippocampus and retina. In vol. 3, *Scanning Electron Microscopy*, edited by A. M. F. O'Hare, 1177-1182. Chicago: SEM, Inc.

Chapter 8

PSYCHOLOGICAL FACTORS IN NUCLEAR WARFARE

G. ANDREW MICKLEY, Ph.D.*

*Lieutenant Colonel, United States Air Force; Behavioral Sciences Department, Armed Forces Radiobiology Research Institute, Bethesda, Maryland 20814-5145

INTRODUCTION

The psychological casualties of a nuclear conflict may seem to be insignificant compared to the casualties from physical trauma, but they can dramatically alter the outcome of a battle. The neuropsychiatric casualties of World War II were 18%–48% of all casualties,[1,2] and they were the largest single cause of lost military personnel strength in that war.[3] The Arab-Israeli Yom Kippur War of 1973 lasted only 3 weeks, but its psychiatric casualties were 23% of all nonfatal casualties.[4] Even if neuropsychiatric trauma from intense combat does not produce a casualty, it can degrade the performance of normal duties. Slightly altered reaction times, attention, or motives may have important consequences in warfare.

DETERMINANTS OF PSYCHOLOGICAL DYSFUNCTION IN CONVENTIONAL WARFARE

Much has been learned about the origins of psychiatric casualties of war. On the most basic level, even visual representations of war evoke significant increases in sympathetic activity as indicated by increased electrodermal activity, decreased salivary function, and marked cardiac changes.[5] These changes in physiology are correlated with higher scores on psychological measures of stress. However, laboratory measurements significantly oversimplify the array of variables that coproduce a particular behavioral and psychological outcome. These variables include the intensity and duration of the battle, the leadership and cohesiveness of the group, the availability of information and ability or inability to communicate it, physical strain, individual expectations, experience, and morale.

Intensity of the Battle

The most important precipitating factor affecting the rate of neuropsychiatric casualties is the battle's intensity or the current degree of stress.[2,6] Combat is usually episodic, but the effect of combat stress is often cumulative. An analysis of three infantry battalions in the Sicilian campaign of World War II revealed that the number of casualties from physical wounds remained relatively constant over the 17 days studied, but the number of psychiatric casualties steadily increased.[2]

Group Characteristics

Morale, group leadership, and cohesiveness are also good predictors of neuropsychiatric casualties.[1] In a study completed after the 1973 Yom Kippur War, the Israelis revealed that 40% of the soldiers with battle shock reported minimal group cohesion and unit identification, as well as a high incidence of interpersonal difficulties with members of their units. In contrast, only 10% of the soldiers not suffering battle shock reported these unit problems.[4] Psychologically impaired persons were also more likely to have changed teams in combat (63%) than were the control population who experienced no psychological difficulties (15%).[7] These data suggest that strong, stable groups play an important role in preserving the individual's psychological stability in combat.

Duration of the Battle

Expectations about the duration of hostilities affect the psychiatric casualty rate. A decided decrease in neuropsychiatric casualties occurred in the European theater of World War II toward the end of hostilities in 1945. Conversely, the low psychiatric casualty rate of the British soldiers has been attributed, in part, to the British policy of long tours of duty. Believing there was little chance of relief, the soldiers knew that they would have to hold on.[2]

Physical Strain

The terms "combat fatigue" and "combat exhaustion," widely used in the past, indicated that a lack of sleep, lack of food, and other fatiguing properties of combat played an important role in psychiatric breakdown. This impression was supported when psychological symptoms were often partially relieved by sleep and food. Although this suggested that physical fatigue precipitates psychiatric illness, it is now clear that fatigue itself is not the primary cause of psychiatric breakdown. Units advancing against slight enemy opposition may continue without sleep or food for several days, and although the unit members may suffer physical fatigue, they rarely show psychiatric symptoms. A low incidence of psychiatric casualties is also associated with long retreats.[2] Finally, typical psychiatric symptoms may appear early in combat or even prior to battle, before the occurrence of appreciable physical fatigue.[8-10]

Consequences of Incapacitation

Neuropsychiatric casualty rates in wartime tend to be low when the soldier perceives that becoming a casualty either causes additional harm or produces no important advantage. This was the case during the German retreat at Stalingrad when the fleeing Germans feared capture by the Russians. Neuropsychiatric casualties frequently occur after rather than during a battle, when the fate of an incapacitated person is uncertain.[2]

Expectations of the Culture

Expectations of the group or the culture may also influence psychiatric casualty rates. The incidence of psychiatric casualties was low in both the American and South Vietnamese armies during the Vietnam War, but the total number of cases admitted (during a 6-month period) to U.S. hospitals was almost double the number admitted to South Vietnamese hospitals, despite the fact that the total population at risk was considerably larger for the South Vietnamese. Some authors have attributed this to the constraints on some psychiatric diagnoses in the Vietnamese culture.[11]

A similar situation occurred in the Korean War. Early in the war, when most Republic of Korea troops and their officers were relatively untrained and new to combat, it was expected that psychiatric casualties would be high. However, this was not the case, because such behavior was not culturally acceptable. Later in the war, when Korean soldiers were integrated into American units, they incurred psychiatric breakdowns with the same frequency and symptoms as their American comrades.[10]

Finally, anxiety states were far less common in Indian soldiers than in British soldiers fighting side by side during the Arakan campaign in Burma in 1943–1944. The Indian soldiers may have felt as anxious as their British comrades, but they could not admit it; their culture dictated that they enjoy battle, and it was a point of honor to do so. The Indian soldier could deal with anxiety only by denying its existence, by using a magical charm, or by self-inflicting a wound (which released him with honor intact). If these methods were not feasible, the Indian soldier might break into exuberant hysterical behavior similar to the accepted religious displays of his culture; this released tension and entailed no social stigma.[3]

Communication

The way in which soldiers respond in any situation depends on how they perceive it; how they perceive it depends on the information they have about it. A person who is uninformed in a complex, chaotic situation will be under great stress. Disruption of communications during warfare may produce sufficient anxiety and fear to degrade performance.[2] Reduced communication can also impose significant psychological stress in a nuclear conflict. [12]

NUCLEAR WARFARE VERSUS CONVENTIONAL WARFARE

The debate continues over the expected differences between the psychological changes produced by conventional war and those produced by nuclear war. Experts at a recent symposium on the psychological effects of tactical nuclear warfare agreed that differences would exist, but there was considerable disagreement over whether the differences would be quantitative, qualitative, or both. With a quantitative difference, more combatants would experience higher levels of fear, stress, and confusion, resulting in a greater number of neuropsychiatric casualties. However, if the differences are qualitative, the soldiers might experience completely different psychological symptoms, and a new and different response to the stress of war might emerge.[13]

Nuclear weapons have the power to produce such devastation that the apparent unreality of the detonation's aftermath may differentiate a nuclear battle from a conventional battle. A modern warhead can produce an explosion measured in megatons. Two megatons is roughly equal to the explosive output of all bombs dropped during World War II.[14] A Japanese survivor of the nuclear detonation at Hiroshima described a scene illustrative of the severity of the nuclear battlefield:

> I had to cross the river to reach the station. As I came to the river and went down the bank to the water, I found that the stream was filled with dead bodies. I started to cross by crawling over the corpses, on my hands and knees. As I got about a

> third of the way across, a dead body began to sink under my weight and I went into the water, wetting my burned skin. It pained severely. I could go no further, as there was a break in the bridge of corpses, so I turned back to the shore, and started to walk upstream, hoping to come upon another way across.[15]

Both nuclear and conventional weapons produce blast and thermal effects, but ionizing radiations are unique to nuclear weapons. Radiation effects may have caused as many as 15%–20% of the deaths at Hiroshima and Nagasaki.[16] The insidious and lethal nature of radiation makes it especially feared. In 1951, Brigadier General James Cooney worried about his soldiers' ability to function in a nuclear battle, because radiation associated with the atomic bomb was believed by many to "cause immediate and mysterious injury or death."[17] Despite our current knowledge about radiation effects, these beliefs are still pervasive. The 1979 nuclear reactor accident at Three Mile Island produced almost no radiation exposure above normal background levels, but the public believed that a radiation hazard was present, which evoked long-term signs of emotional, behavioral, and physiological stress.[18]

The psychological reactions to nuclear warfare have an added dimension, namely, anxiety that the human species will be annihilated. People achieve symbolic immortality by identifying with their children, grandchildren, and larger cultural units, such as their nation or religion.[19] Unlike all the past wars, in a strategic nuclear war we will not be able to sacrifice ourselves so that our children, family, or nation can survive. This loss of assurance of a future for humanity may result in emotional changes that differ from those during a conventional war.[20]

The psychological changes in persons exposed to nuclear weapons will partially coincide with those seen in other disasters. But the magnitude and type of destruction from a nuclear weapon will probably (at least) intensify most psychological reactions. By 1945, the people of Japan were accustomed to destruction from conventional bombing. However, the atomic bomb effects were new and vastly more horrible, eliciting more extreme psychological reactions in the residents of Hiroshima and Nagasaki who responded to the U.S. Strategic Bombing Survey several years later.[21] Still debatable is the question of qualitative differences in the psychological responses to different types of natural disasters and other stressful events. Psychological symptom complexes may differ, depending on the nature of the disaster.[22] In some studies, the psychological morbidity is clearly defined by diagnostic criteria, such as those identified for post-traumatic stress disorder, anxiety, or depression. Other studies address a more nonspecific psychological distress reaction. Symptom clusters and perhaps specific somatic complaints may be specifically related to particular types of disasters.[22] It would not be surprising if in-depth studies reveal that some components of stress reactions are more likely to be expressed during nuclear conflicts than during conventional warfare or natural disasters.[1,23,24]

PSYCHOLOGY IN TODAY'S NUCLEAR MILIEU

When a person is faced with the horror of nuclear warfare, the responses are fairly predictable: fear, dread, and finally denial. It has been suggested that the levels of fear and anxiety in the world's population have been substantially increased by the prospect of nuclear annihilation. In 1984, Gallup surveyed 514 teenagers (ages 13–18), as a representative national cross section, on the likelihood of the occurrence of nuclear confrontations in their lifetimes.[25] Fifty-one percent indicated that it was "somewhat likely" that a nuclear war would be started during their lifetimes, and 15% thought it was "very likely." Other surveys by direct interview or questionnaire have been conducted in the United States, the Soviet Union, and elsewhere.[26-28] Although the methodology of some studies has been questioned,[29] their results indicate that many youngsters, particularly from white-collar families, are troubled by the prospect of nuclear war. They have fears about the future, and view their futures less hopefully than previous generations did.

Adults appear to be much more complacent about the threat of nuclear war.[30] For example, the movie *The Day After*, depicting a nuclear war and its aftermath, was shown on network television in the United States in November 1983. The film received extensive publicity and a large audience viewed it. Mental-health professionals anticipated that the program would generate significant distress in viewers, so they publicized the crisis services that were to be available during and after the broadcast. The Massachusetts Psychological Association had 25 volunteers standing by telephones across the state. Not a single call was received.[20]

Much has been said and written about the apparent apathy of the adult population to the prospect of nuclear self-destruction. Psychic numbing, denial, and other psychological techniques have been proposed as reasons. Despite the horrible possibilities of war, remaining relatively unworried and inactive may not be irrational if people are correct in judging that their activities have no consequence.[31] For example, the citizens of the District of Columbia ("ground zero") decided by referendum in 1982 that devising a civil defense strategy would be a waste of time.[32]

It is often difficult to distinguish between a lack of concern about nuclear war and an active denial of it.[33] Since children worry about nuclear war and adults generally do not, the process of active denial is suggested. Furthermore, nuclear war is easy to deny. It is an abstract concept, and we have no experience of it. Many other urgent, immediate things compete for our attention. People seem less motivated by abstract fears than by immediate benefits (life insurance, for example, is sold not on the basis of fear of the future, but rather on the basis of more security today).[30] Denial as a psychological defense may be comforting, but it has its dangers. This trend, thought by some also to exist in the U.S. military,[24] could significantly affect the way one prepares for and functions in a nuclear conflict.[17]

LIMITATIONS TO THE CURRENT DISCUSSION

The circumstances of a tactical nuclear war will dramatically affect predictable psychological outcomes.[34] A strategic exchange of nuclear weapons would be expected to produce more devastation and cause more dramatic emotional changes in survivors than would a single local detonation. But the psychological changes from a tactical nuclear war are not expected to be simple, straightforward, or minor. One study of predictable troop reactions to a tactical nuclear battle identified specific psychological outcomes to be expected at different times (periods of shock, informal organization, formal organization, and rehabilitation) and distances (zones of destruction, heavy damage, light damage, and periphery) from the nuclear weapon's detonation.[35] The study contains a detailed hypothesis on the spectrum of possible psychological changes in nuclear combatants. This chapter, however, is limited to a general overview of the acute and chronic psychological symptoms that can be expected in soldiers actively involved in a tactical nuclear battle.

No definitive data speak directly to the issue of human psychological responses to radiation exposure or use of nuclear weapons. Experiences of nuclear accident victims have usually been poorly documented regarding mental alterations. Patients who are exposed to ionizing radiation as part of cancer treatment also frequently receive drugs to suppress the side effects and enhance the effectiveness of the radiation. These patients are usually quite sick even before the radiation therapy, so it is difficult to assess the psychological effects of the radiation itself.

A research model for psychological reactions to the nuclear battle has been established by assuming that the reactions are similar to those observed after an intense conventional battle or a natural disaster, such as a flood or earthquake. Although this approach has merit, it also has a number of problems.[36] In particular, the stress of ionizing radiation exposure is missing, with its unique characteristics and implications to those exposed. Persons exposed to radiation on a nuclear battlefield may have little or no initial knowledge of the severity of their radiogenic injuries. This uncertainty, and each individual's interpretation of it, may affect the emotions and ability to perform. These models also ignore the direct radiogenic changes in the CNS, which may also alter the psychological variables.

The data derived from the atomic bombings of Japan are flawed, in part, because the population was predominately civilian. Civilians may or may not react to the use of nuclear weapons in the same way a military force might. Because this was the first use of an atomic bomb, the element of surprise was great. Many of the Japanese citizens were unaware at first that radiation was present. In addition, the radiation doses actually received by persons in Hiroshima and Nagasaki were not well described.

Although the Japanese data are limited, they are too important to ignore. The bombings of Hiroshima and Nagasaki provide the only available data on the combined results of blast, thermal, and radiation insults to a large human population. Some military personnel were present in both cities during the bombings, and provided a few examples of military actions in a nuclear environment.[37] Although data derived from other wars and disasters are not perfect, they can also give clues to the psychological factors in nuclear conflict.

RADIOGENIC CNS CHANGES AND PSYCHOLOGICAL VARIABLES

One aspect of the psychological effects of nuclear weapons that has received little attention is the direct interaction of nervous tissue and radiation. Since the brain is the seat of emotion, ionizing radiation exposure may be capable of directly influencing psychological changes. Especially relevant here are *(a)* data suggesting that the CNS is sensitive to changes induced by ionizing radiation exposure, and *(b)* data suggesting that radiation can change psychological variables in nonhuman animals.

Neurons were once thought to be relatively radioresistant, based on data from studies measuring cell death rather than disruption of cell functioning.[38] More current studies are revising these ideas. Developing cells are particularly sensitive to the lethal effects of ionizing radiation. The adult neurogenesis that takes place in some brain areas in certain animals suggests that these nuclei may be damaged by much lower doses of ionizing radiation (less than 4 Gy) than previously expected.[39] Changes in the amplitude and frequency of EEG recordings occur after 1–4 Gy of X rays,[38] and doses as low as 0.008 Gy can change the spontaneous electrical discharges of hippocampal pacemaker-like neurons.[40] Metabolic alterations of the neurotransmitter dopamine have been reported in the brain after 10 Gy of cobalt-60 radiation.[41] Levels of the putative neuromodulator beta-endorphin also change in irradiated mice and monkeys at doses that do not kill neurons.[42] Neuronal sodium channels may lose their ability to respond properly to stimulation after only 1 Gy of high-energy electrons.[43] Thus, a growing body of evidence suggests that ionizing radiation may alter neural physiology and function at doses substantially below those required to produce morphological changes and neuronal death. It would not be surprising if psychological changes correlate with these changes in brain function.

Acute Psychological Changes

Evidence suggests that emotional variables can be influenced by radiation exposure. It may be possible to study this component of the psychological effects of irradiation by reviewing some of the work done in laboratory animals. The validity of using animals in this kind of work has been detailed elsewhere.[44] This approach has the disadvantage of ignoring (for the moment) some of the psychogenic aspects of a reaction to a nuclear confrontation, but it has the advantage of being able to control the radiation dose and the testing of behavior. The animal data apparently reinforce much of the anecdotal human data from the Japanese experience.

This section addresses the range of psychological phenomena likely to be observed during the first minutes and hours of a nuclear battle, based on both human and experimental animal data. The time course of these acute changes is in question, and the changes may extend for days after the conflict.

Motivation. Motivation may be altered after ionizing radiation exposure. An animal's tendency to perform is governed by a number of factors, including the physical capacity of the animal, rewards or punishments present, and the animal's perception of these reinforcements. If an experimental subject has the capacity to perform in the presence of previously motivating stimuli but does not do so, then it may be inferred that some change in the subject's motivation has occurred. For example, after irradiation, rats will decrease the number of times they press a bar that, when struck, gives them some information about when shock will occur.[45] However, they significantly increase the number of times they press a bar to delay footshock. These data suggest that the animal is fully capable of pressing the bar, but chooses to do so only under certain conditions.

Another study supports this concept. Rats will work in order to receive electrical stimulation of particular brain areas.[46] In one rat, electrodes were implanted into two brain areas (lateral hypothalamus and septum). Before irradiation, the subject pressed the bar at the same rate to activate either site. After irradiation, the animal worked to stimulate only the lateral hypothalamus. Clearly, the animal had the physical capacity to perform the task, but its motivation was altered after irradiation, producing a selective decrease in responding to septal stimulation. These data suggest that motivation may, in some cases, be more radiosensitive than physical capacity.

Some observations have been made about curiosity and investigative behaviors after radiation exposure. Chimpanzees given 3.75–4.0 Gy of gamma radiation made fewer attempts to solve a variety of puzzles. This deficit seems to be independent of changes in capacity, because measures of dexterity and strength were unchanged in these same animals.[47] In another experiment, pairs of monkeys were irradiated with 4 Gy of whole-body X radiation.[48] Twice daily, continuous observations of home-cage behavior were made during a 10-minute period in accordance with a checklist. In order to control for any debilitation factor, the number of instances of each category of behavior was divided by the total number of times that any identifiable behavior occurred in that same period. In these animals, a reliable deficit in curiosity was measured by the reduced relative frequency of manipulating inanimate objects. The monkeys exhibited relatively more cage-directed movements (toward well-known stimuli) and less attention and orienting to incidental novel noises. They selected food in their central line of sight, rarely chosing food from the periphery. Furthermore, when attempts were made to distract them, they were less likely to orient to the stimuli than were the controls. Because this procedure attempted to factor out general malaise, the results suggested reduced levels of curiosity and attention in the animals.[49,50] These observations agree with others in which irradiated monkeys showed increased performance of tasks that placed a premium on attention to a known site of food reward. Conversely, the monkeys showed reduced performance of tasks that required attention to stimuli in the periphery of vision.[48]

The data from Hiroshima and Nagasaki suggest that a similar change in motivation may occur in humans exposed to the trauma of a nuclear detonation. The defensive mechanism of "psychic numbing" or "psychic closing off" was observed in the atomic bomb victims.[19] One writer described this scene:

> Those who were able walked silently toward the suburbs in the distant hills, their spirits broken, their initiative gone. When asked whence they came, they pointed toward the city and said "that way;" and when asked where they were going, pointed away from the city and said, "this way." They were so broken and confused that they moved and behaved like automatons.
>
> Their reactions astonished outsiders who reported with amazement the spectacle of long files of people holding stolidly to a narrow, rough path when close by was a smooth, easy road going in the same direction. The outsiders could not grasp the fact that they were witnessing the exodus of a people who walked in the realm of dreams.[51]

These data are consistent with others from Hiroshima reporting "fatigue," "mental weakness," "spiritual desolation," or "closing off."[37] Certainly, in the case of these atomic-bomb survivors, this change in motivation cannot be solely attributed to a dose of radiation. These people had just witnessed the devastation of their homes and, in many cases, the deaths of family members. Thus, it is very likely that these behavioral and psychological changes may have a psychogenic component, which may compound the radiation-induced alterations described above in laboratory animals.

Despite the emotional deadening and "mental weakness" reported by almost everyone influenced by the bombing of Hiroshima, it is remarkable how much physical activity was exhibited by some of the survivors. Some of this activity seemed ill directed:

> There was no organized activity. The people seemed stunned by the catastrophe and rushed about as jungle animals suddenly released from a cage. Some few apparently attempted to help others from the wreckage, particularly members of their family. . . . However, many injured were left trapped beneath collapsed buildings as people fled by them in the streets.[52]

This account of frantic activity raises the issue of panic. Was there mass panic after the dropping of the atomic bomb? Probably not. Although several isolated instances of aimless and hysterical activity have been reported, these did not seem to be typical behaviors. Disaster victims are extremely concerned about how the disaster will affect the things and persons they value. They want to know what has happened to those they hold dear, and they want to help them if necessary. This concern often leads to a great deal of activity, which may appear to an observer as irrational and disorganized. Thus, the very rational and deliberate flight of people from an area of danger (a highly adaptive behavior) is often mistakenly described as panic.[35] Reports from the U.S. Army (which interviewed the survivors of the bombing)[21] did not support the claim that a sizable portion of the population behaved in an ineffective, nonsocial, or nonrational way.[53] The report also clearly indicated that many people felt terrified or fearful, even though they did not exhibit panic reactions. In only a few cases can one surmise from interviews that individuals might have exhibited uncontrolled emotional behavior. Instead, compliant, subdued behaviors were more prominent, perhaps mediated in part by some radiogenic CNS effects or other injuries:

> Many, although injured themselves, supported relatives who were worse off. Almost all had their heads bowed, looked straight ahead, were silent, and showed no expression whatsoever.[52]

It seems that a depressed motivational state, rather than panic, was a typical reaction to the disaster.

Obviously, either a chaotic or an apathetic response

to a bombing would not be adaptive in a military environment. Some evidence exists that inhabitants of Hiroshima who had a specific job to perform or a goal to meet tried valiantly to do so after the bombing. A group of wounded soldiers was observed gamely attempting to struggle out of the disaster area in military formation:

> At Misasa Bridge, they encountered a long line of soldiers making a bizarre forced march away from the Chugoku Regional Army Headquarters in the center of the town. All were grotesquely burned, and they supported themselves with staves or leaned on one another.[37]

One account of a young Japanese soldier is particularly relevant here:

> We were under military order to return to our unit immediately in case of any attack or emergency, so I returned almost without thinking.... At first I couldn't get through . . . so in the evening I started out again. This time I didn't try to help anyone but just walked through them. I was worried about the Army camp because according to what people told me, it had simply gone up in flames and disappeared. I was also a bit ashamed about having taken such a long time to return. But when I finally got back to camp, just about everyone was dead—so there was no one to scold me.... Next thing I did was to look for the ashes of the military code book—since we had a military order to look for this book even if it were burned, as it was a secret code which had to be protected. Finally I located the ashes of the book, and wrapped them in a furoshiki and carried this around with me. I wanted to take it to the military headquarters as soon as possible, but when I finally did take it there in the morning, the officer scolded me for doing such a stupid thing. . . I was fresh from the Military Academy and my head was full of such regulations.[54]

Some of these phenomena may be explained by *attentional focusing*, a behavior similar to that which was exhibited by irradiated laboratory animals. These people tended to focus on a particular aspect of their environment and to pursue it, sometimes to an illogical or inappropriate end. The soldier above pursued his assigned task, ignoring the fact that the nuclear detonation had totally changed his world (a behavior that would not necessarily be discouraged by military commanders). Thus, although a generalized decrease in motivation may have occurred in much of the Hiroshima population, some behaviors directed toward a well-defined goal apparently persisted after the catastrophe.

Fear and Terror. The main reaction of the Japanese populace in the atomic-bomb target areas was "unqualified terror," fed by the horror of the destruction and suffering either witnessed or experienced by the survivors.[21] Sixty-three percent of all respondents to the U.S. Strategic Bombing Survey reported either generalized terror or fear for one's own life. Some experiences cannot be described by cold figures:

> People were running toward our place with terrible burns. That night they slept on the road everywhere. Some collapsed during the day due to the effects of burns. People would stop by and ask for water, which was the most urgent need of these people. They were so upset that they couldn't think of food. It was a horrible sight—crying and screaming. I can't describe the burns that were on these people, and the odor of burning flesh was in the air, and it was so awful you have to see it before you can actually describe it or even talk about it. It's hard to comprehend. Some father with his entire family dead would be yelling to die, so that he would not have to live alone.[21]

Social Relations. It is of psychological and social importance that, in the extreme trauma after the atomic explosions in Japan, most people behaved in a manner compatible with established social norms.

> To Father Kleinsorge, an Occidental, the silence in the grove by a river, where hundreds of gruesomely wounded suffered together, was one of the most dreadful and awesome events of his whole experience: The hurt ones were quiet; no one wept, much less screamed in pain; no one complained; none of the many who died did so noisily; not even the children cried; very few people even spoke. And when Father Kleinsorge gave water to some whose faces had been almost blotted out by flash burns, they took their share and then raised themselves a little and bowed to him in thanks.[37]

With the disruption of individual motivation, people seemed most likely to pursue the goals established by others. Attention to leaders did not seem to be jeopardized after the detonation. For example, a victim of Hiroshima recounted:

> All the people were going in that direction and so I suppose I was taken into this movement and went with them. . . . I couldn't make any clear decision in a specific way . . . so I followed the other people. . . . I lost myself and was carried away.[54]

Various cultures may differ on the issue of conformity. But if we can generalize from these data, we can expect the social structure to be maintained after a nuclear conflict.

Learning and Memory. The results of animal studies are consistent with the hypothesis that functions of learning and memory may be altered by some doses of radiation. For example, rabbits learned to associate a tone and a light with apnea produced by inhaling ammonia vapor.[39] Once this classically conditioned response was established, the tone and light alone produced apnea. However, after irradiation (15 Gy), the conditioned response was absent or considerably reduced in duration. In contrast, the apnea produced by the ammonia itself was enhanced after radiation exposure (confirming that the animal was still capable of this response). Retrograde amnesia has also been reported in rats exposed to rapid, low doses (0.1 Gy) of electrons.[55]

Interviews with people exposed to radiation at Hiroshima indicated few cases of acute retrograde amnesia in the population.[52] However, 5 years after the detonation, deficits in memory and intellectual capacity were noted in persons who had experienced radiation sickness.[56] Acute radiogenic impairments of memory in the human have also been reported in the Soviet literature.[57]

Chronic Psychological Reactions

The initial reactions to a nuclear weapon detonation may be quite different from reactions that occur after weeks, months, or years. Psychogenic changes in emotionality, personality, and somatic effects usually take a period of time to be expressed fully. Studies of psychological symptoms in various cultures after the death of a loved one reveal that reactions to grief are seldom completed in less than 1 or 2 years. The more severe or complicated the loss or injury in a disaster, the more extended the reaction time may be.[58] These data suggest that significant chronic psychological dysfunctions may occur in nuclear combatants.

Psychoses. Serious psychological derangements involving distorted perceptions of reality and thought were rare after the atomic-bomb detonations, just as they were after the large-scale conventional bombings of World War II.[59] The incidence of psychosis (mainly schizophrenia) in military populations is similar in peace and war.[10] This is confirmed by evidence that a variety of traumatic situations are not associated with an increased rate of psychosis. For example, massive aerial bombardment of population centers in England, Germany, and Japan during World War II did not produce an increased number of psychoses, as indicated by mental-hospital admission records. Similarly, psychoses do not usually result from spontaneous civil disasters (such as hurricane, tornado, or fire).[60] It appears that psychoses are not the result of external danger. When units new to combat are exposed to severe battle stress, they frequently exhibit severe behavioral disorganization and disorientation, hallucinations, and even mute, catatonia-like states. These conditions are transient and usually subside in 1–3 days to become typical cases of neurosis.

Neuroses. Neurotic reactions to the traumas of nuclear combat are to be expected. Among 7,297 patients exposed to ionizing radiation during the atomic bombings of Japan, 533 patients had neurosis-like symptoms.[56] The patients were divided into two groups: those with symptoms of atomic-bomb radiation illness and those without. Neurosis-like symptoms were twice as common in the former group as in the latter. The Japanese researchers pointed out that some of these cases were recognizable as "pure neuroses" caused by psychogenic factors (other than the bombings), but that others could be caused by functional disorders of brain or body due to radiation. Not surprisingly, the more severe the symptoms of atomic-bomb radiation illness, the stronger the neuropsychiatric aftereffects. The common symptoms included weariness, lack of spirit, a tendency toward introversion, and poor memory.

Post-Traumatic Stress Disorder. Seeing large numbers of burned, cut, and maimed bodies was a major source of emotional trauma after the bombing of Hiroshima. Many survivors located a short distance from the center of the explosion received two emotional shocks: the first from the physical impact of the explosion, and the second after they ran out into the streets and saw so many casualties. Among those at the periphery who escaped the full physical violence of the explosion, the first emotional impact seems to have occurred when they saw the streams of injured victims pouring out of the destroyed areas. Apparently, it was not only the large number of casualties but also the specific character of the injuries (particularly the grossly altered physical appearance of persons with severe burns) that produced emotional disturbances in the people who saw them.[54] For example,

> I walked past Hiroshima station . . . and saw people with their bowels and brains coming out. . . I saw an old lady badly burned and carrying a suckling infant in her arms . . . I saw many children . . . with dead mothers. . . . I just cannot put into words the horror I felt.[54]

Post-traumatic stress disorders (PTSD) are seen after a variety of natural disasters[61] and should be expected after the shock of a nuclear conflict.[62] The full PTSD syndrome is a cluster of symptoms occurring after exposure to unpredictable life-threatening environmental trauma.[63] Sufferers of chronic PTSD continue to live in the emotional environment of the traumatic event, with prolonged vigilance for and sensitivity to external threat. The five principal features of PTSD are *(a)* persistence of startle responses and irritability, *(b)* proclivity to react explosively, *(c)* fixation on the trauma, *(d)* constriction of the general level of personality functioning, and *(e)* an atypical dream life.

A numbing of responsiveness, reduced involvement with the external world, and constricted affect are part of the diagnostic criteria established for PTSD.[64] Long-term depressive reactions with these characteristics have been reported to occur after catastrophic natural disasters, such as floods.[65] Depression is one of the prominent symptoms observed in soldiers during the extreme stresses of combat.[2] Although acute depression (evidenced by weakness and lethargy) characterized much of the Hiroshima population for a few days after the bombing, it is difficult to say if significant numbers of people experienced chronic depression. Although individual questionnaire responses from Hiroshima residents seemed to describe a depressive reaction in many cases, statistical analyses revealed no greater incidence of depression there than in other Japanese cities.[52] This may be misleading, however, because postwar apathy seemed to characterize most of the population of Japan. Chronic depressive reactions have been known to follow a variety of traumas, so they are not exclusive characteristics of nuclear disasters.

Anxiety and Phobias. In view of the horrors of the nuclear detonations in Japan, it is not surprising that severe anxiety persisted for many days and sometimes for weeks and months, according to various sources.[21] One of the most frequent types of sustained emotional disturbance appears to have been a phobia-like fear of exposure to another traumatic disaster. This reaction consisted of strong feelings of anxiety and exaggerated efforts to ward off new threats. A physician in Hiroshima wrote:

> Whenever a plane was seen after that, people would rush into their shelters. They went in and out so much that they did not have time to eat. They were so nervous they could not work.[52]

Another author described the following: "It began to rain. . . . The drops grew abnormally large, and someone [in the evacuation area] shouted, 'The Americans are dropping gasoline. They're going to set fire to us!' "[37]

Further indications of sustained apprehension in Hiroshima came from the anxiety-laden rumors reported to circulate during the postdisaster period.[52] For example, one woman reported:

> I heard that people who had not been wounded and seemed to be all right would begin feeling out of sorts and all of a sudden drop dead. It made me panicky. Here I was bustling around now, but I might go off myself.[52]

Most of the survivors had never heard of radiation sickness and were unprepared for its manifestation. During the weeks following the atomic explosions, many survivors began to exhibit signs of organic pathology: loss of hair, high fever, excessive fatigue, hemorrhagic spots under the skin, and other severe symptoms of what we now recognize as ARS. Witnessing the agonizing deaths of children and relatives probably touched off or reinforced rumors and sustained the fear reactions created by the disaster.[52]

Rumors may play a significant part in any future nuclear combat. Communication on the nuclear battlefield will be disturbed by electronic warfare tactics and by the spreading of deliberate misinformation by the enemy. Negative rumors can be expected in any population if radiation is a perceived threat.[66]

Survivor Guilt. Although the adherence to social customs seemed to be strong after the atomic bombings, not everyone acted in a completely altruistic fashion. It was impossible to do so, given the sheer number of casualties. Some people fought fires and fed the hungry, but most people (especially those who did not work in the helping or service professions) restricted their assistance, when they could give it, to people they knew: "Under many houses, people screamed for help, but no one helped; in general, survivors . . . assisted only their relatives or immediate neighbors, for they could not comprehend or tolerate a wider circle of misery."[59] As one survivor summarized, "The idea of 'love thy neighbor as thyself' that I always believed in, had disappeared some place. I guess it was too much for any of us."[67] Persistent survivor guilt may be an inevitable consequence of atomic bombing. People in the heart of the city were able to survive only by running away from the fires without stopping to rescue others. People who were in a position to give aid could not simultaneously perform all the duties and obligations of rescuing the wounded, rushing to their own families, assisting neighbors, carrying out their civil defense assignments, saving valuable materials at the offices or factories where they worked, preserving treasured household articles, and so on. Although independent observations indicate that some survivors experienced temporary guilt reactions following the atomic bombings, no satisfactory evidence supports the claim that such reactions persisted in large numbers of survivors or for very long periods of time.[52]

Psychosomatic Symptoms. Some patients may have had a psychosomatic "atomic bomb neurosis," in which the survivor's identification with the dead and maimed initiates a vicious psychosomatic circle.[36] Such a survivor is likely to associate the mildest everyday injury or sickness with possible radiation effects, and anything that could relate to radiation effects becomes associated with death:

> Frankly speaking, even now I have fear.... Even today people die in the hospitals from A-bomb disease, and [when I hear about this] I worry that I too might sooner or later have the same thing happen to me. . . . I have a special feeling that I am different from ordinary people . . . that I have a mark of wounds—as if I were a cripple. . . . It is not a matter of lacking something externally, but rather something like a handicap—something mental that does not show—the feeling that I am mentally different from ordinary people . . . so when I hear about people who die from atomic bomb disease or who have operations because of this illness, then I feel that I am the same kind of person as they. . . .[54]

Thus, combatants involved in a nuclear battle may "share" physical symptoms of radiation sickness. This adoption of symptoms may be due, in part, to not understanding their disorders and also to anxiety about the lethal effects of radiation exposure. Physicians may be caught in a conflict between the humanitarian provision of medical care and the danger of encouraging the development in survivors of hypochondria, general weakness, and dependency.

SUMMARY OF PSYCHOLOGICAL EFFECTS

Although the atomic bomb experience in Japan is the best model available, it is difficult to determine how much information this model and correlated animal data can provide on the psychological changes in a military nuclear confrontation. All psychological effects (like all physiological effects) are dependent on the dose of radiation received; the distance from ground zero (and correlated blast and thermal effects); and the indefinable personal, psychological, and social background of the potential nuclear victim. However, if we can assume a certain degree of congruity between the psychological response of the Japanese and the expected response of military personnel, the following summary may apply.

With ionizing radiation exposure will come alteration of CNS physiology, which in turn may bring about acute behavioral and psychological changes, such as a generalized reduction of motivation. There may also be symptoms of lethargy and fatigue, which will inhibit the likelihood of generalized panic. Persons will still be able to take direction, but the capacities to learn and remember may be changed. The horrible wounding and destruction produced by a nuclear weapon could be expected to have immediate psychological effects on the military personnel who observe them. If they react like the citizens of Hiroshima, they will be fearful and anxious, perhaps even more so than during a conventional conflict. These symptoms may be heightened by rumor and by any misinformation about the threat. Group cohesion will contribute to the likelihood of altruistic behaviors, but self-preservation may be a more compelling need for many. Social order (military protocol) will probably remain intact in many cases. Longer-term psychological reactions may include phobias, PTSD, depression, and various psychosomatic symptoms. Guilt concerning questions of personal survival and inadequacies in performance could contribute to the development of neurotic symptoms, as will the severity of physical wounding. Psychotic reactions are probably less likely to occur.

PREDICTION OF NEUROPSYCHIATRIC CASUALTIES

It is important to know how severely these psychological changes will affect the performance of military units or the outcome of a nuclear battle.[8,2,68] The distribution of the psychological effects of a nuclear disaster may be consistent with a normal curve.[62] Here, as in other disasters, most survivors (about 75%) would manifest a few of the symptoms described above. About half of the remaining survivors would be almost totally unaffected, and the others would show many or a high degree of acute and chronic psychological changes. If tactical nuclear weapons are used in combination with the extensive conventional arsenals that are available, then the predicted neuropsychiatric casualties in a nuclear battle would exceed those expected in a conventional conflict. Since the psychological casualties of high-intensity conventional warfare may be 18%–48% of the total casualties under certain circumstances, it can be expected that psychological factors will play a substantial role in determining the outcome of a nuclear battle.

CARE OF PSYCHOLOGICAL CASUALTIES

Some of those with minor emotional symptoms will never be seen clinically. However, the literature suggests that those who do find their way to psychological treatment should be handled in conventional ways.[2] These techniques involve the principles of *proximity*, *recency*, and *expectancy*. Individuals respond better if they receive therapy as soon as possible and as near as possible to the scene of the battle. Medical personnel should calmly accept the person's problems and regard them as a temporary incapacity, with recovery expected after a brief rest. The condition of persons with situationally induced, acute psychological disorders will worsen or improve, depending on what is expected from them by the providers.[3] In World War I, military psychiatrists came to recognize that the "shell shock" syndrome was fostered by prolonged hospitalization and then evacuation to the zone of the interior.[8] However, some British officers noticed that if the shell-shocked soldiers were treated quickly and near the front line, 70%–80% soon returned to full duty.[69] When soldiers are evacuated from the combat area, a vicious circle may be set in motion.[70] Removal from the front and admission to a hospital confirm their belief in the seriousness of their condition. Then they discover (unconsciously or consciously) that their illness is an asset that keeps them out of combat. Under these conditions, symptoms may become fixed and the soldiers may become incapacitated for further combat duty. The practice of forward therapy was developed from these observations. If combat soldiers who become neuropsychiatric casualties are not long separated from their groups and are quickly treated in the vicinity of the fighting, they can frequently rejoin their units in a few hours or days. The treatment includes some simple therapy with an interview, rest, perhaps sedation, and individual or group psychotherapy, followed by a return to duty accompanied by friends. This is combined with assurances from the medical personnel that their symptoms are natural ones that may break out in almost any soldier under enemy fire.[71] Although some of these techniques have been recently questioned,[72] they were proven to be useful as recently as the Israeli war experiences of 1973 and 1982, in which a few aggressive teams returned 95% of battle-shock cases to duty with their units.[4]

This conventional approach to treatment is effective, but a nuclear conflict will present special problems to medical personnel. One problem is the uncertainty of personal injury. Most people now realize that radiation exposure can be lethal even though initial effects may be minimal. This uncertainty about one's health after irradiation will increase the medical treatment load. It has been shown in previous studies of disasters that threats or dangers that cannot be reliably perceived by the senses can cause considerable psychological disturbance. For example, a mass poisoning of bootleg whiskey in Georgia resulted in a large number of people seeking emergency medical treatment. When tested, about 40% were unaffected by lethal alcohol; some confessed that they did not know if they were affected, but they wanted to be checked.[73] Under a current military plan, each soldier will be provided a dosimeter the size of a wristwatch before a nuclear battle, but it will be possible to read the dose only by using a heavy, bulky device at the unit's headquarters.[24] After a nuclear attack, many soldiers will wish to be reassured that they have not been exposed to appreciable levels of radiation.[73] The situation may be similar to one in World War I in which mustard and phosgene bombardments (both of which have delayed effects) were first used. For every true case of gas exposure evacuated to the field hospitals, two soldiers were evacuated who only believed they had been gassed.[24] Without information, combatants are more likely to overestimate the danger and to succumb to rumor and hysteria. This could add to the chaos that may already exist at the treatment centers.

Knowing that medical care is available has always provided comfort to combatants, but the Japanese experience[70] as well as current estimates[23,74] suggest that medical facilities will be stressed, if not overwhelmed, after a nuclear conflict. For example, burn cases place a great strain on medical personnel. Using evidence from the English experiences of World War I, the British Army Operational Research Group estimated an average time of 52 minutes for three persons to simply dress a burned hand.[75] Extrapolations from their data suggest that the requirement for treating 1,000 serious burn cases would be 5,000 health professionals and 235 tons of supplies. Based on a case in which a 38-year-old man was accidentally exposed to 2 Gy of cobalt-60 radiation, others have conservatively estimated that the cost of treating such a person would be $22,000 (in 1982 dollars). It is doubtful that such extensive care could be guaranteed to large numbers of battlefield casualties. If the medical load becomes too extensive and reasonable care cannot be given to casualties, morale will suffer. The detrimental effect of inadequate medical care on morale was noted in the Hiroshima experience, in which many medical facilities were destroyed. The care was so limited that it may have been a factor in some acute depressive reactions and feelings of helplessness following the bombing.[37,76]

In addition, the concept of removing combatants from the field for psychological treatment and then returning them better prepared to deal with the stresses of combat may be less useful in a nuclear conflict. Removal from the conventional battle allows psychological and physical healing. However, in some cases, the progressive physical radiation effects may continually erode the individual's ability to perform a task that is necessary for the success of a military mission. The efficacy of removing psychologically impaired irradiated soldiers from the battlefield with any expectation of their return is questionable.

An ethical dilemma may present itself with soldiers who are believed to have received intermediate doses of radiation that may kill them, but who can almost certainly be saved by treatment in a secure hospital setting.[24] A researcher writes,

> Should he be evacuated, and [the unit] lose a potentially effective soldier during the latent phase? Or should he be returned to duty, knowing that he has a greatly increased risk of death from disease or injury, even if not killed by enemy action, due to impaired blood clotting, wound healing, and resistance to infection?[24]

These are difficult issues. They deserve our attention now, before a nuclear weapon is used again.

PREVENTION OF PSYCHOLOGICAL CASUALTIES

Steps are available to reduce psychological problems after a nuclear confrontation. Proper training and preparedness apparently provide some degree of protection. The benefits of training are confirmed by the remarkable experiences of nine persons who survived the Hiroshima bombing and then fled to Nagasaki in time for the second atomic bomb.[15] They remembered very well what they had done that allowed them to live, and they quickly instructed others in Nagasaki:

> Yamaguchi's lecture on A-bomb precautions, he pointed out later, was not lost upon his colleagues. With the young designer's words still fresh in their minds [at the time of the second bombing] they leaped for the cover of desks and tables. "As a result," said Yamaguchi, "my section staff suffered the least in that building. In other sections there was a heavy toll of serious injuries from flying glass."[15]

In the most beneficial type of training, emphasis should be on *(a)* realism, in order to reduce the psychological shock of a nuclear confrontation, *(b)* accurate information about the threat, and *(c)* information that not only can be readily comprehended and assimilated by the average person but also can be directed toward self-preservation.[2] Recent recommendations have called for the use of a nuclear simulator in order to desensitize soldiers to the unique destructiveness of a nuclear battle.[24] The following training may help to prevent psychological casualties in a nuclear war:

> First, every soldier should be trained in methods of individual protection against atomic attack, for both the actual protection and the self-confidence which such knowledge will give. . . .
>
> Second, individual soldiers should be given training designed to enable them to reorient themselves after atomic attack. This should include training in methods of determining whether the attack involved an air or ground burst, in methods of estimating their own location with reference to the center of the disaster area, and in the use of instruments for the measurement of radioactivity.
>
> Third, individuals should be taught that they are not defenseless against atomic attack, but that they should not expect to survive such an attack without suffering severe shock effects and seeing many of their own forces killed or wounded.
>
> Fourth, individuals of all ranks should be impressed with the importance of offering all the resistance of which they are capable to ground

> assault following an atomic attack, no matter how hopeless and ineffective it may seem.
>
> Fifth, indoctrination should teach soldiers that the role of troops subjected to atomic bombing will very likely be that of delaying the enemy ground assault at all costs until relatively unharmed reserves can establish an effective defense or launch a coordinated counterattack.
>
> Sixth, all personnel should be impressed with the importance of giving absolute priority to traffic moving towards the front following an atomic attack, no matter what their own reasons for moving toward the rear may be.[35]

The forces of social cohesion will also influence the psychological and performance variables after a nuclear weapon detonation. The single most important factor that sustains soldiers in combat is the powerful psychological support of their fellows—the squad, platoon, company, and so on.[2] Isolation increases stress and also reduces the soldier's capacity to resist the effects of that stress. Various historical accounts have suggested that an isolated soldier is more likely to surrender than another member of the group who is in the same tactically hopeless situation but is still bound by the continuous ties of fighting, eating, and sleeping next to fellow soldiers.[2] Also, a significant relationship exists between a group's cohesion, its confidence in combat skills, and measures of its actual performance. The Israelis reported almost no psychiatric casualties in their elite (and cohesive) airborne forces, regardless of the intensity of combat in the 1973 Yom Kippur War.[1] The ability of the primary group to resist disintegration will greatly affect the capacity of its members to withstand the stress of a nuclear confrontation. However, we should recognize that disruption of the primary group by loss of personnel and leadership, breaks in communication, and deterioration of supply and medical care are more likely to occur in nuclear combat than in conventional confrontations.[2]

Much of the current training promotes hopelessness in our military forces and drives them further into avoidance and denial.[24] More work needs to be done to meet the training needs outlined above and to prepare for the expected psychological reactions to the use of nuclear weapons.

REFERENCES

1. Marlowe, D. H. 1982. Cohesion, anticipated breakdown, and endurance in battle: Considerations for severe and high intensity combat. Paper prepared at Walter Reed Army Institute of Research, Washington, DC.

2. Vineberg, R. 1965. *Human factors in tactical nuclear combat* [TR65-2 (Contract DA 44-188-ARO-2)]. Alexandria, VA: Human Resources Research Office, George Washington University.

3. Mandelbaum, D. G. 1954. Psychiatry in military society. *Human Organiz.* 13: 5-15.

4. Belenky, G. L.; Tyner, C. F.; and Sodetz, F. J. 1983. Israeli battle shock casualties: 1973 and 1982 [WRAIR Report Number NP-83-003; NTIS AD-A133-359-0]. Washington, DC: Walter Reed Army Institute of Research.

5. Steele, K., and Cox, T. 1986. Psychological and physiological reactions to visual representations of war. *Int. J. Psychophysiol.* 3: 237-252.

6. Vineberg, R. 1987. A preliminary model for predicting probable effects of stress on performance on the tactical nuclear battlefield. In *Proceedings of the Defense Nuclear Agency Symposium/Workshop on the Psychological Effects of Tactical Nuclear Warfare* [DNA-TR-87-209; NTIS AD-A194-754-8-XAB], edited by R. W. Young, 3.1-3.12. Washington, DC: Defense Nuclear Agency.

7. Gal, R. Yesterday's conventional warfare—tomorrow's nuclear warfare? Lessons from the Israeli experience. In reference 6, 6.1-6.66.

8. Glass, A. J. 1951. Combat exhaustion. *U.S. Armed Forces Med. J.* 2: 1471-1478.

9. Glass, A. J. 1956. Psychological considerations in atomic warfare. *U.S. Armed Forces Med. J.* 7: 625-639.

10. Glass, A. J. 1957. Observations upon the epidemiology of mental illness in troops during warfare. In *Proceedings of the Symposium on Preventative and Social Psychology*, 185-189. Washington, DC: Walter Reed Army Institute of Research, 185-198.

11. Bourne, P. G. 1970. *Men, stress and Vietnam.* Boston: Little, Brown and Co.

12. Green, T. E. A description of the nuclear battlefield. In reference 6, 1.1-1.21.

13. Young, R. W., ed. 1987. *Proceedings of the Defense Nuclear Agency Symposium/Workshop on the Psychological Effects of Tactical Nuclear Warfare* [DNA-TR-87-209; NTIS AD-A194-754-8-XAB]. Washington, DC: Defense Nuclear Agency.

14. Sagan, C. 1983. The nuclear winter. *Parade,* 30 October: 4-7.

15. Trumbull, R. 1957. *Nine who survived Hiroshima and Nagasaki.* New York: E. P. Dutton and Co.

16. U.S. Strategic Bombing Survey. 1946. *The effects of atomic bombs on Hiroshima and Nagasaki.* Washington, DC: U.S. Government Printing Office.

17. Cooney, J. P. 1951. Psychological factors in atomic warfare. *Can. Army J.* (January): 19-22.

18. Baum, A. ; Gatchel, R. J.; and Schaeffer, M. A. 1983. Emotional, behavioral, and physiological effects of chronic stress at Three Mile Island. *J. Consult. Clin. Psychol.* 51: 565-572.

19. Lifton, R. J. 1982. Beyond psychic numbing—a call to awareness. *Am. J. Orthopsychiatry* 54: 619-629.

20. Lotto, D. 1986. The analytic response to the threat of nuclear war. *Am. J. Psychoanal.* 46: 191-202.

21. U.S. Strategic Bombing Survey. 1947. *The effects of strategic bombing on Japanese morale.* Washington, DC: U.S. Government Printing Office.

22. Raphael, B. 1985. Mental and physical health consequences of disasters. *Med. J. Aust.* 143: 180-181.

23. Black, S. Psychological effects on the nuclear battlefield. In reference 6, 5.1-5.9.

24. Stokes, J. W. Psychological aspects of nuclear defense. In reference 6, 2.1-2.51.

25. Gallup, G. 1984. The Gallup youth survey. *Associated Press,* 17 October.

26. Beardslee, W. R., and Mack, J. E. 1983. Adolescents and the threat of nuclear war: The evolution of the perspective. *Yale J. Biol. Med.* 56: 79-91.

27. Chivian, E.; Mack, J. E.; and Waletsky, J. P. Soviet children and the threat of nuclear war: A preliminary study. *Am. J. Orthopsychiatry,* in press.

28. Mack, J. E. 1984. Resistance to knowing in the nuclear age. *Harvard Educ. Rev.* 54: 260-270.

29. Gold, P. 1987. Psyche watching in the atomic age. *Insight,* 4 May, 48-50.

30. Leaning, J., and Leaf, A. 1986. Public health aspects of nuclear war. *Annu. Rev. Public Health* 7: 411-439.

31. Fiske, S. T. 1986. Adults' beliefs, images, feelings, and actions regarding nuclear war: Evidence from surveys and experiments. In *Proceedings of the Institute of Medicine, U.S. National Academy of Science, Symposium on Medical Implications of Nuclear War,* 444-466. Washington, DC: National Academy Press.

32. Marshall, E. 1987. Armageddon revisited. *Science* 236: 1421-1422.

33. Breznitz, S. Hope and denial of stress in the nuclear age. In reference 31, 467-473.

34. Marlowe, D. H. Human endurance on the nuclear battlefield: Thoughts on prediction and prophecy. In reference 6, 10.1-10.23.

35. Logan, L., and Killian, L. K. 1953. *Troop reactions to atomic attack: A preview* [Technical Memorandum ORO-T-205]. Chevy Chase, MD: Operations Research Office, Johns Hopkins University.

36. Lifton, R. J. 1982. Psychological effects of the atomic bombings. In *Last Aid*, edited by E. Chivian, S. Chivian, R. J. Lifton, and J. E. Mack, 48-68. New York: W. H. Freeman and Co.

37. Hersey, J. 1981. *Hiroshima.* New York: Alfred A. Knopf Co.

38. Kimeldorf, D. J., and Hunt, E. L. 1965. *Ionizing radiation: Neural function and behavior.* New York: Academic Press.

39. Gueneau, G.; Drouet, J.; Privat, A.; and Court, L. 1983. Neurogenesis and reactivity in the subgranular zone of the rabbit dentate gyrus as seen with 3H-thymidine radioautography and gamma-irradiation. In *Proceedings of the Seventh International Congress of Radiation Research,* D2-07. Amsterdam: Martinus-Nijhoff.

40. Peimer, S. I.; Dudkin, A. O.; and Swerdlov, A. G. 1986. Response of hippocampal pacemaker-like neurons to low doses of ionizing radiation. *Int. J. Radiat. Biol.* 49: 597-600.

41. Hunt, W. 1987. Personal communication at Armed Forces Radiobiology Research Institute, Bethesda, MD 20814-5145.

42. Mickley, G. A.; Stevens, K. E.; Moore, G. H.; Deere, W.; White, G. A.; Gibbs, G. L.; and Mueller, G. L. 1983. Ionizing radiation alters beta-endorphin-like immunoreactivity in brain but not blood. *Pharmacol. Biochem. Behav.* 19: 979-983.

43. Wixon, H. N., and Hunt, W. A. 1983. Ionizing radiation decreases veratridine-stimulated uptake of sodium in rat brain synaptosomes. *Science* 220: 1073-1074.

44. Mickley, G. A. Psychological phenomena associated with nuclear warfare: Potential animal models. In reference 6, 7.1-7.35.

45. Burghardt, W. F., and Hunt, W. A. 1985. Characterization of radiation-induced performance decrement using a two-lever shock-avoidance task. *Radiat. Res.* 103: 149-157.

46. Mickley, G. A., and Teitelbaum, H. 1978. Persistence of lateral hypothalamic-mediated behaviors after a supra-lethal dose of ionizing radiation. *Aviat. Space Environ. Med.* 49: 868-873.

47. Davis, R. T. 1965. The radiation syndrome. In vol. 2, *Behavior of Non-Human Primates,* edited by A. M. Schrier, H. F. Harlow, and F. Stollnitz, 495-524. New York: Academic Press.

48. Brown, W. L., and McDowell, A. A. 1962. Some effects of radiation on psychologic processes in rhesus monkeys. In *Response of the Nervous System to Ionizing Radiation,* edited by T. J. Haley and R. S. Snider, 729-746. New York: Academic Press.

49. Davis, R. T.; Elam, C. B.; and McDowell, A. A. 1958. *Latent effects of chronic whole-body irradiation of monkeys with mixed source radiation* [Report No. 57-59]. Brooks Air Force Base, TX: School of Aerospace Medicine.

50. McDowell, A. A.; Davis, R. T.; and Steel, J. P. 1956. Application of systematic direct observational methods to analysis of the radiation syndrome in monkeys. *Percept. Mot. Skills* (Monograph Suppl. 3) 6: 117-130.

51. Hachiya, M. 1955. *Hiroshima diary,* translated by W. Well. Chapel Hill: University of North Carolina Press.

52. Janis, I. L. 1951. *Air war and emotional stress.* New York: McGraw-Hill Book Co.

53. Quarentelli, E. L. 1954. The nature and conditions of panic. *Am. J. Sociol.* 60: 267-275.

54. Lifton, R. J. 1967. *Death in life: Survivors of Hiroshima.* New York: Random House.

55. Wheeler, T. G., and Hardy, K. A. 1985. Retrograde amnesia produced by electron beam exposure: Causal parameters and duration of memory loss. *Radiat. Res.* 101: 74-80.

56. Nishikawa, T., and Tsuiki, S. 1961. Psychiatric investigations of atomic bomb survivors. *Nagasaki: Medical Journal* 36: 717-752.

57. Furchtgott, E. 1963. Behavioral effects of ionizing radiations: 1955-61. *Psychol. Bull.* 60: 157-199.

58. Horowitz, M. J. 1985. Disasters and psychological responses to stress. *Psychiat. Ann.* 15: 161-167.

59. Von Greyerz, W. 1962. *Psychology of survival.* New York: Elsevier Publishing Co.

60. Sessions, G. R. Human emotional responses in tactical nuclear warfare: Literature review and current considerations. In reference 6, 9.1-9.44.

61. Madakasira, S., and O'Brien, K. F. 1987. Acute postraumatic stress disorder in victims of a natural disaster. *J. Nerv. Ment. Dis.* 175: 286-290.

62. Ross, W. D. 1952. The emotional effects of an atomic incident. *Cincinnati J. Med.* 33: 39-41.

63. Kardiner, A. 1941. *The traumatic neuroses of war.* New York: P. Hoeber.

64. American Psychiatric Association. 1980. *Diagnostic and statistical manual of mental disorders.* 3d ed. Washington, DC: American Psychiatric Association.

65. Gleser, G. C.; Green, B. L.; and Winget, C. 1981. *Prolonged psychosocial effects of disaster.* New York: Academic Press.

66. Donnelly, C. 1982. The Soviet attitude to stress in battle. *J. Royal Army Med. Corps.* 128 (2): 72-78.

67. Nagai, T. 1958. *We of Nagasaki.* New York: Meredith Press.

68. Levin, S. G. Prediction of neuropsychiatric casualties in the nuclear battlefield. In reference 6, 8.1-8.37.

69. Gillespie, R. D. 1942. *Psychological effects of war on citizen and soldier.* New York: W. W. Norton and Co.

70. Appel, J. W., and Beebe, G. W. 1946. Preventative psychiatry. *JAMA* 131: 1469-1475.

71. Ranson, S. W. 1949. The normal battle reaction: Its relation to the pathologic battle reaction. *Bull. U.S. Army Med. Dept.* (Suppl) 9: 3-11.

72. Palinkas, L. A., and Coben, P. 1987. Psychiatric disorders among U.S. Marines wounded in action in Vietnam. *J. Nerv. Ment. Dis.* 175: 291-300.

73. British Medical Association, Board of Science and Education. 1983. *The medical effects of nuclear war.* Chichester: John Wiley and Sons.

74. Abrams, H. L. 1984. Medical resources after nuclear war: Availability vs. need. *JAMA* 252: 653-658.

75. Gellhorn, A. The immediate medical response. In reference 36, 181-201.

76. Thomas, L. 1983. *Late night thoughts on listening to Mahler's Ninth Symphony.* New York: Viking Press.

Chapter 9

LONG-TERM AND LOW-LEVEL EFFECTS OF IONIZING RADIATION

THOMAS L. WALDEN, Jr., Ph.D.*

*Radiation Biologist, Radiation Biochemistry Department, Armed Forces Radiobiology Research Institute, Bethesda, Maryland 20814-5145

INTRODUCTION

Ionizing radiation damages biological tissues by exciting or ionizing their atoms and molecules.[1] Additional indirect damage is caused by the formation of free radicals in water, which makes up 75%–80% of the mass of living systems. The primary products of water radiolysis are the hydroxyl radical, hydrogen radical (hydrogen atom), and hydrated electron; hydroperoxy radicals and hydrogen peroxide are also formed in the presence of oxygen. The production of lysosomal enyzmes and biological mediators, such as histamine and prostaglandins, is another biological response to radiation exposure.[2,3] Depending on the radiation dose and the biochemical processes altered, damage may be prompt (expressed minutes to weeks after exposure) or delayed (expressed several months to years later) (Figure 9-1). Some radiation-induced injuries may not become apparent until they are passed on to succeeding generations.

Radiation doses to biological tissues are measured in three ways. *(a)* The exposure dose of gamma or X rays in air is expressed in *roentgens* (R). *(b)* The dose of any type of radiation absorbed by the tissues was, at one time, expressed by the *rad*, which is equivalent to 100 ergs of energy per gram of tissue. The international measure of absorbed dose is now the *gray* (Gy), which is equal to 100 rads (conversely, 1 rad equals 1 cGy). *(c)* Finally, because the biological responses to radiation exposure may vary with the type of radiation, dose equivalents are expressed by the *rem*, which equals 1 joule per kilogram, or by the *sievert* (Sv), which is an international unit equaling 100 rem. The Sv allows effects from radiations with differing LET values to be compared, since 1 Sv of neutron radiation has the same biological effects as 1 Sv of low-LET gamma or X radiation. Comparisons cannot be made among absorbed-dose measures of different kinds of radiation (for example, 1 Gy of neutron radiation will not have the same effect as 1 Gy of gamma or X radiation).

Low-level radiation exposure is generally considered to be less than the dose that produces immediate or short-term observable biological effects. In the human, low-LET gamma or X radiation doses of less than 0.5 Gy do not produce any prodromal symptoms or the hematopoietic subsyndrome;[4,5] however, low-level radiation exposure does increase the probability that delayed effects will occur.[6-13] Three primary delayed effects—somatic, genetic, and teratogenic[6-9]—can be observed and are already present in the population and in the gene pool.[7,8] Irradiation enhances the naturally occurring frequency of the effect, and in some cases produces the observable end point by a process different from those of natural selection. Certain biological responses have such low thresholds that they are statistically indistinguishable, in many cases, from normal incidence.[7,8,10] Even so, current radioprotection guidelines state that all exposures to radiation should be avoided if possible and that exposure should be kept as low as is reasonably achievable.[14]

BACKGROUND RADIATION

Living organisms are continually exposed to ionizing radiation in nature as well as from nuclear weapons testing, occupations, consumer products, and medical procedures.[7,8,15] The radiation from all of these sources together is called *background radiation*, and is estimated to measure 180–200 mrem/person/year. Medical procedures contribute most whole-body background radiation (Figure 9-2).[7,8] In addition, large doses of partial-body radiation may be delivered to the lung by radon gas (radon-222 and radon-220), produced from the natural decay of radium and thorium.[16] High concentrations of radon gas escape from soil and are released from marble and granite, accumulating in buildings with poor air circulation.[16] Radon exposure is a health concern because its solid daughter products, polonium-214 and -218, decay by alpha-particle emission in the human body near the lung tissue and may increase the incidence of lung cancer.[16]

Extraterrestrial radiation includes solar-flare and cosmic radiation. Most cosmic radiation is absorbed

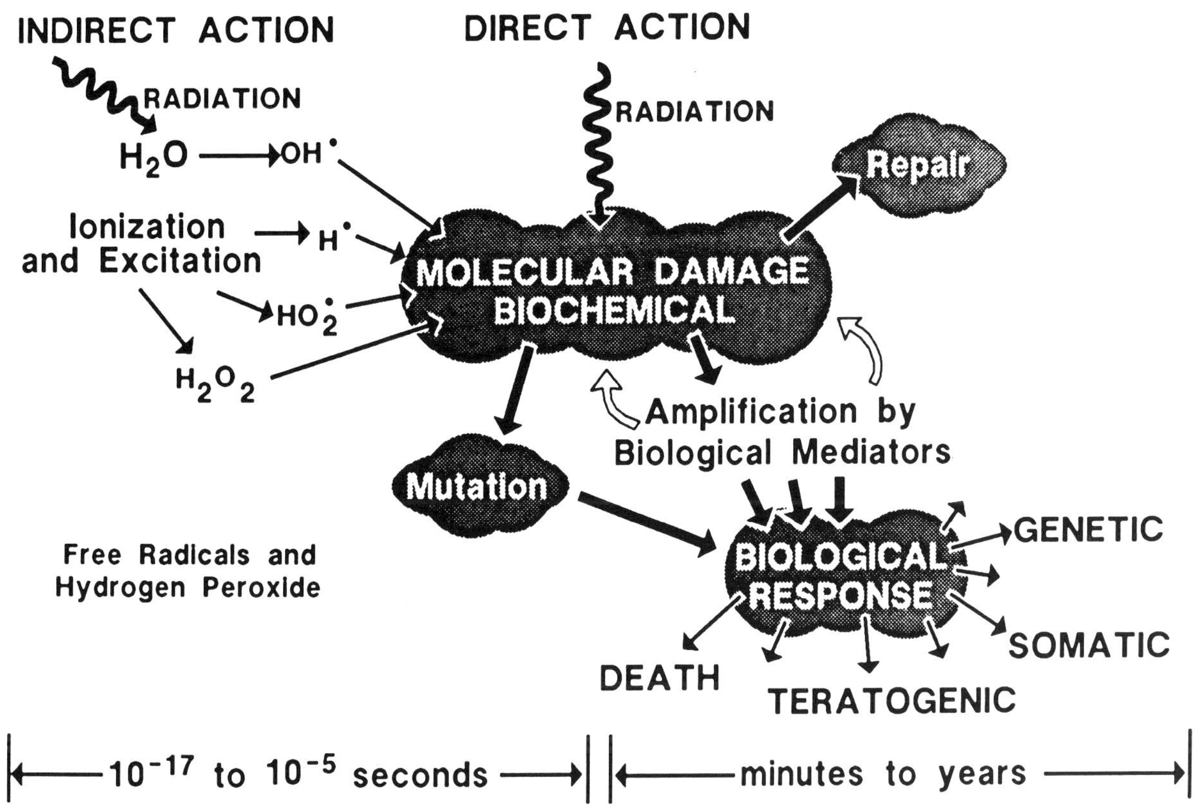

Fig. 9-1. Physical and biological responses to ionizing radiation. Ionizing radiation causes damage either directly by damaging the molecular target or indirectly by generating free radicals, which attack the molecular target. Physical steps leading to energy deposition and free radical formation occur within femtoseconds to microseconds, while the manifestation of actual biological damage may require seconds to years.

by the dense atmosphere before it reaches the earth's surface. A person's exposure to cosmic radiation increases at higher latitudes or altitudes, as the atmosphere becomes less dense.[7,8] A resident of the higher-altitude city of Denver receives approximately 100 mrem more radiation exposure than does a resident of Washington, D.C. A cross-country airplane flight increases individual exposure by 0.2 mrem/hour because the level of cosmic radiation is greater at 36,000 feet than at sea level.[7] As humans venture farther from the protective atmosphere, either in supersonic air carriers or in spaceflight, their background occupational exposures to cosmic radiation will increase. The British Concorde supersonic transport maintains radiation-monitoring equipment so that it may drop to lower-altitude flight routes if increases in solar or cosmic radiation are detected.[8] Spaceflight increases exposure to solar and cosmic radiations; *Apollo* astronauts traveling to the moon received an average of 275 mrem over 19.5 days.[8]

On earth, naturally occurring radioactive elements contribute to background radiation.[7,8] External exposure sources include potassium-40, which may be concentrated in concrete, and radon gas. Internal radiation comes primarily from radioactive isotopes of naturally occurring elements in biological systems, such as potassium-40 and sodium-24. In some areas of Brazil and India, large concentrations of monazite, a mineral containing thorium, are present in the soil or sand. Background-radiation exposures there range from 0.008 to 0.17 Gy/year.[8]

Fallout from nuclear weapons testing peaked in 1964, after seventy-seven atmospheric detonations occurred in 1962. Of the total fallout, 69% was from carbon-14, 4% was from cesium-137, and 3% was from strontium-90. The remaining 24% was from radioactive isotopes of plutonium, rubidium, barium, iodine, iron, manganese, krypton, americium, tritium, and

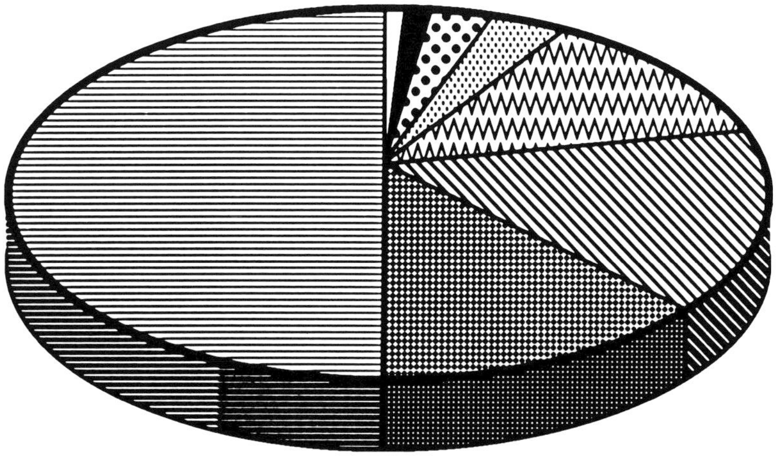

Fig. 9-2. Major contributors to average background radiation in the United States

zinc.[8] Carbon-14 will be a long-term contributor to background radiation because it has a half-life of 5,700 years. Nuclear fallout has decreased because of the total ban on atmospheric testing by the United States, Great Britain, and the Soviet Union, although several other countries continue atmospheric testing.

Radiation is also emitted from consumer products, such as color television sets (averaging 0.3–1.0 rem/hour of use), video terminals, smoke detectors (which contain an alpha emitter, usually americium-241), and dinnerware that uses uranium for an orange color.[7,15] Ophthalmic glass, used in prescription lenses, contains trace impurities of thorium-232, and uranium is added to dental porcelain to give dentures a natural fluorescent quality.[15] The latter may result in an alpha radiation dose of 60 rem/year to the gums.[15]

SOMATIC EFFECTS

Delayed somatic effects of ionizing radiation result from somatic mutations and accumulated damage, and include impaired circulation, necrosis, fibrosis of skin and muscle tissue, loss of hair, loss of taste, impaired bone growth, susceptibility to disease, immunodeficiency, aplastic anemia, cataracts, and increased incidence of cancer.[6-9,12]

Some organs are more radioresistant than others. Radiation doses exceeding 15–50 Gy must be received before damage to the liver or heart is detected.[6,8] Other tissues, such as the lens and the sperm, show some detriment from doses as low as 0.15–0.30 Gy.[7,8,10,17] Delayed somatic effects of intermediate- or high-level exposures include cataract formation, skin abnormalities, and sterility.

Cataract Formation

The lens tissue of the eye is particularly radiosensitive, and radiation exposure can result in its increased opacity.[7,8,18-22] Radiation cataractogenesis is the most common delayed radiation injury,[21] and is thought to result from damage to the anterior equatorial cells of the lens's epithelial tissue.[23] These cells normally divide and migrate to the posterior portion of the lens, where they gradually lose their nuclei and become lens fibers.[8,23] The lens tissue, like that of the testes and the brain, is separated from the rest of the body by a barrier system.[8] As a result, it has no direct blood supply, no macrophages for phagocytosis, and no way to remove accumulated damage. In a study of 446 survivors of the Nagasaki atomic bomb, 45% of the 395 persons who were 0.1–2.0 km from the hypocenter of the bomb developed cataracts by 1959 (whereas only 0.5%, or 2 out of 395, had severe visual impairment).[19-21] Four of the remaining fifty-one persons (7.8%) who were 2–4 km from the bomb hypocenter developed mild cataract impairment. Even survivors exposed to small doses of radiation were at increased risk for cataract formation. By 1964, the incidence of cataract formation among atomic-bomb survivors who received 0.01–0.99 Gy of radiation was 1.5% in Hiroshima compared to 1.0% in the control population, and 2.0% in Nagasaki compared to 0.9% in controls (Figure 9-3).[22] Higher doses tend to increase the degree of opacity and shorten the latency period.[7,8] There is a 10% risk of developing a severely impairing cataract following a single exposure to 2.4 Gy of low-LET radiation, and a 50% risk for a dose of 3.1 Gy.[10] The estimated dose for 50% incidence of cataract formation increases from 3.1 Gy to 9.3 Gy by lowering the dose rate or extending the exposure period.[10] The latency period for cataract formation in humans has been estimated to be 6 months to 35 years; however, fractionation or protracted exposure lowers the incidence and prolongs the latency.[7,8]

Small radiation doses may increase the opacity, but visually impairing cataract formation results from an accumulation of dead or injured cells, and therefore has a threshold. For low-LET radiation, this threshold is 2 Gy.[7,8] High-LET neutrons have thresholds of less than 0.2 Gy.

Other parts of the eye are not as radiosensitive as is the lens. The threshold for corneal edema is 10 Gy of low-LET radiation; for atrophy of the lacrimal gland, it is 20 Gy.[8,10] Doses of less than 0.1 Sv/year are not thought to present appreciable risk for detectable visual impairment. The International Commission on Radiological Protection (ICRP) has recommended an occupational exposure limit of 0.15 Sv for the eye.[24]

Sterility

Males. Germ cells of the human testes are very radiosensitive.[7,8,25] Temporary sterility may occur after 0.1-Gy whole-body or local irradiation, with 50% incidence following 0.7 Gy.[7,8,10] Sperm cells become more resistant as they develop; spermatogonia are more radiosensitive than spermatocytes, which are in turn more radiosensitive than spermatids.[26] The regenerating spermatogonial stem cell (A_S) is more radioresistant than the developing spermatogonia (B). The ED_{50} for damage to spermatogonia is 0.11 Gy of low-LET radiation.[27] The spermatid is also fairly radioresistant, requiring X-ray doses of 6 Gy to show visible damage.[26]

Radiogenic aspermia is caused by a maturation-depletion process similar to that observed for hematopoietic cells after irradiation. Radiation kills stem cells or delays mitosis, so that differentiating cells continue to divide without being replaced. The latency period for aspermia after radiation exposure is approximately 2 months,[26] and the time for recovery is several months to years. Chronic and protracted exposures produce greater testicular damage than do acute large exposures. This damage is reflected in the duration of aspermia,[7,8,25] and is thought to result from cycling of the radioresistant A_S spermatogonia to the more radiosensitive B spermatogonia.[7,8,25] A dose of about 0.35 Gy produces a 50% incidence of aspermia after a protracted exposure of 1–10 days.[10] At low dose rates, the recovery period depends on the total dose received:

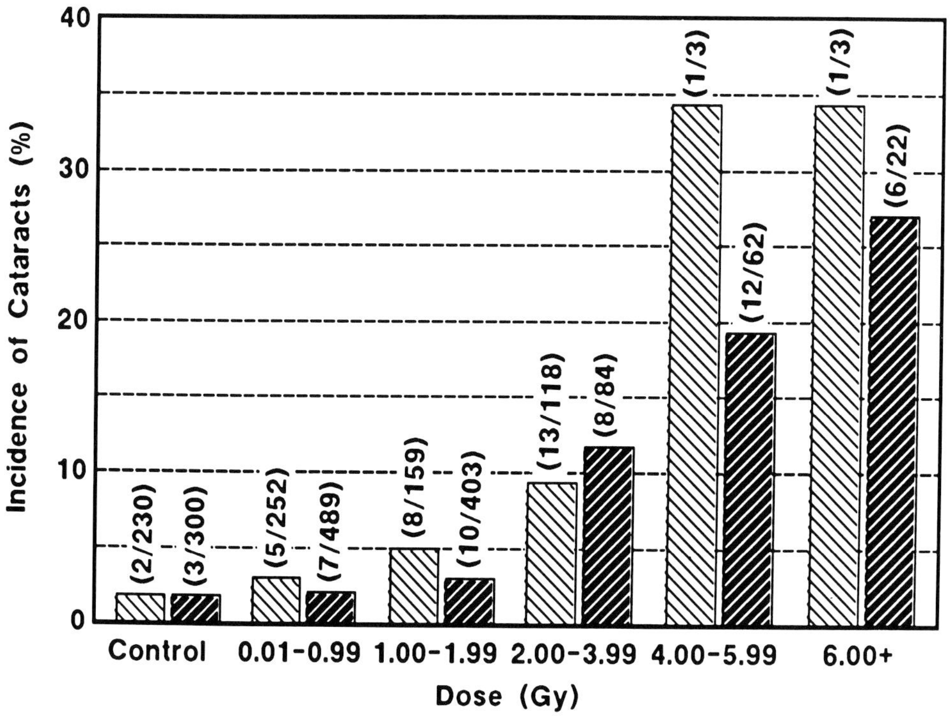

Fig. 9-3. Incidence of severe cataracts in atomic-bomb survivors, according to radiation dose received. Cataracts were detected by examinations in 1963–1964 for populations of Nagasaki and Hiroshima. Numbers in parentheses are the actual numbers of cataracts observed per number of persons examined who received that dose of radiation. Radiation doses are based on Oak Ridge National Laboratory (ORNL) calculations, which contain a lower neutron dose estimation in the Hiroshima population than originally estimated. Based on the 1965 tentative dose relationship (T65D) estimate, the average total dose for the 600+ Hiroshima group is 7.783 Gy, including 2.343 Gy of neutrons. Using ORNL dosimetry, the average dose for this group is 8.514 Gy, with 0.74 Gy of neutrons. Dosimetry was recently revised based on new information on explosion characteristics. Risks will be revised by scientific advisory boards when these new estimates (DR86) become available.

Source: References 107 and 108

approximately 1 year following a 1-Gy exposure, 3 years for 2–3 Gy, and up to 5 years for 6 Gy.[26] A fractionated dose of 2–3 Gy may require up to 14 years for recovery.[28] Doses of 0.08 Gy do not significantly affect sperm count or alter plasma follicle stimulating hormone (FSH) levels.[26] Radiation doses of up to 6 Gy do not alter plasma levels of testosterone, but do decrease the levels of urinary hormone. Decreased production of testosterone by the Leydig cells has been observed in humans receiving 6 Gy of X rays. Plasma levels are not affected because there will be a compensating increased number of Leydig cells 3 months after irradiation.[26] Following the onset of aspermia, there is a three- to fourfold increase in urinary gonadotropin, plasma FSH, and luteinizing hormone. Elevated levels return to normal when spermatogenesis resumes.[26]

Permanent male sterility may occur after 2 Gy (local or whole-body exposure) but generally requires doses between 5 and 9.5 Gy.[8] These doses are within the lethal range for whole-body exposure.[7]

Females. The ovary is not as sensitive to radiation-induced temporary sterility as is the testis, but it is more sensitive to permanent sterility.[7,8,25] These distinctions are based on differences in the stages of development of the two germ cell groups. Shortly before birth, the oogonia stop multiplying and proceed to prophase I of meiosis.[29] After puberty, meiosis resumes for individual cells by ovulation. Oocytes lose the ability to renew after birth and are unable to replace stem cells that have been damaged or killed by radiation. The oocyte is most radiosensitive as a proliferative stem cell during the fetal stage of gestation, prior to ceasing mitosis and entering meiosis.[7,8]

Temporary sterility may be induced in females by acute radiation doses of 1.5–6.4 Gy.[8,10] Permanent sterility results from doses of 2–10 Gy, and depends on the woman's age at the time of irradiation.[8,10,25] Older women, particularly those close to menopause, are particularly radiosensitive for sterilization. Two Gy of low-LET radiation may result in permanent sterility of 50% of the exposed female population over 40 years of age, compared to an estimated 3.5 Gy for women under 40.[10] This is simply due to the numbers of oocytes present at the time of irradiation.[7,8,25] Women have about one-half million oocytes at puberty, which are almost depleted through atresia at menopause.[29]

Higher radiation doses of 3.6–20.0 Gy are required for sterilization when the exposures are prolonged or fractionated.[8,10] From the 1920s through the 1950s, radiation exposure was occasionally prescribed to treat infertility and sterility.[30] One-third of the women referred for this treatment had amenorrhea. Each woman received a total dose of 0.65 Gy to the ovaries and 0.75 Gy to the pituitary gland, divided in three fractions over 2 weeks. In one study, this technique had a 55% success rate: 351 of 644 patients treated were able to conceive.[30] The treatment has been discontinued because of the concern for associated risks of genetic and somatic damage. Higher doses of low-LET radiation (1.25 Gy) can result in a delay of the menstrual cycle.[10]

Radiation Effects on Skin and Hair

Soon after Roentgen's discovery of X rays,[31] researchers and radiologists became aware of the skin's sensitivity to radiation damage.[32-36] Eight months after the discovery of X rays in 1896, a German scientist reported a case of dermatitis and alopecia on the face and back of a 17-year-old man who had been exposed to these rays for 10–20 minutes a day for 4 weeks during an investigation.[33] Interestingly, the accompanying erythema, which resembled a burn, was painless, whereas chronic radiation dermatitis following repeated exposure is usually extremely painful.[35-37]

In another 1896 case, a man received an hour-long X-ray exposure during an examination for a kidney stone.[37] The patient experienced nausea (a prodromal symptom) 3 hours after irradiation. Following a second exposure lasting 1.5 hours, the patient developed a radiation sequela leading to ulcer formation at the site of exposure, which was not responsive to skin grafting.

An 1897 case study initiated the popularity of X-radiation treatment for dermatological ailments. A Viennese doctor administered X radiation in two hour-long treatments per day for 10 days to depilate a nevus pilosis birthmark covering the back of a 5-year-old girl.[34] Epilation occurred 11 days after the initiation of treatment.

Before the introduction of the roentgen in 1928 as a unit to measure exposure dose, the *skin erythema dose* (SED) was commonly used.[38] The SED is the radiation dose required to produce a given degree of erythema. It depends on the quality, energy, and exposure time of the radiation. For X radiation, the SED is about 8.5 Gy. In 1925, it was proposed that the exposure of radiologists and X-ray machine operators not exceed 1/100th of the SED in a 30-day period.[38]

During a radiation incident, skin may be exposed either by direct blast irradiation or by *beta burn* from the direct deposition of particulate fallout.[5,39] The degree of radiation-induced skin damage depends on a number of factors, including the type of radiation; the dose and dose rate; the area of skin irradiated; and skin-quality characteristics, such as texture, age, color, thickness, and location.[7,8,10,40-45] The neck is the most radiosensitive area because its skin is thin and usually not protected by clothing.[46,47] Additional trauma through burn, abrasion, exposure to ultraviolet light, or extreme temperature variations will increase the damage.[45,46,48] Environmental factors or inadequate clothing may contribute to hyperthermia, and wool or other coarse fabrics may further abrade the damaged skin. An illness like diabetes[43] or a genetic disease like ataxia telangiectasia[8,40,44] may also make the skin more radiosensitive. Alpha radiation is of little concern for skin damage because the average penetrated dose is usually absorbed by the dead corneocytes of the stratum corneum. However, it may present a problem at sites where the skin is thinner and the radiation can penetrate to the basal level.[41]

Beta particulates in fallout may contain extremely high radiation dose rates (tens of Gy per hour). When they land on the skin, their energy may penetrate to the germinal basal cells.[5,39,41,49] This radiation damage (beta burn) was observed in the atomic-bomb survivors and the Marshall Islanders (Figure 9-4) who had been exposed to nuclear fallout.[5,39,50,51] The threshold dose of beta radiation for skin damage depends on the average energy of the beta particle, the total absorbed dose, and the dose rate.[49] The average penetrating

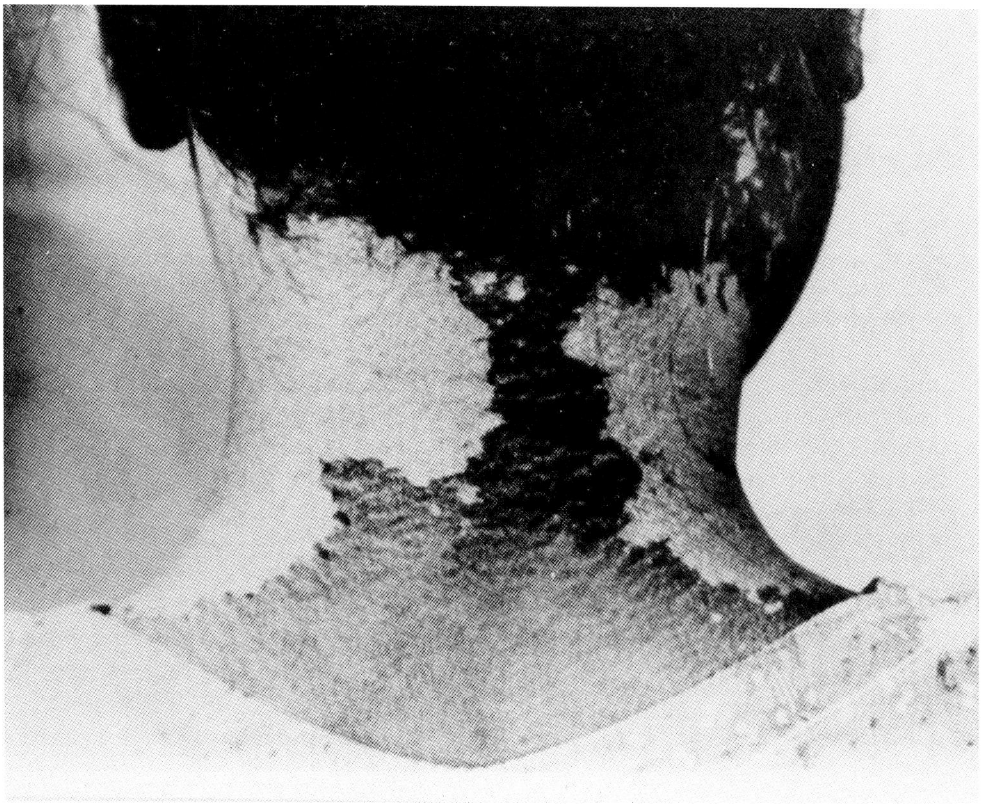

Fig. 9-4. Beta burn on neck of Marshall Island woman 1 month after exposure to fallout radiation from a nuclear weapon. Note discoloration of skin on left and right sides.

range of a beta particle is proportional to its energy; thus, higher-energy beta emitters, such as strontium-90 (0.61 MeV average), require lower surface doses to produce wet desquamation than do lower-energy beta particles, such as those from cobalt-60 (0.31 MeV average).[49] The surface threshold doses for transepidermal injury in the skin of pigs is 15 Gy for strontium-90, 40 Gy for cobalt-60, and 200 Gy for sulfur-35.[49] The exposure from each of these radioisotopes delivers approximately the same tissue dose to the basal germ cells. Lower-energy beta particles like sulfur-35 (0.17 MeV energy) are not capable of penetrating to the dermis and cannot induce chronic radiation dermatitis.[49] Beta injuries from fallout can be minimized by decontamination and washing.

Radiation damage to the dermis has a threshold dose of about 20 Gy,[52] with 50% incidence at 60 Gy.[53] Five progressive categories of radiation damage are observed in skin: erythema, transepithelial injury (moist desquamation), ulceration, necrosis, and skin cancer.[32,38-43,45,54]

Radiation-induced erythema occurs in two stages: *(a)* mild initial erythema, appearing usually within minutes or hours on the first day after irradiation (occurring earlier with higher doses), and *(b)* the main erythema, appearing at 2–3 weeks and persisting for longer periods.[10,45,54] In some cases, a third erythema may occur at 6 weeks.[45] Radiation-induced erythema is a threshold phenomenon.[8,45,54] A dose of 6 Gy of low-LET radiation received in less than 1 day, or 10 Gy in 10 days, will induce erythema in 50% of exposed persons.[8,10] The threshold for neutron radiation is 2 Gy.[8] Because of these variables, and the fact that the threshold dose decreases with an increase in the surface area exposed, erythema is not a good biological dosimeter.[8,10,45,49,54] Early erythema arises from the release of mediators and from increased capillary dilation and permeability.[48] It is equivalent to a first-degree burn or mild sunburn, subsiding within 2 or 3 days.[45,54] Although indomethacin or other prostaglandin-synthesis inhibitors have been used topically to prevent or reduce erythema caused by sunburn or ultraviolet light,[52] they have not been widely used to treat radiation-induced erythema. (One study suggested that systemic and topical applications of prostaglandin inhibitors may be useful in minimizing late damage and necrosis from large radiation doses.)[53] When early erythema subsides, it will be latent for 2–3 weeks, depending on the dose.

The second onset of erythema is attributed to impaired circulation in the arterioles and capillaries, producing inflammation and edema[8,45,48] and accompanied by dry desquamation of the epidermal corneocytes. Low radiation doses induce mitotic delay,[45,55] with subsequent sloughing of epidermal layers. Higher radiation doses extend the duration of mitotic delay but do not alter the rate of cell sloughing at the skin surface. Upper cells are sloughed or abraded off, exposing cells that are not completely keratinized. Cell death and moist desquamation ensue.

Both dry and wet desquamation occur about 1–4 weeks after irradiation.[37,45,54] Regeneration of the stratum corneum requires 2 months to 4 years,[44] and this regenerated tissue will be more sensitive to other skin-damaging agents.[45,46] The new skin may be thinner than the original, with greater sensitivity to touch and pain.[45,49] Reduction or loss of the dermal ridges making up the fingerprint has occurred from large or chronic exposures.[45]

Epidermal basal cells are thought to be the targets of early radiation damage,[45,54] and further damage to the surrounding vasculature is an important factor in late radiation injury and necrosis.[8,32,41,45,46] The blood vessel damage may lead to telangiectasia, and fibrosis and alterations in connective tissue may appear.[8,42,45,46] Hyper- or hypopigmentation may occur after radiation exposure: low doses activate melanocytes and produce hyperpigmentation, and higher doses may result in death of melanocytes and hypopigmentation.[45,56]

Dermal necrosis from radiation results from cell death in the dermis, and is equivalent to third-degree thermal burns.[10,42,53] Ulceration is seen with doses greater than 20 Gy;[44] some muscular atrophy may occur with highly penetrating radiation.[44,46] When the proliferation rate of basal cells is depressed for long periods, fibrotic repair may surpass the basal cell repair, leading to reduced tonicity and resiliency and the formation of scar tissue.[44,45] Figure 9-5 shows the general pattern of skin damage of a patient who received large doses of radiotherapy. Ulceration with scar-tissue formation occurs after 30 Gy,[44] and severe fibrosis after 55 Gy.[56] Ulcerations may require corrective surgery, because the underlying tissue may maintain the ulcer and the recovery of the immediate surrounding tissue may be slow.[45] Chronic radiation exposure (chronic radiodermatitis) can also lead to increased fibrosis and to ulceration.[42,45] Skin cancers may be evident after months or years.[42,45,49,54] They may result from either acute or chronic exposure, but are not generally associated with increased mortality.[7,8,45]

Radiation induces a bluish-brown pigmentation of the fingernails in persons of dark-skinned races.[39] The threshold dose has not been determined. Fingernail pigmentation was observed in the Marshall Islanders, who received an average estimated whole-body gamma-radiation dose of 61 rem. The bluish-brown pigment was slowly eliminated by normal fingernail growth over the first 6 months after irradiation.[39] Cracking or shedding of the nails may occasionally occur.[45]

The first report of epilation caused by X rays was written in 1896.[57] As a way to test the machine's ability to make a photograph of the skull (in preparation for locating a bullet in the head of a child who had been accidentally shot), the author exposed the head of a colleague to X radiation for 1 hour. The photograph did not turn out, and 3 weeks later, the colleague developed a 2-inch bald spot on his scalp.[57]

Generally, epilation occurs about 2 weeks after irradiation with doses greater than 2–3 Gy.[10,42,54] This loss is temporary, with regrowth occurring in 2–6 months. The returning hair may be thinner, with either different pigmentation or loss of pigmentation. Permanent epilation occurs with doses greater than 6 Gy.[54] Epilation results from a combination of mitotic delay, interphase death, and reproductive death of the hair cell.

Cancer

Two months after their discovery, X rays were being used to treat cancer.[58,59] The earliest radiotherapy was performed in 1896 for breast carcinoma[58] and stomach tumors.[60,61] However, with the increasing use of radiotherapy came reports that radiation actually induces cancer.[51,58,59,62,63] One of the earliest radiation-induced cancers occurred in the laboratory of Thomas Edison, whose assistant died in 1904 from skin cancer contracted while working on the development of a fluorescent light using an X-ray tube.[58] By 1907, eleven mortalities were attributed to cancer induced by X radiation.[62] The first investigator to demonstrate that X radiation causes cancers in laboratory animals used a fractionated radiation schedule to induce spindle-cell carcinomas in rats.[64] Many early radiologists, researchers, and workers experienced chronic radiodermatitis, increased incidence of cancers, and other damage before the dangers of radiation were clarified and protective measures were initiated.[7,51,63] Now, the National Academy of Sciences considers cancer induction to be the most important somatic effect of low-dose ionizing radiation.[7]

Cancer Induction. Cancer development is thought to be a multistep process, in which the initial damage leads to a preneoplastic stage, followed by selection

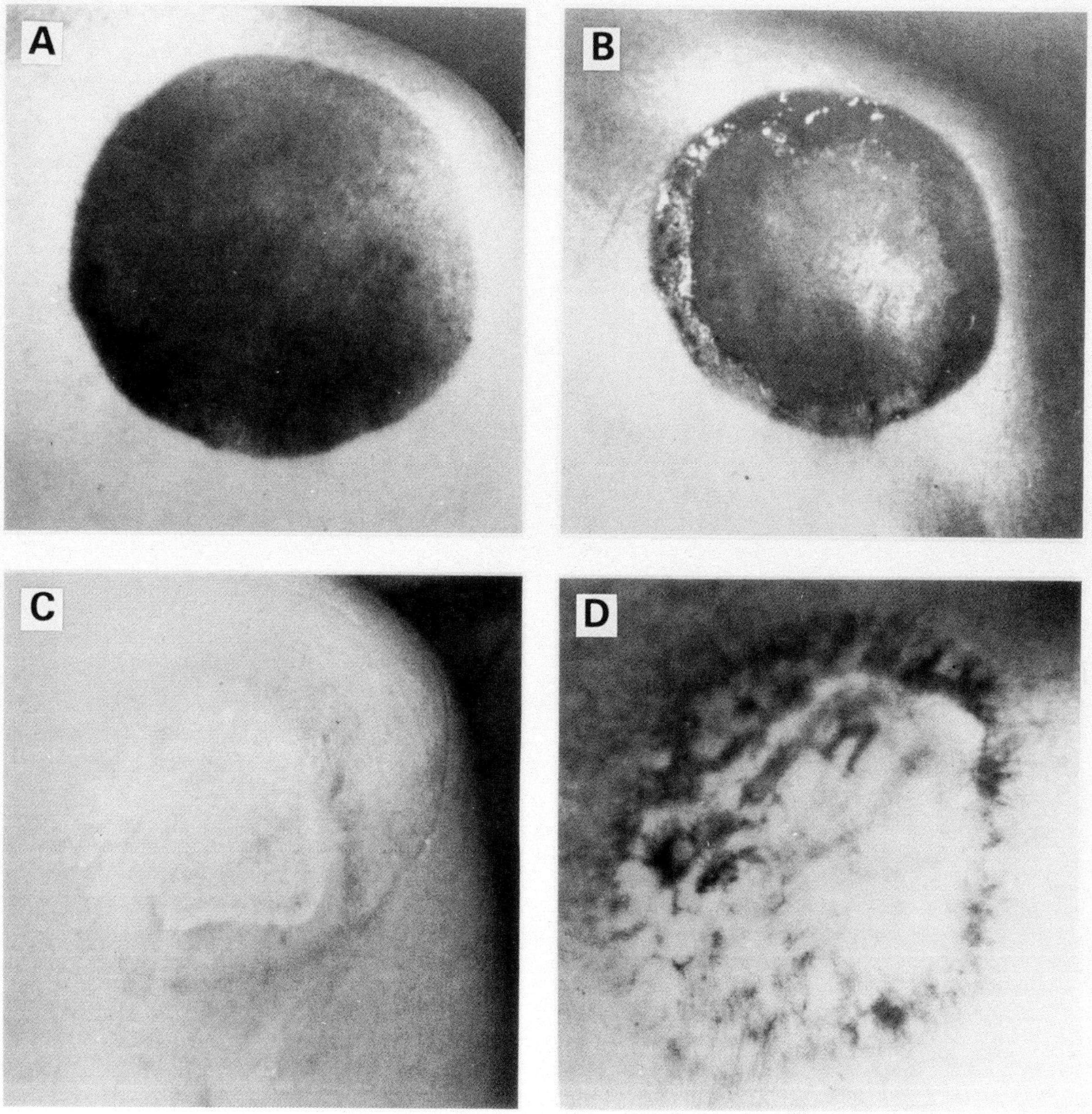

Fig. 9-5. Clinical course of radiation damage to the skin of a radiotherapy patient: (A) erythema, (B) erosion, (C) ulcer, (D) scar.
Source: Reference 45

and proliferation of the neoplastic cell.[6-8,65-68] Chromosomal and enzymatic analyses indicate that all of the cancer cells of a tumor and its metastases are derivatives or clones of a single cell.[69-71] A neoplasm is characterized by unrestrained growth, irregular migration, transformation, and genetic diversity.[67]

The three stages in cancer formation are *initiation*, *promotion*, and *latency* (Figure 9-6).[7,65] During initiation, fixation of the somatic mutational event occurs, which leads to the development of a neoplasm. Damage can be initiated by various agents, including exposure to radiation or another environmental or chemical carcinogen.

During the promotion stage, the preneoplastic cell is stimulated to divide or is given preferential selection. A *promoter* is an agent that by itself does not cause cancer, but once the initiating carcinogenic event has occurred, it promotes or stimulates the cell containing

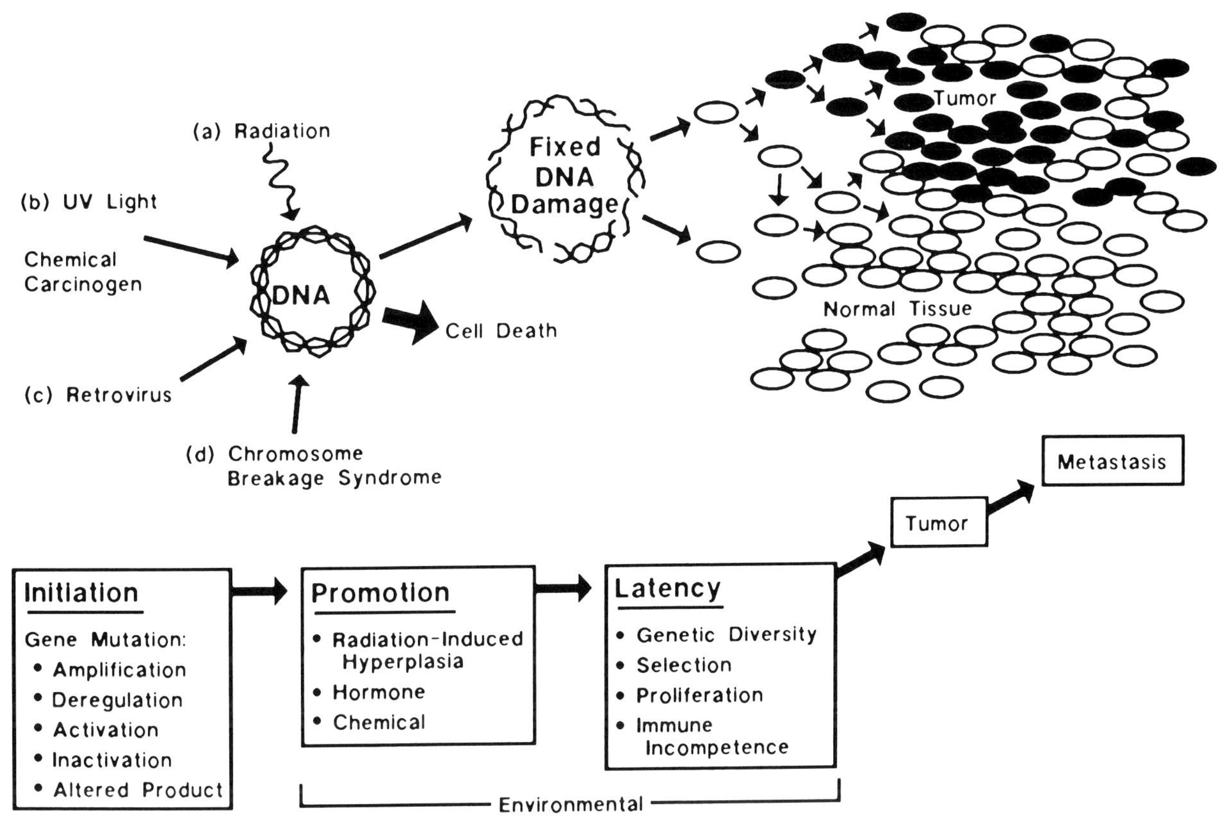

Fig. 9-6. Sequential steps in the development of cancer. Cancer originates from a single cell (clone) through a multistep process. Initiation by one of four methods (a-d) leads to repair of damage, or cell death, or fixation of DNA damage, which may predispose the cell to transition into a neoplastic state. Chromosome-breakage syndromes (also called genetic syndromes, such as xeroderma pigmentosum and ataxia telangiectasia) are associated with deficiencies in DNA repair and genetic instability. Environmental or host factors may play roles in cancer promotion and latency. End products of these steps are the tumor and its potential metastases.

the original damage.[65] The National Toxicology Program lists 148 chemical agents and groups known to be carcinogenic in humans, including asbestos, benzene, vinyl chloride, nickel, soots, tars, formaldehyde, DDT, saccharin, and urethane.[72] Unlike most carcinogens, radiation may act both as an initiator by inducing somatic mutation, and as a promoter by stimulating cell division as a result of recovery and repair processes.[6,7] Some chemotherapeutic alkylating agents (including cyclophosphamide and nitrogen mustard) initiate biochemical damage similar to that caused by radiation, and are called *radiomimetic* agents. Like ionizing radiation, they are useful for chemotherapy but are also carcinogenic. Some hormones may act as promoters by stimulating the growth of target tissues.[7] For example, estrogen may function as a promoter of breast cancer, and thyroid-stimulating hormone (TSH) may act as a promoter of thyroid cancer. Conjugated and unconjugated estrogens have been identified as carcinogenic in human populations.[72]

Radiation may also affect latency, which is the third (and last) stage of cancer development. During latency, the transformed cell produces a number of different phenotypic clones through continued genetic diversity, although not all clones will be neoplastic.[65,67,68] Eventually, one phenotype acquires the selective advantage of evading the host's defense systems and metastasizing (Figure 9-6). The primary contributions of radiation in latency are the immunosuppression and alteration of biological mediators released in the surrounding tumor microenvironment.

Environmental and host factors have roles in cancer

TABLE 9-1

LOWEST CANCER INCIDENCE RATES FROM SELECTED WORLD REGISTRIES*

Type or Site of Cancer	Connecticut Registry	Lowest Incidence Worldwide	Location of Incidence
Lung	325.8	9.0	Rural Norway
Colon	137.2	13.7	Ibada, Nigeria
Prostate	92.3	5.3	Miyagi, Japan
Stomach	66.2	28.0	New Mexico, United States
Leukemia	57.9	40.8	Miyagi, Japan
Myeloma	15.1	1.8	Miyagi, Japan
Thyroid	12.4	3.6	Southern metro region, United Kingdom

*Per million males younger than 65 years

Source: Condensed from reference 73

promotion.[6,7] The contribution of environmental agents can be estimated by comparing high and low cancer incidences in different populations of the world.[73] As many as 80% of cancer deaths in the United States may be linked to environmental factors that could have been avoided.[73] The incidence of lung cancer in males in the state of Connecticut in 1968–1972 was 325.8 cases per million males under 65 years old, compared to nine cases per million in rural Norway (Table 9-1).[73] Similar differences occur for the incidences of prostate cancer and myeloma in the populations of Connecticut and Miyagi, Japan. Environmental factors that may promote cancer are the use of tobacco, alcohol, and food additives; other dietary factors; sexual behavior; occupation; air pollution; industrial products; medicines and medical procedures; bacterial and viral infections; and geophysical factors.[73] Tumor registry studies have shown higher incidences of colon cancer in the United States than in Japan, while higher incidences of stomach cancer occur in Japan.[74] Japanese immigrants in the United States have a higher incidence of colon cancer than those living in Japan, indicating that environmental factors and dietary changes may influence its development. One environmental agent of increasing importance is the human immunodeficiency virus (HIV), implicated in the cause of acquired immune deficiency syndrome (AIDS).[75] This virus selectively attacks and destroys a subclass of T-cells (T-4 lymphocytes) that is responsible for monitoring the immunity of the spontaneously developing neoplastic cells. Impairment of the immune system may, therefore, promote cancer growth.

The differing incidences of cancer for males and females (Table 9-2) may be the result of hormonal, environmental, or behavioral factors. Leukemias and lung cancer are more prevalent in men. Their higher incidence of lung cancer may be due to the greater percentage of males who smoke. Thyroid cancers are more prevalent in women.[73] Genetic studies have shown that family tendencies for developing certain cancers are associated with several genetic syndromes, including xeroderma pigmentosum, ataxia telangiectasia, Fanconi's anemia, Bloom's syndrome, Gardner's syndrome, and Li-Fraumeni's syndrome.[6-8,51,69,76] These diseases are associated with increased cellular mutation rates, sensitivity to environmental and chemical mutagens, and exposure to ionizing radiation. Chromosomal translocations are observed more frequently in cells from persons with these diseases, and specific defects in the repair of deoxyribonucleic acid (DNA) have been identified for most of these syndromes. These hereditary syndromes may increase susceptibility to cancer by providing the genetic diversity that is necessary for its development.[69,76]

TABLE 9-2

UNITED STATES CANCER MORTALITY RATES IN 1968-1972*

Type or Site of Cancer	Number of Males	Number of Females
Lung	288.0	71.3
Colon	85.2	74.9
Prostate	25.5	—
Leukemia	43.4	3.0
Stomach	37.5	18.2
Thyroid	1.8	2.1
Breast	1.3	174.0

*Per million males or females younger than 65 years

Source: Condensed from reference 73

Specific gene mutations and chromosomal aberrations are associated with particular cancers.[65-67,69,77] Research in this area has been stimulated by the discovery in recent years of *oncogenes*, *proto-oncogenes*, and *antioncogenes*.[66,67,78,79]

Oncogenes are genes that induce the transformation of cells in culture when incorporated into the DNA of otherwise normal cells.[67] These genes have been found to have structural similarity to normally occurring genes that are present in nontransformed, noncancerous cells.[67,80] About forty different oncogenes have been identified.[79] Their functions are diverse; however, many of their gene products bind to DNA or promote cellular proliferation.[67,79,80]

The normally occurring counterpart of the oncogene is the proto-oncogene. Very few natural functions of the proto-oncogenes are known, although similarity exists between the v-sis oncogene and the gene coding for the platelet-derived growth factor-2 peptide.[80,81]

Most oncogenes were first isolated from avian leukemia retroviruses, and later research identified oncogenic and normal counterparts in laboratory animals and in humans.[78] The viral oncogene is referred to as v-onc. One of the most commonly studied v-onc genes is v-myc.[67,79,80] Its homologous cellular gene (c-myc) is amplified in several different forms of cancer, including Burkitt's lymphoma in humans.[69,79,80,82] Another oncogene (ras) codes for a G-protein that regulates cell receptor activity by controlling adenyl cyclase activity.[83] Up to 40% of the surgically removed human colon cancers contain an activated ras oncogene.[84] Radiation-induced skin tumors in rats and mice have been found to have activated forms of the c-myc, k-ras, and ras oncogenes as well as amplification of the c-myc gene.[85-87] A mouse lymphoma induced by radiation was shown to have an activated c-k-ras oncogene that differed from the normal gene by a single point mutation, resulting in incorporation of aspartic acid instead of glycine into the corresponding protein.[87]

Oncogenic activation by itself is not necessarily a carcinogenic event because these genes have important normal cell functions.[67,69] They are thought to participate in initiating a neoplasm state by either quantitative or qualitative changes in their specified gene product as a result of amplification, mutation, or deregulation.[67,69,77] Some antioncogenes help repress cancer induction.[68,88] The deletion, inactivation, or presence of that gene in a homozygous recessive state may predispose or permit cancer development.[69,89] Hybridization experiments using normal cells and cancerous cells show that the cancerous actions of some oncogenes are repressed by the presence of the normal chromosome in the new hybrid.[69,90] An activated raf-oncogene has been implicated in the radioresistance of a human laryngeal cancer cell line[91] and also in radioresistant benign skin fibroblasts from a patient with Li-Fraumeni's syndrome.[76]

Radiation is known to induce chromosomal aberrations, and specific chromosomal aberrations are shown by many cancers. The most common translocations and trisomic conditions observed in human cancer involve chromosomes 1, 8, and 14.[69] The c-myc and c-mos genes are located on chromosome 8.[92,93] Translocation of chromosome 8 to 14 is present in 80% of patients with Burkitt's lymphoma and is associated with amplification of the c-myc gene.[77,92] A similar translocation occurs in 10%–20% of patients with acute T-cell leukemia.[77] The Philadelphia chromosome that is present in 90%–95% of patients with chronic myeloid leukemia is a translocation of a portion of chromosome 9 to chromosome 22,[94-96] and it is thought to involve the c-abl proto-oncogene.[77,95-97] A transformation is thought to arise by random selection in the tumor cell due to its greater genetic diversity. Once present, the transformation provides a selective growth advantage that allows the cell possessing that modification to predominate.[65,66,69,98,99]

Models for Predicting Cancer Incidence. With few exceptions, radiation may induce cancer in any organ of the body.[7,8] Radiation-induced cancers cannot be distinguished from spontaneous cancers.[6,7,100] The possibility of radiation induction is based on a person's history of exposure to large doses, and is influenced by a number of variables, including total dose, dose rate, and radiation quality.[7,8] As with other somatic effects, genetic changes, and *in utero* effects, high-LET radiation and high dose rates have a greater probability of initiating or promoting cancer than does low-LET radiation. Most leukemias and cancers of the thyroid, breast, lung, liver, and bone are induced at higher rates by high-LET radiation, but the incidence is not large enough to allow accurate determination of the RBE in human populations. Low dose rates permit partial or complete cell repair of the radiation damage. In contrast, with high dose rates, the rate of cell damage may be faster than the repair rate, resulting in damage accumulation. Fractionation of the dose permits repair of a potential neoplasm and decreases the incidence of carcinogenesis for leukemia, but does not appear to be as important in reducing the incidence of breast and thyroid cancers. The latency and total risks for breast, lung, intestinal, stomach, and thyroid cancers vary with the age at exposure. In general, persons who are younger at the time of exposure are at increased risk for most cancers. For breast and thyroid cancers, persons younger than 20 years at the time of exposure are more radiosensitive, whereas they are less radiosensitive for stomach cancer and leukemia. The minimum latency periods are 2–3 years for leukemia and 5–40 years for solid tumors.

The probabilities of developing cancer as a result of exposure to high doses of either low- or high-LET radiation are fairly well established, but the risks of low-level exposure are not.[6-8] Insufficient data exist to accurately determine the risks to humans.[7,8,11,12] The risk for low-level exposure is extremely small and may be nonexistent.[7] Epidemiological analyses for determining the role of radiation exposure in carcinogenesis are made difficult by the small numbers of irradiated populations and the even smaller chance that a specific cancer resulting from a specific radiation exposure can be detected in a population.[7,8,11-13,101-103] Epidemiology is also clouded by the contributions of other carcinogens, differences in health factors, inappropriate control populations, and (in retrospective studies) possible death certificate inaccuracies, missing data in the records, and poor or biased memories.[11,102-104] The most recent estimates for the incidences of cancers resulting from 1 cGy of low-LET radiation are shown in Table 9-3.[11]

Within the limitations described above, the scientific community has attempted to derive risk estimates for low-level radiation exposures that may be used by legislative bodies to prescribe occupational and public safety standards. Four research models are used: *linear*, *linear-quadratic*, *quadratic*, and *pure quadratic with cell killing*.[6-8,13,101-103] Each model may exist with or without thresholds. Two of these models, linear and quadratic (nonlinear), are shown in Figure 9-7. A linear model is more likely to overestimate the incidence of cancer for lower doses. If the initial rate of increase is shallow for the lower doses, then a threshold essentially exists for the lower doses of a nonlinear model (Figure 9-7) because the incidence is extremely low in proportion to the dose. Different cancers may fit one model better than another. For some cancers, the confidence limits of the curve fit may not permit the selection of one model over another with any degree of accuracy. Figure 9-8 shows the degree of fit to the incidence of leukemia in the Nagasaki atomic-bomb survivors.[102] The data are best predicted by a linear-quadratic model,[6,11] although either model is applicable. The radiation-induced incidences of breast cancer and thyroid cancer are best described by linear models.[11] The cell-killing component of the pure-quadratic-with-cell-killing model refers to the fact that some incidence curves decrease at the higher radiation doses. Lower radiation doses increase the incidence of cancer cell induction, whereas the accumulated damage from higher doses is more likely to kill the cell, thus eliminating potential neoplasms.

TABLE 9-3

RISK ESTIMATES FOR RADIATION-INDUCED INCIDENCE OF CANCER PER MILLION PERSONS EXPOSED PER cGy (rad) OF LOW-LET RADIATION

Type or Site of Cancer	Age at Exposure	Years at Risk After Irradiation	Absolute Risk Male	Absolute Risk Female
Leukemia*	0–9	5–26	1.73	1.10
	10–19	5–26	0.85	0.54
	20–34	5–26	0.85	0.54
	35–49	5–26	1.05	0.67
	50+	5–26	1.56	0.99
Lung	10–19	10–33	0.30	0.30
	20–34	10–33	0.56	0.56
	35–49	10–33	0.86	0.86
	50+	10–33	1.20	1.20
Breast	0–9	10–35	—	3.80
	10–19	10–35	—	7.60
	20–29	10–35	—	4.90
	30–39	10–35	—	4.90
	40–49	10–35	—	1.30
	50+	10–35	—	0.80
Thyroid	0–9	10–34	1.50	5.00
	10–19	10–34	1.50	5.00
	20+	10–34	0.50	0.50
Colon	20–34	10–30	0.21	0.21
	35–49	10–30	0.34	0.34
	50+	10–30	0.89	0.89
Stomach	10–19	10–30	0.16	0.16
	20–34	10–30	0.31	0.31
	35–49	10–30	0.51	0.51
	50+	10–30	1.34	1.34
Liver	20+	10–30	0.28	0.28

*Except chronic lymphocytic leukemia

Source: Condensed from reference 11, Table VI-1-A

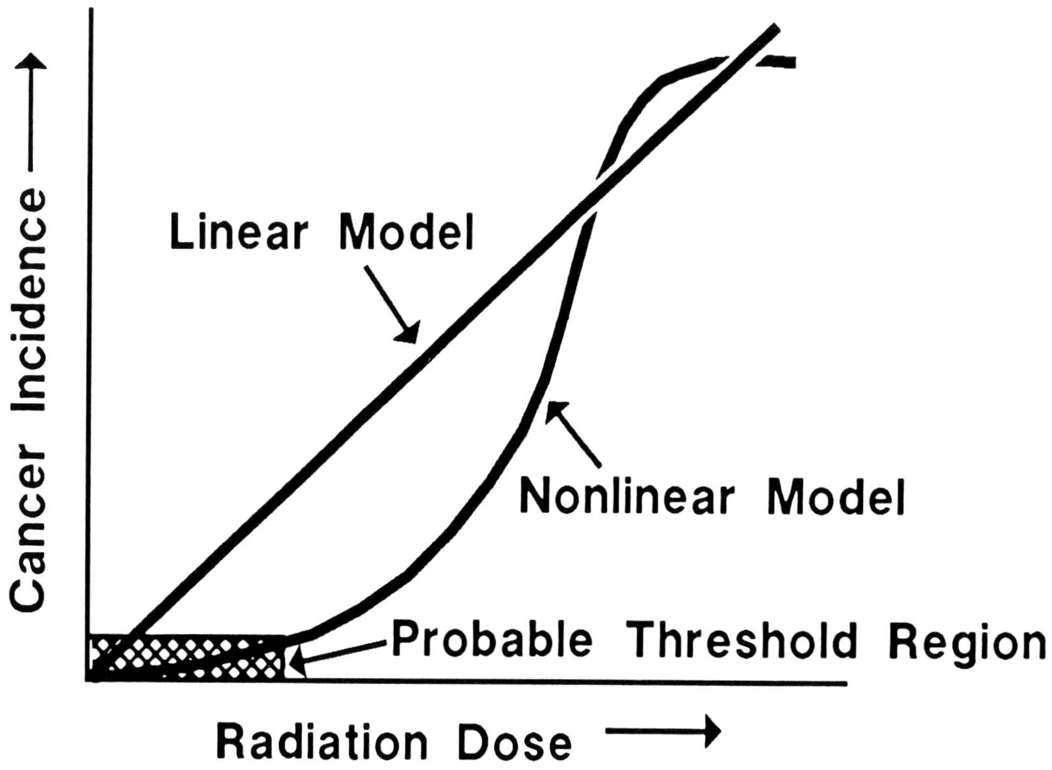

Fig. 9-7. Mathematical models for radiation dose and incidence of cancer. Four models estimate the effects of low-level radiation on incidence of cancer: linear model with threshold, linear model without threshold, nonlinear model with threshold, and nonlinear model without threshold. A "quasi" or probable threshold may exist in the nonlinear model (shaded area), where an increase in incidence within that region is so low that a threshold essentially exists.

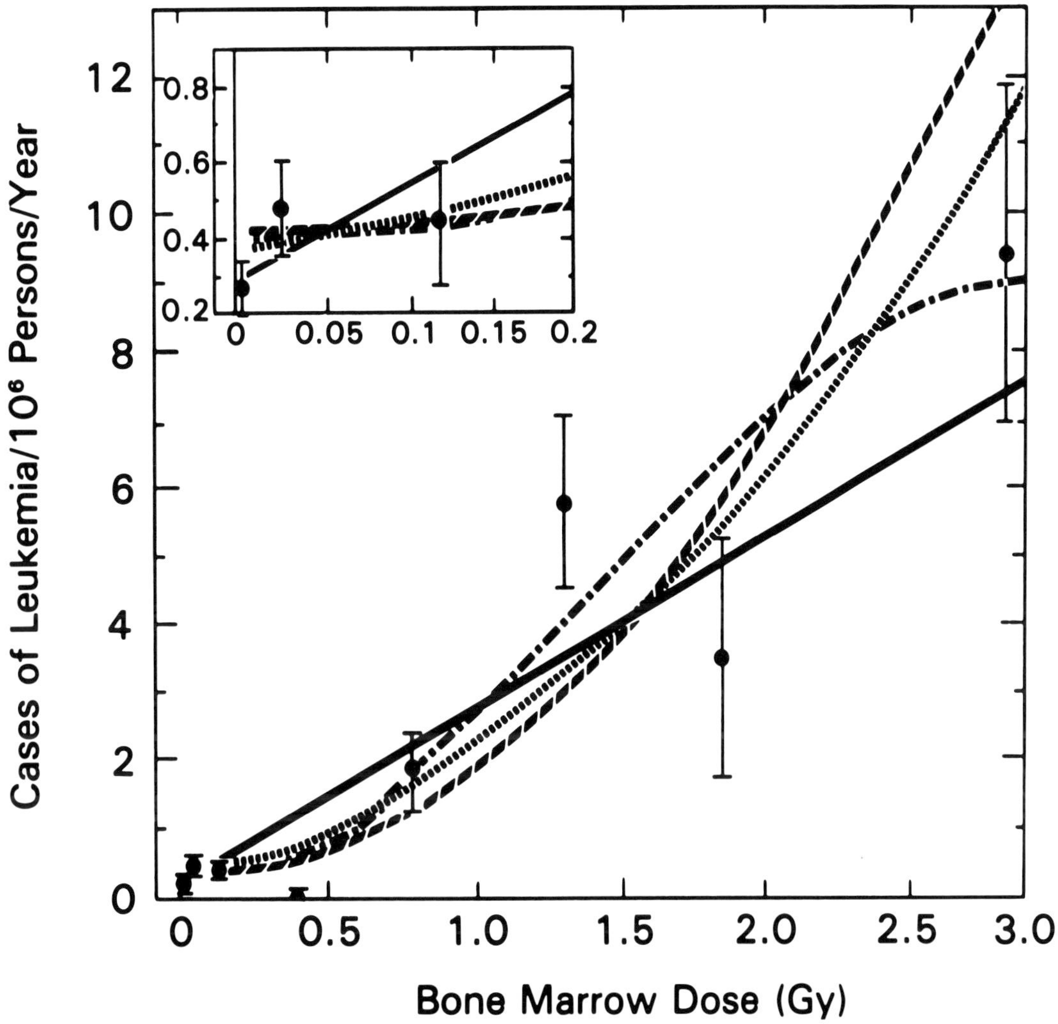

Fig. 9-8. Incidence of leukemia in Nagasaki atomic-bomb survivors through 1972. Bone-marrow doses have been adjusted for differences in age at time of exposure, and 50% confidence intervals are provided. Relative fits of four different mathematical models to data are shown: pure quadratic with cell killing (–•–•–), pure quadratic (– – – –), linear-quadratic (••••••••), and linear (——). Insert is enlargement of the dose range (< 0.2 Gy).

Source: Redrawn from reference 102

HUMAN DATA BASE

Data from the human population on the effects of low-level radiation come from four sources (Table 9-4): atomic-bomb survivors, medical exposures, occupational exposures, and epidemiological comparisons of geographic areas containing high background radiation.[7,8]

The 92,231 survivors of the atomic detonations in Hiroshima and Nagasaki are being monitored by the Radiation Research Foundation for possible radiation-induced health effects.[105] Of the 24,000 deaths in this population through 1982, 6,720 were attributable to radiogenic and nonradiogenic cancers. The foundation is also following 27,000 children of the survivors who were conceived after the detonations to determine if genetic damage was induced in their parents and passed on to them.[106] Radiation doses received by a majority of the survivors were first determined in 1965,[107] and were recalculated in 1986 after more information on the explosions became available.[108] Earlier differences in the biological responses of the Hiroshima and Nagasaki populations were thought to be attributable to the larger neutron exposure and, hence, the greater RBE in the Hiroshima explosion;[7,8] however, reestimation of the radiation doses indicates less contribution from neutrons and a greater influence from gamma radiation in the Hiroshima bomb.[108] This necessitates revising the risk estimates for low-LET radiation exposure and may increase the potential risk estimates by 50%.[105]

The largest medically irradiated population for which dosimetry is available comprises the 14,111 patients in the United Kingdom who received spinal irradiation for treatment of ankylosing spondylitis.[8,13,109-111] Ankylosing spondylitis is a rheumatoid disease primarily affecting the spine and characterized by destruction of the cartilage and ossification of the vertebral joints. The patients received their radiation treatments sometime between 1935 and 1954. In the most recent study, they were monitored through 1970.[110] An increased incidence of leukemia has been observed in this population. Other medically irradiated groups with increased cancer incidence are children who received head radiation for treatment of tinea capitis,[112] and patients who received routine fluoroscopy examinations for postpartum mastitis[113] or during treatment of tuberculosis.[114,115]

The third category includes occupational groups with very low radiation doses (averaging less than 1 rem/year); the medical, scientific, and industrial professions; and victims of radiation accidents. In the early 1900s, workers in a number of occupations received large or chronic exposures to ionizing radiation because of inadequate safety standards and ignorance of its long-term biological effects. Three groups with a high incidence of radiation-induced cancer were the early radiologists, the radium-dial painters of the 1920s,[7,8] and uranium miners.[116,117]

Leukemia

Leukemia is one of the most frequently observed radiation-induced cancers.[7,8,118] It accounts for one-sixth of the mortality associated with radiocarcinogenesis, with equal numbers of cancers of the lung, breast, and gastrointestinal tract.[7,8,11] Leukemia may be acute or chronic, and may take a lymphocytic or myeloid form. With the exception of chronic lymphocytic leukemia, increases in all forms of leukemia have been detected in humans exposed to radiation and in irradiated laboratory animals.[6-8,51] More acute than chronic leukemias are induced, although the latencies are roughly equal.[51] Characteristic chromosomal aberrations induced by radiation have been identified in patients with either acute lymphocytic leukemia[119] or chronic myelogenous leukemia.[77,97] The most common aberration is the Philadelphia chromosome, found in approximately 95% of patients with chronic myelogenous leukemia.[76,94-96]

Leukemia first appeared in the atomic-bomb survivors 2–3 years after the nuclear detonations, and reached a peak incidence 10–15 years after irradiation.[7,8,51] The data for the Nagasaki atomic-bomb survivors best fit a linear-quadratic model (Figure 9-8), although the number of observations is so small that, statistically, either model fits well.[102] The average latency period for leukemia is thought to be 2–20 years.[7,8,11] The mean time from exposure to death was 6 years in the ankylosing spondylitis patients [109,110] and 13.7 years in the atomic-bomb casualties (Table 9-5).[51] The difference between the two groups may reflect the larger radiation dose (averaging 3.21 Gy) received by the bone marrow of the ankylosing spondylitis patients, compared to an average dose of 0.27 Gy in the atomic-bomb survivors. Table 9-5 shows the large numbers of observed leukemias in five irradiated populations compared to the predicted numbers. Between 1950 and 1972, sixty-three excess leukemia deaths occurred among the 92,000 survivors of the

TABLE 9-4

SOURCES OF DATA ON RADIATION EXPOSURE TO HUMANS

Atomic-Bomb Detonation Exposures
Survivors
Offspring of survivors
Medical Exposures
Treatment of tinea capitis
X-ray treatment of ankylosing spondylitis
Prenatal diagnostic X rays
X-ray therapy for enlarged thymus glands
Fluoroscopy (treatment for tuberculosis)
Thorotrast treatment
Occupational Exposures
Radium dial painters (1920s)
Uranium miners and millers
Nuclear dockyard workers
Nuclear-materials enrichment and processing workers
Participants in nuclear weapons tests
Construction workers
Industrial photography workers
Radioisotope production workers
Reactor personnel
Civil aviation and astronautic personnel
Phosphate fertilizer industry workers
Scientific researchers
Diagnostic and therapeutic radiation medical personnel
Epidemiological Comparisons of Areas with High-Background Radiation

atomic bombs.[51,118,120] Results from a group of women in Scotland treated for metropathia hemorrhagica with pelvic X radiation are also shown in Table 9-5.[121] These patients received an average radiation dose of 1.34 Gy to the bone marrow, and have experienced increased incidences of leukemia and cancers at the site of irradiation (intestines, rectum, and uterus).

Thorotrast is a contrast medium that contains thorium-22 and decays by alpha emission (Table 9-5). It was used in diagnostic radiological procedures between 1928 and 1955.[7,8,51] An increased incidence of leukemia and liver cancer was observed in patients in whom thorium had concentrated in the liver and bone. The mean radiation dose to the bone marrow from Thorotrast ingestion was 3.5 Gy.[51] The estimated incidence of leukemia from 1 cGy of internal alpha radiation from Thorotrast is 32 persons per million, compared with 11.4 per million in the ankylosing spondylitis patients, who received 1 cGy of low-LET X radiation.[51] The alpha particle releases so much energy into a small area that most of the local tissue is destroyed before neoplasia occurs, thereby reducing the RBE for neoplasia. Although the risk of inducing cancer increases with an increasing dose, the accumulated damage results in the death of the cell before it can express its cancer potential. The RBE for leukemia induction by neutron radiation is estimated to be 1–25, according to data from the atomic-bomb survivors.[122]

The incidence of leukemia is influenced by age at the time of exposure (Figure 9-9). The younger the person at the time of exposure, the shorter the latency and the risk period for developing leukemia.[7,8] The

TABLE 9-5

LEUKEMIA STATISTICS FOR POPULATIONS EXPOSED TO RADIATION

Population	Average Exposure (Gy)	Follow-up Period (years)	Mean Latency to Death (years)	Number of Persons Exposed	Leukemia Cases Observed*
Atomic-bomb Survivors	0.27	27	13.7	82,000	84 (21)
Ankylosing Spondylitis Patients	3.21	20	6.6	14,109	31 (6.5)
Pelvic Irradiation Patients	1.34	19	12.4	2,068	7 (2.3)
Marshall Island Residents	0.60	28	—	240	1 (—)
Thorotrast Patients (26 ml average)	3.50	27	—	4,594	60 (6)

*Numbers in parentheses are predicted cases of leukemia

incidence of leukemia decreases with increasing age at the time of exposure; however, this individual is at increased risk for a greater period of time (Figure 9-9). Conversely, as the leukemia risk decreases, the risk of developing a solid tumor increases. For radiation doses of less than 0.2 Gy, there appears to be a threshold region in which increasing radiation doses carry slightly increased risks for leukemia induction.[102] This may simply be due to the sigmoid shape of the curve in the low-dose region, but the result is a quasi-threshold effect. Apparently no difference exists in the incidences of leukemia in females and males at any age or at any dose.[7,8,11]

Over 200,000 U.S. military and civilian personnel have been involved in the testing of nuclear weapons since 1945.[104] This number includes military personnel who were permitted to view a nuclear detonation from a safe distance. Later U.S. weapons testing occurred at the Nevada test site and at the Pacific Proving Ground in the Marshall Islands. The average doses received by the participants in those tests were 0.5 rem of gamma radiation and 0.005 rem of neutron radiation.[104] These doses were then and are now considered to be safe; Nuclear Regulatory Commission regulations permit persons in occupations with radiation exposures to receive 3 rem in any calendar quarter or 5 rem per year.[123] At the request of the Department of Defense, the National Research Council conducted a study of mortality among participants of nuclear weapons tests. The study included 46,000 of the approximately 200,000 test participants and, of these, 5,100 deaths occurred from all causes.[104] No increased incidence of leukemia was observed. Significantly fewer circulatory deaths occurred than expected (1,723 versus 2,541) as well as fewer cancer deaths (1,046 versus 1,243). The study concluded that "there is no consistent or statistically significant evidence for an increase in leukemia or other malignant disease in nuclear test participants."

However, a person who was present at the 1957 nuclear test shot (code-named SMOKY) developed leukemia 19 years later.[124] A follow-up study found a statistically significant increase of 8–10 cases of leukemia in the SMOKY test participants, compared with 3.5 leukemia cases expected in a general population of that size.[124,125] The increase could be due to chance alone because of the small population size or because

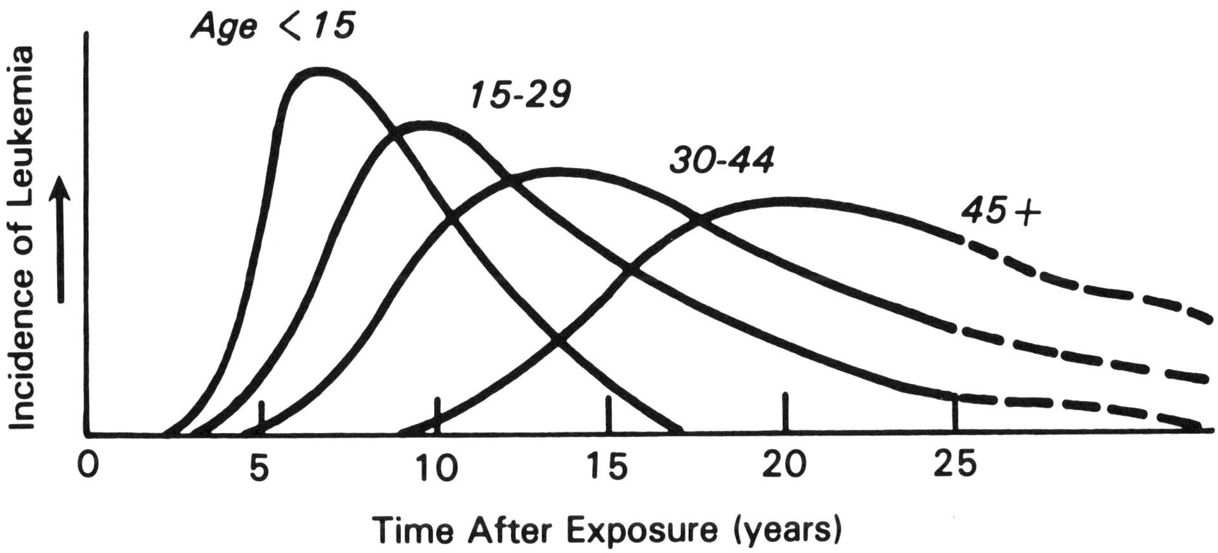

Fig. 9-9. Effect of age at time of radiation exposure on incidence of leukemia in atomic-bomb survivors. Radiation-induced risks are shown for all forms of leukemia (combined) relative to age at time of atomic-bomb explosions, based on 1977 data. Chronic lymphocytic leukemia is not included because increased incidence has not been observed in any exposed human population.

Source: Reference 118

of statistical fluctuation resulting from the *healthy worker effect*. The healthy worker effect states that in a small employed population, some change in mortality will occur if there is better health care, and this factor statistically sets that population apart from the general population. If mortality in one category decreases, then incidences in the other categories also shift. In-depth investigations by the Center for Disease Control and the National Research Council show that a healthy worker effect is present in the SMOKY test participants.[102,126] Fewer circulatory-related deaths occurred in the SMOKY participants (103 versus 139 expected in the general population) as well as fewer respiratory-related deaths (9 versus 17 expected).[126] Although the incidence of leukemia increased, the total incidence of cancers did not.

Thyroid Cancer

Thyroid cancer is also a concern for low-level exposure and late radiation effects (Figure 9-10), possibly accounting for 6%–12% of the mortality attributed to radiation-induced cancers.[7,8,11]

Radiation-induced thyroid cancer is 2.0–3.5 times more prevalent in women than in men (Figure 9-10 and Table 9-3).[7,8,11,127-132] Female atomic-bomb survivors had 3.5 times more thyroid cancer than male survi-

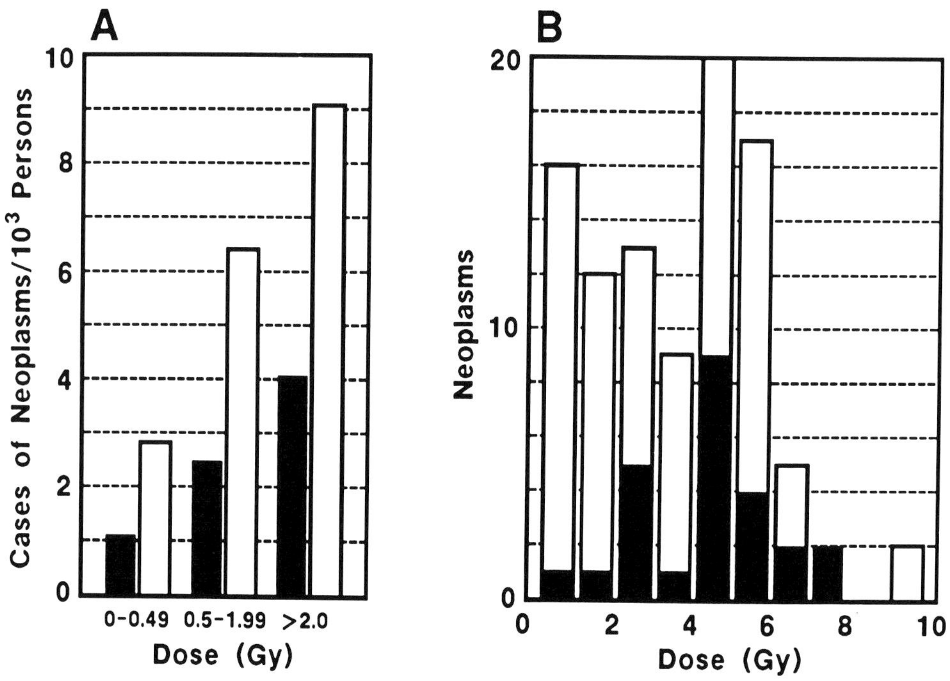

Fig. 9-10. Incidence of thyroid cancer in atomic-bomb survivors. (A) Incidence of thyroid cancer as a function of dose and gender (male □, female ■). Data were obtained in a 1964 study of thyroid neoplasms. (B) Incidence of benign (□) and malignant (■) thyroid neoplasms in persons who had received therapeutic radiation for tinea capitis.

Source: (A) redrawn from reference 130; (B) redrawn from reference 128

vors,[11,129] and as much as 5 times more cancer in one clinical study.[128] The difference in thyroid tumor inductions in males and females is most likely due to hormonal influences on thyroid function.[8,133] Depressing TSH levels in irradiated rats by supplementing their diet with thyroxine reduces the incidence of thyroid cancer.[133] In the Marshall Islanders, the incidence of hypothyroidism is associated with elevated levels of TSH and closely matches the incidence of benign thyroid nodules.[50,134]

Variations also exist for ethnic groups. One study examined thyroid neoplasms in Jewish and gentile women who received radiotherapy during infancy for enlarged thymus glands.[128] The thyroid was in the exposure field during treatment and received a mean dose of 3.99 Gy. The risk of thyroid cancer in women of Jewish background was 163 per million women exposed to 1 cGy of low-LET radiation; in the gentile women studied, the risk was 48 per million.[120] Their risk was 16.5-fold greater than that for men in the same study. Persons of North African ancestory may also be at increased risk.[135]

A study on the atomic-bomb survivors,[129] two studies of 11,000 Israelis irradiated for tinea capitis,[127,135] and a study of patients treated by X-ray epilation for tinea capitis[112] indicate that the incidence of thyroid nodules is affected by the age at exposure. The risk is greater during the first two decades of life (Table 9-3).[11,127,135] Within this age range, children in the Israeli study who were younger than 6 years at the time of radiation treatment had a 1.6–2.3 times greater risk than their older counterparts.[135] The average dose received during treatment was less than 0.09 Gy.[136] Fourteen thyroid tumors occurred in 3,762 persons younger than 6 years at the time of exposure, compared with fifteen tumors per 7,080 persons 6–15 years old.[135] However, not all studies support an age effect.[59]

Thyroid neoplasms induced by radiation are the papillary (89%) and follicular (11%) forms.[7] These forms are usually benign and slow growing, with an associated mortality rate of 5% (Figure 9-10).[7] In a 20-year follow-up of patients who received X radiation during infancy to shrink an enlarged thymus gland, 68% of the thyroid neoplasms were benign.[128] Of the surgically removed thyroid nodules that developed in the Marshall Islanders as a result of their fallout exposure, thirty-six out of forty-five (80%) were benign adenomas, and nine were malignant tumors consisting of seven occult papillary carcinomas and two papillary carcinomas.[50] Doses for these persons were 1–8 Gy. Malignant thyroid nodules tended to develop or to be detected earlier than the benign.[50,128,134] The latency period for benign thyroid nodules is 5–34 years; for thyroid malignancies, 10–34 years.[7,11,128] In a follow-up investigation, an increase in thyroid neoplasms was observed in persons receiving X radiation in childhood for treatment of tinea capitis. The thyroid doses were 0.043–0.113 Gy with a mean of 0.09 Gy.[136] The dose response for thyroid cancer fits a linear pattern.[11] External radiation has a higher incidence of thyroid cancers than internal radiation.[137]

Irradiation of the thyroid may produce other responses, including hypothyroidism and thyroiditis. Hypothyroidism may occur in individuals receiving large sublethal radiation doses from external exposures. Threshold estimates for hypothyroidism in humans may vary by a factor of 25, from 2 Gy to 50 Gy, depending on whether the exposure source is external or internal.[10,137] Higher thresholds exist for internal irradiation (50 Gy), where the concentration of radioactive iodine by the thyroid may pose a problem.[137] Lower thresholds exist for children: 0.2 Gy for internal iodine-131 exposure and 1 Gy for external exposure. In the younger Marshall Island population exposed to 9 Gy, a high incidence of hypothyroidism occurred, characterized by elevated TSH levels. Above this dose, increasing incidence of hypofunction was associated with decreased carcinoma. Ten percent of persons with internal exposures of 200–300 Gy to the thyroid from radioactive iodine in fallout will develop symptoms of thyroiditis. At the upper end of that range estimate, thyroid ablation is likely.[137]

Breast Cancer

Breast cancer is the major concern for women exposed to low-level radiation because of its high incidence (Table 9-3) and 40% mortality rate.[7,8,11,138] In the United States, one in eleven women will get breast cancer.[139] The incidence of mortality from breast cancer is almost nonexistent in men.[7,8,140,141] Because of their increased incidences of thyroid and breast cancer, women are also at greater risk of developing these cancers as a result of radiation.[7,8]

The risk of breast cancer associated with radiation exposure is age dependent (Table 9-3).[6,7,113-115,138,140,142] The absolute risk for women 10–19 years old at the time of exposure is 7.6 cases per million women per cGy of low-LET radiation; for persons over 40 years old, the risk is 0.8–1.3 cases per million.[11] In female adolescents, cancer does not become manifest until after puberty. Studies indicate increased incidence of breast cancer in atomic-bomb survivors who were younger than 10 years at the time of exposure.[140,143] Previous studies detected no increase in numbers of females of that age group.[144] Increases in breast cancer have been observed in women who received radiotherapy during infancy for treatment of enlarged thymus glands.[145]

The latency period for breast cancer is 5–40 years.[7,11,138,140,146] Women younger than 25 years have longer latencies than do older women, and in general, an increased incidence manifests itself in a woman's thirties and forties.[7,8,11,138,140,144] The mean latency period varies from 18 years in the atomic-bomb survivors[51,144,146] to 27 years in one medical study.[114] Estrogen may promote breast cancer because a woman's age at exposure is associated with increased risk, and because few breast cancers occur until age 30.[7,51,140] This is supported by the fact that incidence of breast cancer does not increase in men following irradiation.[7,51,140,141] Several investigators have proposed that the actual period in which estrogen is present as a promoter is the important factor in determining cancer incidence and latency.[7,51,140] Women irradiated after menopause are less likely to incur radiation-induced breast cancer.[7,8,11,138,142] A decreased incidence of breast cancer was seen in women who received X-radiotherapy to the ovaries for metropathia hemorrhagica, although the incidence of radiation-induced leukemia did increase, as expected.[121] The radiotherapy induced an artificial menopause, with a corresponding decrease in estrogen production.

Breast cancer appears to fit a linear model.[7,11,51,146] If a threshold exists, it is in the range of 1 cGy, although a small increase in breast cancer occurred in atomic-bomb survivors who received exposures of less than 0.5 Gy.[7,51] The estimated dose of radiation required to double the naturally occurring incidence of breast cancer is 0.8 Gy.[138] A 1950–1977 study of 23,318 Canadian women who received less than 1 Gy from fluoroscopy during treatment of tuberculosis 20 years earlier showed no significant increase in risk of breast cancer,[138] but in another study, increases in breast cancer were observed in women who received multiple fluoroscopic examinations during tuberculosis treatment.[114] In another group of multiple fluoroscopy patients who received average doses of 0.66 Gy, no increase in cancer incidence was found.[147] These differences might be attributed to lower radiation doses and older age at exposure in the negative group.

Dose fractionation does not appear to reduce the incidence of breast cancer.[7,8,113-115] Damage in breast tissue tends to accumulate rather than to be repaired, so the risk from acute exposure (such as the atomic detonations) is the same as the risk from chronic exposure (such as small daily doses from fluoroscopy or treatment for postpartum mastitis) (Figure 9-11).[113] The data from medical studies and atomic-bomb survivors are very similar in their dose responses.[146]

Other Systemic Cancers

Cancers of the stomach, colon, liver, pancreas, salivary glands, lungs, and kidneys are also induced by radiation.[6-8,11] The incidences of these neoplasms fit a linear-quadratic response model. Like most solid tumors, they have a latency of 10–30 years, and no difference exists in the absolute risks for males and females.[11] With the exception of liver cancer, the radiation-associated risks depend on the age at exposure and increase with age.[6-8,11,51] The greatest risks are for induction of lung or stomach cancer in persons over age 50 at the time of exposure.[7,11] An association between radiation exposure and induction of brain tumors has been reported in two studies of children who received 1.4 Gy of X radiation as treatment for tinea capitis.[148,149] In the combined studies totaling 13,100 children, twenty-four tumors were observed, compared to three of 17,800 in the control population.

In the 1920s, workers who hand-painted the fluorescent dials on wristwatches with radium-based paint achieved the necessary fine detail by moistening the tip of the brush into a point with their tongues; in so doing, they ingested small amounts of the radium. Because radium is a bone-seeking element with a half-life of 1,600 years, these workers had a higher incidence of bone sarcomas. Increased incidences of breast cancer were also observed.[7, 148, 149]

Digestive System Cancers. Significant increases in cancers of the digestive tract, including the esophagus, stomach, and colon, have been observed in the atomic-bomb survivors[105] and in patients following therapeutic irradiation.[6-8,11] These cancers are ranked in order of descending radiation-induced cancer mortality as follows: *(a)* stomach, *(b)* colon, *(c)* pancreas, *(d)* esophagus, and *(e)* rectum.[11] This order reflects an averaging of the data; dose responses for rectal and pancreatic cancer are not significant in the atomic-bomb survivors.[105] Recent estimates by the National Institutes of Health indicate that stomach, colon, and esophageal cancers occur with greatest incidence in persons over 50 years old at the time of exposure (Table 9-3). The combined estimates in persons between 20 and 34 years old at the time of exposure for these three cancers is 1.068 excess cancers per million persons per year for each cGy of radiation. They will incur an increased risk for at least 20 years, beginning about 10 years after exposure, producing a total excess of 21 cancers. Although an estimate for 1 cGy was used, there is no statistical evidence demonstrating that these cancers can be induced by a dose this low. Environmental contributions from dietary and other sources may also influence the development of cancers of the digestive tract (Table 9-1).[73,74]

Tumors of the parotid gland have been observed 13–25 years after medical irradiation with doses as low as 0.9 Gy, and they may be either benign or malignant. In radiotherapy patients, large doses of radiation to the parotid and other salivary glands may result in atrophy, with subsequent difficulty in chewing food and swallowing due to loss of lubrication from saliva secretions.

Data on radiosensitivity of the liver are conflicting.[7,10,11] Several updated studies of the atomic-bomb survivors have failed to demonstrate a radiation dose-related increase in liver cancer.[105,120,152] Increased incidence of liver cancer is observed in patients treated with Thorotrast, although doubt exists about the origin of the disease in these patients.[7,51] There are three possibilities for cancer induction by Thorotrast: *(a)* alpha radiation exposure, *(b)* chemical toxicity from thorium dioxide, and *(c)* metal toxicity from several grams of thorium estimated to accumulate in the liver.[7,11] It is not likely that liver cancer is induced by alpha radiation from internal contamination with plutonium from fallout.[7] Estimates for liver cancer range from 5.6 to 15 deaths per million persons per cGy of external low-LET radiation.[7,11] Radiation hepatitis and cirrhosis of the liver may occur after large doses; may be acute, intermediate, or chronic; and may appear in some radiotherapy patients at 1–3 months after irradiation.[152,153] Sclerosis and blood-vessel narrowing appear to be primary factors in its development. Hepatitis has been observed following doses as low as 4 Gy, although most clinical cases occur after 40–67 Gy.[153] Chronic radiation hepatitis is characterized by atrophy of the liver. Postnecrotic cirrhosis of the liver is two times greater in atomic-bomb survivors who received doses of less than 0.5 Gy, compared with the control population.[152]

Respiratory System Cancers. The induction of cancers may be affected by environmental factors,

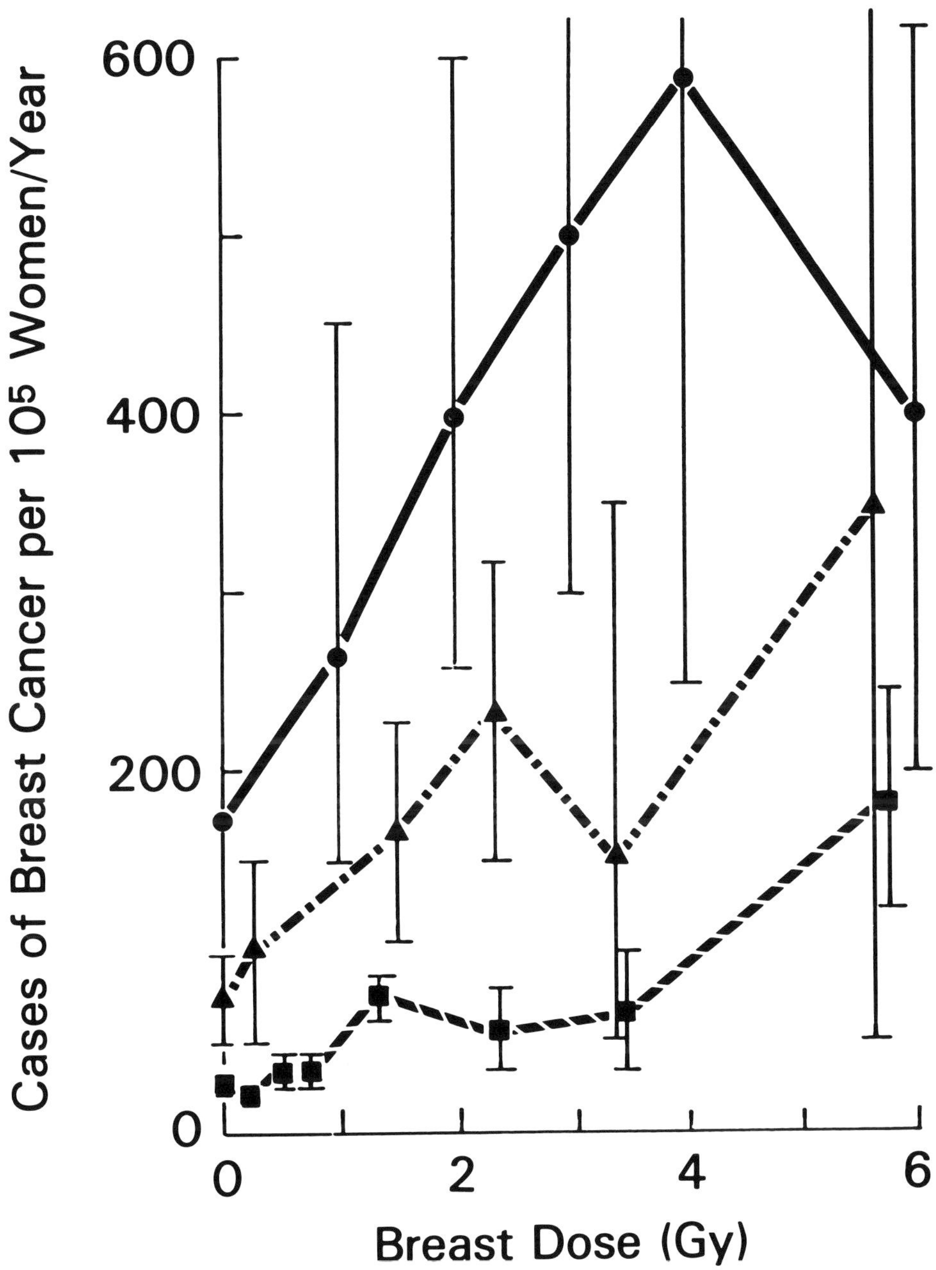

Fig. 9-11. Incidence of breast cancer as a function of fractionated versus acute radiation exposure. The incidence of disease appears to be similar (within statistical limits) whether women received a single acute exposure, as in atomic-bomb survivors (■), or a fractionated series of smaller doses, as in mastitis patients (●) and fluoroscopy patients (▲).

Source: Redrawn from reference 142

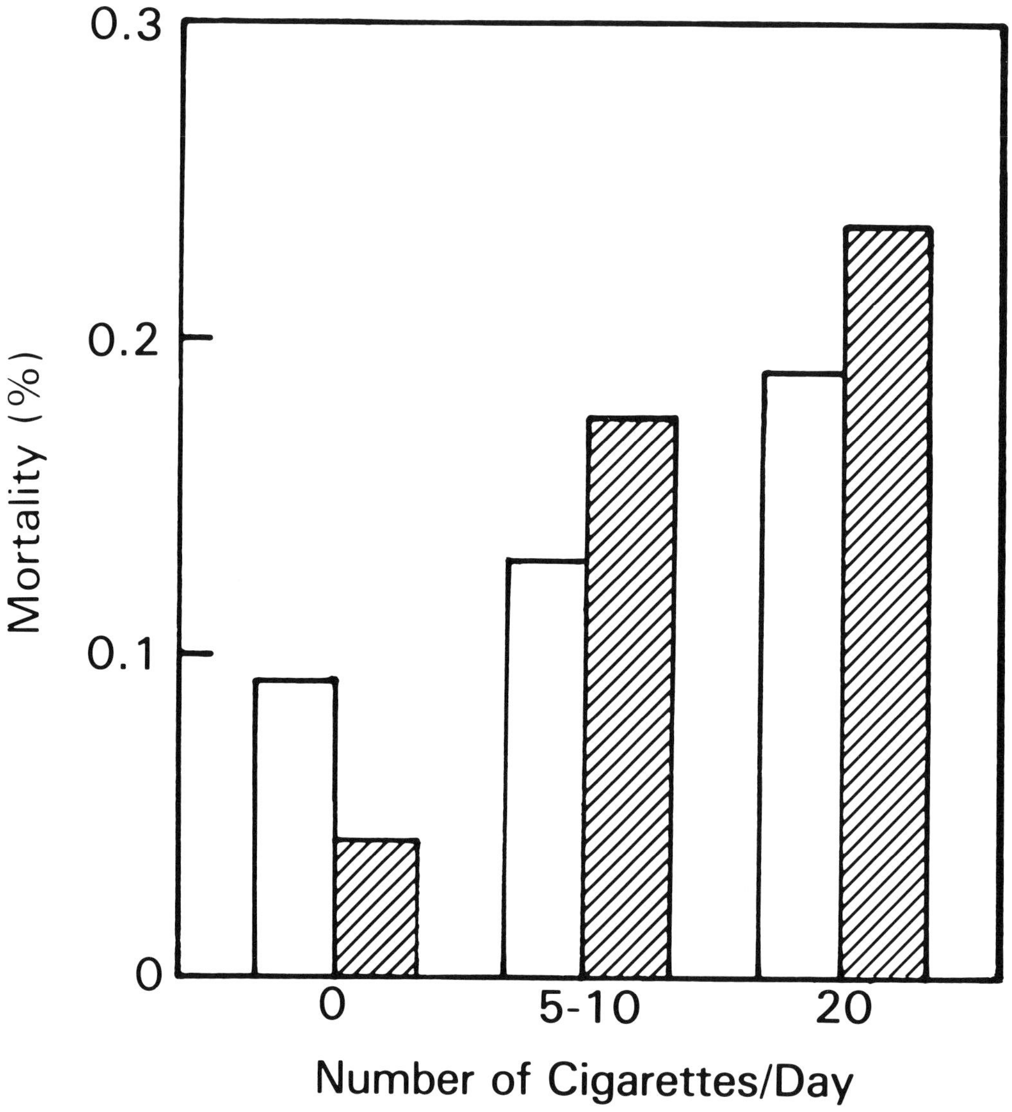

Fig. 9-12. Mortality rate from lung cancer related to cigarette smoking in atomic-bomb survivors. Mortality in 1965–1978 is for persons exposed to 0–0.09 Gy (☐) and >1 Gy (▨).

Source: Redrawn from reference 120

including occupational risks and personal habits, such as smoking (Figure 9-12).[7,11,73,85,154-156]

Workers in uranium mines and mills receive concentrated, high-LET alpha radiation from breathing uranium dust and concentrations of radon gas that seep into the mines from the surrounding rock.[7,51,120,121] Ore dust becomes trapped in the bronchi and alveoli and releases large amounts of radiation to the surrounding tissue, which leads to a higher incidence of lung cancer in this population.[16] In some areas, high radon concentrations in homes and buildings appear to contribute to lung cancer.[16]

In miners and atomic-bomb survivors, smoking has been shown to be an important contributing factor in lung cancer (Figure 9-12).[73,154-157] Risk estimates for radiation-induced lung cancer are four times higher for persons who smoke 1–10 cigarettes per day and twenty-four times higher for persons who smoke 40 cigarettes.[11] Increased cancer in smokers may result from the inhalation of volatile polonium-210, which is concentrated in the lungs and circulatory system.[155-157] Contributing factors are complicated, because the incidence of lung cancers induced by polonium-210 exposure can be enhanced in laboratory animals by the co-administration of saline.[158] Hamsters receiving 40 nCi of polonium-210 by intratracheal administration followed by saline had a 5% incidence of lung tumors, compared with 0% for hamsters receiving polonium-210 alone. In addition, cigarette smoke contains other carcinogens that may be important contributors to cancer development.[60,159]

Radiation pneumonitis will occur 1–7 months after irradiation in persons who survive large whole-body or upper-body exposures.[160] Studies of patients receiving single exposures for radiotherapy indicate that the threshold for this response is 7.5 Gy to the lung.[160] Since this dose is in the lethal range for the hematopoietic subsyndrome from whole-body exposure, the occurrence of pneumonitis will be limited, but it may be important as a late effect in patients receiving a bone-marrow transplant because of the larger radiation doses. A 5% incidence of radiation-induced pneumonitis is expected after a dose of 8.2 Gy, and a 50% incidence is expected at 9.3 Gy.[160] Characteristic symptoms include dyspnea, tachypnea, and coughing. Severe cases may result in death. Radiation pneumonitis is usually followed within 6–12 months by persistent pulmonary fibrosis.[161]

Reproductive System Cancers. A significant increase in malignant and benign tumors of the ovaries occurred in the atomic-bomb survivors between 1965 and 1980.[162] The latency period was 15 years, and a greater frequency was observed in women who were younger than 20 years at the time of exposure.

Cancers of Negligible Risk

Several types of cancer have a low or negligible risk of induction from radiation exposure. No increase in chronic lymphocytic leukemia has been observed to date in irradiated populations,[7] and increases in hairy cell leukemia are low or nonexistent.[11] Cancers of the uterus, cervix, testis, mesentery, prostate, and mesothelium also have a low or nonexistent risk.[7,154] Some cancers are thought to be relatively insensitive to induction by radiation yet still have a small probability of occurrence, such as cancers of the larynx, nasal sinuses, parathyroid, nervous tissue, and connective tissue.[7,105]

In the most recent mortality study of the atomic-bomb survivors, the frequency of cancer of the rectum, gallbladder, pancreas, uterus, lymph glands, and nervous system was not statistically increased.[105] Cancers with a low probability of induction are not observed following low-level radiation because of the apparent long latencies.[7,105]

GENETIC EFFECTS

In 1927, radiation was conclusively shown to damage cells.[163] *Drosophila melanogaster* (fruit fly) sperm were irradiated, and radiation-induced increases were seen in *(a)* mutations leading to mortality and *(b)* mutations of characteristic morphological and phenotypic traits, such as wing shape and eye color. Since then, radiation-induced genetic damage has been consistently demonstrated in plant and animal species, leading to the conclusions that *(a)* radiation is a potent mutagenic agent, *(b)* most radiation-induced mutations are considered to be detrimental, and *(c)* radiation-induced genetic damage is thought to have no threshold, so even very small doses of radiation carry potential risk.[7,8,164-167] The natural incidence of genetic disorders is one in ten for live births and five in ten for spontaneous abortions. Background radiation (200 mrem per person per year) may account for up to 5% of the spontaneous genetic damage in the general population. Radiation causes genetic damage by either *gene mutations* or *chromosomal damage*.[7,8,164-169]

Gene Mutations

Gene mutations are alterations in a single gene locus, which is the smallest amount of genetic information that can code for a single protein. The gene is composed of DNA (Figure 9-13), which is made up of four bases: adenine, guanine, cytosine, and thymine. A group of three bases on a single strand of DNA represents a *codon*, coding for the insertion of one of twenty different amino acids into the protein to be synthesized. A change in one of the three bases within a codon changes the blueprint for the amino acid to be incorporated into the protein at that position.

Radiation may cause point mutations, deletions, insertions, and inversions.[7,8,165,167] The mutation may

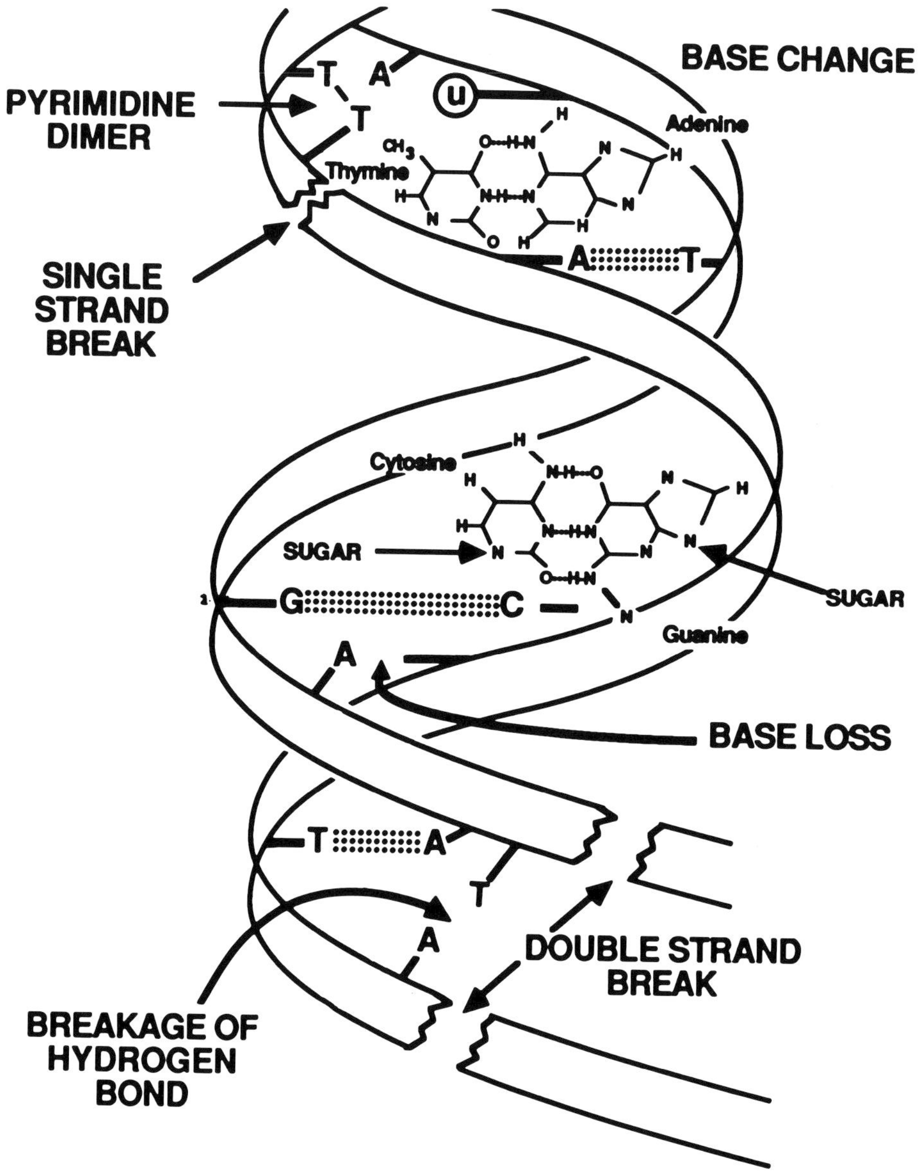

Fig. 9-13. General structures of the four bases of DNA. Three hydrogen bonds occur between cytosine (C) and guanine (G), and two between adenine (A) and thymine (T). Several types of radiation damage to DNA are shown.

Source: Redrawn from reference 247

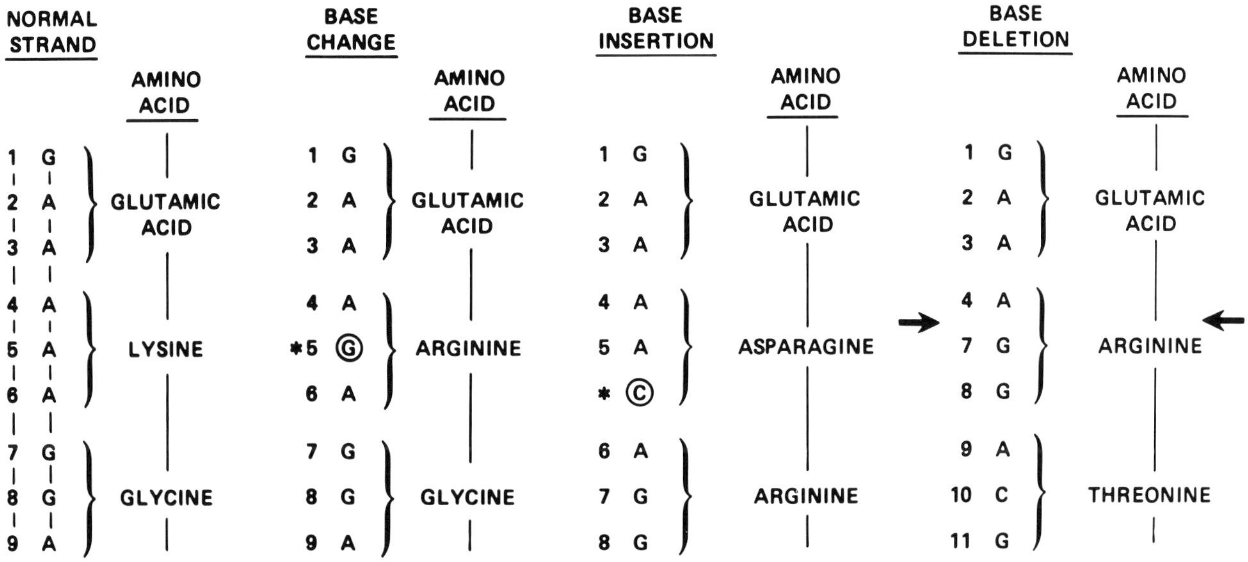

Fig. 9-14. Types of mutations in the gene. One normal strand of DNA (illustrating nine bases within the strand) is shown on the left. These nine bases code for three amino acids within a longer peptide chain. A base change at position 5 from adenine to guanine changes the code for the second amino acid from lysine to arginine. The intercalation of cytosine between positions 5 and 6 changes the codes for the second and third amino acids and for every amino acid in the chain coming after them. Deleting bases 5 and 6 and closing the gap between positions 4 and 7 change the coding for the second and third amino acids and for each amino acid coming after them. Mutations may also occur by inversions (not shown).

occur in either the DNA sequence coding for the protein itself or in one of the regions regulating gene transcription. Mutations in the regulatory region of the gene may modify or shut off a transcription. Some oncogenes, such as the myc-c oncogene, may induce a precancerous state and increased cell proliferation by *(a)* mutation in the promotor region, or *(b)* a translocation that places the gene in a constant state of activation and transcription.[66,82,98] A point mutation occurs through a change in a single base within the gene (Figure 9-14). By changing one base, the codon is altered to represent a different amino acid and may affect the function of the protein. Sickle cell anemia, for example, is a disease resulting from a single point mutation. One form of the ras oncogene has been found to differ from the normal by a point mutation, and this change in one base now codes for a protein that transforms cells in culture to a neoplastic state.[98]

A major concern for radiation genetics is the induction of a dominant gene carrying a trait that results in increased mortality or severe impairment.[7,8,10,165,168,169] Examples of autosomal dominant genes are shown in Table 9-6, although many more exist.[8] As a random mutagenic agent, radiation may induce mutation in any gene. There are no radiation-specific mutations; radiation simply increases the incidence of those that occur naturally.[7,8] The examples in this section should not be regarded as those of radiation-specific mutations occurring after radiation exposure, but rather as particular classes of mutations (dominant or recessive). Of particular concern is the induction of genes that do not become expressed until after the individual has reached reproductive age.[7,8,165,168,169] An example of such a genetic disease occurring in the natural population is Huntington's chorea, a neurological degenerative disease that does not become symptomatic until individuals reach their twenties or thirties.

Recessive radiogenic gene mutations are of less concern since they require homozygosity in order to be expressed. Recessive genes are of more concern when they are located on the X chromosome. Since only one copy of the genes on the X chromosome exists in males, those genes are dominant in their expression. Hemophilia, for example, is a recessive trait on the X chromosome in the natural gene pool that may be expressed as a dominant condition in males (Table 9-6).

TABLE 9-6

INCIDENCE OF SELECTED GENETIC DISORDERS

Disorder	Incidence per 10,000 Live Births
Autosomal Dominant	
Huntington's chorea	5.0
Osteogenesis imperfecta	0.4
Marfan's syndrome	0.4
Familial hypercholesterolemia	20.0
Autosomal Recessive	
Cystic fibrosis	5.0
Phenylketonuria	1.0
Neurogenic muscular distrophy	1.0
Sex-Linked Recessive	
Duchenne's muscular dystrophy	2.0
Hemophilia	1.0
Chromosomal Disorders	
Down's syndrome (trisomy 21)	12.0
Edward's syndrome (trisomy 18)	1.0
Klinefelter's syndrome (XXY)	5.0

Chromosomal Damage

Radiation may also induce genetic damage by chromosomal changes.[7,8] The expression of a number of genes may be altered by damaging a portion of or a whole chromosome. Chromosomal changes may arise either as *chromosomal aberrations* or by *nondisjunction*, resulting in an unequal number of chromosomes.[7,8] Chromosomal aberrations are changes in the size, morphology, or number of chromosomes, and include dicentrics, acentrics, fragments, translocations, inversions, insertions, and deletions (Figure 9-15).[7,8,165,168,169] The most common chromosomal damage induced by radiation is *reciprocal translocation*.[8] In this process, two different chromosomes experience double-stranded DNA breaks, and the two fragments rejoin to different chromosomes rather than those to which they were originally attached. By rejoining to a chromosome containing a centromere, the translocated piece may be transferred into the new gamete during division rather than be lost as an isolated fragment.

Chromosomal aberrations can be produced in both somatic and germ cells, and their frequency is proportional to the dose of radiation received.[170,171] Acentric and dicentric fragments are the most lethal because they may not properly separate at meiosis or mitosis and thus may halt those cellular processes. As a somatic mutation, the percentage of chromosomal aberrations in the lymphocytes of irradiated humans has been used to estimate the dose received. Such damage persisted in the lymphocytes of the atomic-bomb survivors 23 years after their exposure.[172]

The gain or loss of an entire chromosome through nondisjunction occurs less frequently and is more likely to result in mortality.[7,8] Mammalian studies have been unable to demonstrate increased incidence of trisomies in the offspring of irradiated animals.

Factors Affecting Mutation

A number of factors affect the ability of radiation to induce mutations, including rate of biological repair, dose rate, shielding, and number of exposures.[7,8,165,168,169,173] Several enzyme systems constantly monitor and repair the DNA, recognizing specific kinds of base damage and initiating repair.[174] During excision repair, for example, enzymes recognize the damaged part and split the DNA strand to remove it. The other strand then serves as a template to reincorporate the proper bases in the excised site, followed by action of a DNA ligase that reseals the strand. Breaks in the DNA strands may also be reconnected, although proper rejoining (if it occurs at all) becomes more difficult if a break has occurred in both DNA strands.[174,175] Other enzymes repair specific base damage, such as alkylations. Fractionation of the radiation dose can reduce the damage by allowing repair to occur between exposures. If the rate of damage exceeds the rate of repair, then the mutation rate will increase. Experiments in mice show that mutation rates do not further decrease at dose rates below 8 mGy/minute.[166] Dose rates in this range are about one-third as effective as high dose rates of gamma radiation in producing specific locus mutations in mice. High-LET radiations, such as neutrons, impart more energy per unit distance traveled through a biological material than do low-LET radiations. More energy deposited in the area of the DNA is more likely to produce more damage, increasing the likelihood of breaking both strands of the DNA.

Some DNA bases undergo spontaneous deamination. Deamination of cytosine produces uridine, which occurs in ribonucleic acid (RNA) but not in DNA. Unless the deamination product is enzymatically cor-

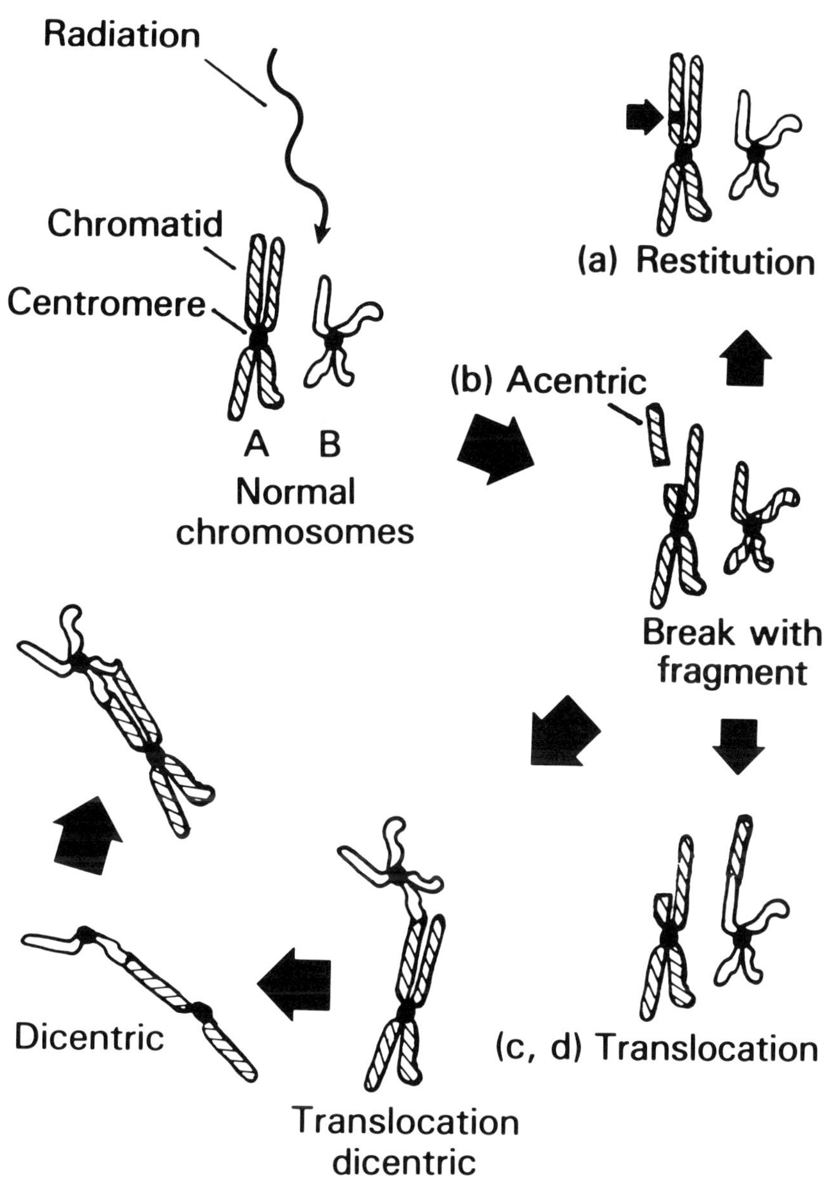

Fig. 9-15. Radiation-induced chromosomal aberrations in two typical chromosomes (A and B). When a chromosome breaks, one of four events occurs: *(a)* the chromosome is restored to its original state (restitution), or the break is rejoined, with no apparent damage; *(b)* the fragment is not replaced and may be lost in subsequent divisions; *(c)* the fragment rejoins the original free end, but in an inverted position; and *(d)* the fragment may be translocated onto a nonhomologous chromosome.

rected before replication, it can be mispaired, producing a base substitution in the newly replicated strand. Spontaneous deamination can be accelerated by increases in temperature.

Six genetic syndromes are known to be more sensitive to ultraviolet light or X-radiation damage to cells in culture, and they are associated with increased incidence of cancer.[7,8,69] These include xeroderma pigmentosum, Down's syndrome, ataxia telangiectasia, Fanconi's anemia, Bloom's syndrome, and Cockayne's syndrome.[8] Most have associated defects in DNA-repair capability and increases in chromosomal aberrations. Age and gender are important secondary determinants for mutagenesis; for instance, studies show that the mother's age at the time of conception is an important factor in the incidence of Down's syndrome. The natural rate of chromosomal abnormalities is eight times higher in children whose mothers were 40 years old at the time of conception than in children whose mothers were 20 years old.[176] Paternal age at time of conception is also of concern, because the risk for a dominant gene mutation in the germ cells of men 30 years old and older is at least eleven times greater than in men who are younger than 30 years at the time of conception.[177]

Internalized radionuclides of hydrogen, carbon, and phosphorus may present special genetic damage, because these elements are the basic elements found in DNA.[178] The radionuclides may damage the DNA when they release their energy through beta decay and as they undergo transmutation, resulting in structural damage at the molecular site of incorporation.[7,178,179] Carbon-14 located in a sugar or base of the DNA decays to nitrogen-14. Tritium (hydrogen-3) decays to helium-3, and phosphorus-32 decays to sulfur-32. Transmutation of the phosphorous-32 in the sugar phosphate DNA chain can produce a strand break.

Plutonium-239, an alpha emitter, has induced genetic damage in mice following internalization.[7,8] Other alpha and beta emitters from internalized fallout will present similar problems. The RBE in mice following injection of plutonium-239 citrate ranges from four for specific locus mutations to fifty for translocations.[7]

Radiation-Induced Damage in Humans

Evidence is lacking for radiation-induced genetic mutation in humans, although mutations of human cells in culture have been shown.[7,8] Based on current risk estimates, the expected increase of genetic damage in the atomic-bomb survivors is so low that it would not be detectable within the larger normal spontaneous incidence.[7,8,10] In screening twenty-eight different protein loci (498,000 loci tested) in the blood of 27,000 children of atomic-bomb survivors, only two children presented mutations that might be related to the radiation exposure of the parents.[106]

Early studies on the survivors' children examined whether radiation exposure caused an increase in sex-linked lethal genes that would result in increased prenatal death of males or alteration of the gender birth ratio.[180] Data did not support that hypothesis. Twelve studies have examined a possible increase in the incidence of Down's syndrome as a result of maternal irradiation,[8,165] but only four of the studies showed statistical significance,[181-184] and the hypothesis has not received widespread acceptance. Irradiation of the human testes has been shown to produce an increase in the incidence of translocations,[185] although no additional chromosomal aberrations have been detected in children of the atomic-bomb survivors.[8,186]

Estimating Genetic Risks

The *genetically significant dose* (GSD) is the dose of ionizing radiation to the gonads that may result in increased incidence of genetic mutations in germ cells.[7,8] Estimation of the GSD takes into account the number of persons of reproductive age in a particular group in determining a collective dose. In the United States, the GSD from background and generated radiation sources is 122 mrem per person (Table 9-7).[7] The GSD from occupational exposure in the military service is less than 0.04 mrem per person, which is less than that received in a national research laboratory (< 0.2 mrem/year) or a nuclear power plant (< 0.15 mrem/year) Most occupational exposures are less than those received from consumer products over the same period.

Another method of estimating radiation-induced genetic damage is the calculation of the *doubling dose*, or radiation dose required to double the spontaneous mutation rate.[7,8] The spontaneous mutation rate in humans is 5 x 10^{-6} per locus, and 6.7–15.1 x 10^{-4} per gamete for chromosomal anomalies.[7] The doubling dose is 0.5–2.5 Gy of low-LET gamma or X radiation, and 1 Gy is commonly used for calculation purposes.[8] The doubling dose for specific locus mutations in mice with low dose rates (< 8 mGy/minute) of low-LET gamma radiation is about 1.1 Gy.[185]

The effects of radiation exposure on the human population have been examined by several national and international scientific committees, including the National Academy of Sciences Committee on Biological Effects of Ionizing Radiation;[7] the United Nations Scientific Committee on Effects of Atomic Radiation;[8,51] and the International Commission on Radiological Protection (ICRP).[187] These groups arrived at similar estimates for the effects of low-level exposure to ioniz-

TABLE 9-7

CONTRIBUTORS TO GENETICALLY SIGNIFICANT DOSES

Source		Mrem per Year
Natural		82.0
Man-made		40.0
Selected Man-made Contributors		
Medical	20.0	
Nuclear power	< 1.0	
Consumer products	4.5	
Weapons testing or fallout	4.5	
Military occupational applications	< 0.004	
Total		122.0

Source: Data from reference 7

ing radiation (Table 9-8, Table 9-9).

The National Academy of Sciences estimates that for an exposure of 1 cGy to the present generation, there will be 5–65 additional genetic disorders per million births in the succeeding generation resulting from increases in autosomal dominant mutations and sex-linked dominant mutations. If a population is continually exposed to an increased radiation dose of 1 cGy for each generation, an equilibrium will be reached between the induction of new genetic disorders and the loss of the earlier induced disorders. In this equilibrium, an additional 60–1,100 genetic disorders would be expected in the population, with the majority contributed by autosomal dominant and sex-linked recessive mutations and a large contribution from irregularly inherited genes. Irregularly inherited genes make up family tendencies for diseases and situations of incomplete dominance (where phenotypic expression is neither the recessive trait nor the dominant trait, but a blend of the two). Chromosomal damage and recessive mutations are thought to make minor contributions to the equilibrium rate. Chromosomal damage and loss are generally either lethal or selected out, while recessives are expressed only in the homozygous condition. The National Academy of Sciences does not provide a confidence interval or a geometric mean for its 60–1,100 range of additional genetic disorders in the next generation per million births.[7,10]

The ICRP estimates that for every million individuals receiving 1 cGy of radiation in the present generation, 125 additional cases of serious genetic disorders will occur over the next two generations.[187] Approximately half will come from dominant, sex-linked, and irregularly inherited mutations. Of the 125 cases, 89 will occur in the first generation. If a doubling dose method is used, then (assuming a doubling dose of 1 Gy) 1,500 autosomal dominant and gender-linked diseases per million live births would be observed in the first generation, and 10,000 (approximately the normal incidence) would be observed in succeeding generations exposed to 1 Gy at equilibrium. The total incidence of genetic disorders, one in ten live births, would not be reached in equilibrium with a 1-Gy doubling dose, since the doubling dose cannot approximate the irregularly inherited component.[8,10] Table 9-8 does not contain an estimated contribution for the irregularly inherited disorders in the first generation. The large variation within the equilibrium category is responsible for the large range (60–1,100) of total disorders expected in the equilibrium generation.

Using the doubling-dose method, the U.N. com-

TABLE 9-8

BEIR III ESTIMATES OF INCIDENCE OF GENETIC DAMAGE*

Genetic Disorder	Current Incidence in Liveborn Offspring (per million)	Increased Incidence in Liveborn Offspring** (per million)	
		First Generation	Equilibrium
Autosomal dominant and X-linked	10,000	5–65	40–200
Irregularly inherited	90,000	5–65	20–900
Recessive	1,100	5	<10
Chromosomal aberrations	6,000	<10	<10
Total	107,100	5–65	60–1,100

*Committee on Biological Effects of Ionizing Radiation of the National Academy of Sciences

**When every individual in preceeding generation receives 1 extra rem

Source: Data from reference 7

TABLE 9-9

ESTIMATED EFFECT OF 1 Gy BY DOUBLING DOSE METHOD OF UNSCEAR*

Genetic Disorder	Current Incidence in Liveborn Offspring (per million)	Increased Incidence in Liveborn Offspring (per million)	
		First Generation	Equilibrium
Autosomal dominant and X-linked	10,000	1,500	10,000
Irregularly inherited	90,000	450	4,500
Recessive	2,500	slight	slow
Chromosomal Diseases			
Structural	400	240	400
Numerical	3,000	small	small
Total	105,900	2,190	14,900

*United Nations Scientific Committee on Effects of Atomic Radiation

Source: Data from reference 8

TABLE 9-10

ESTIMATED INCIDENCE OF HUMAN GENETIC DAMAGE PER Gy*

Genetic Damage	Spermatogonia	Oocytes
Dominant mutations	16–400	0–180
Balanced reciprocal translocations	220–8,750	0–875
Unbalanced translocations	440–17,500	0–5,250
X-chromosome loss	negligible	0–500

*Unbalanced translocations of chromosome fragments
Source: Data from reference 8

mittee predicts that after exposure to 1 Gy, a total of 2,190 additional genetic disorders and an equilibrium of 14,900 will occur per million live births in the first generation after exposure (Table 9-9). Assuming a linear response, the U.N. committee estimates a mean of 22 disorders per million live births compared to the 5–65 disorders per million live births predicted by the National Academy of Sciences for a population exposed to 1 cGy. The U.N. committee extended its estimates to the detrimental effects of radiation exposure on the general population. The average dominant mutation in children of parents receiving a 1-Gy radiation dose would result in 25 years of impaired life, with death occurring 13 years prematurely. Overall, a 1-Gy exposure to parents would result in a total of 53,800 years of impaired life per million births from all causes of radiation-induced genetic damage, and a loss of 47,200 years of life in the succeeding generation. Through natural selection, the gene pool has the capacity to absorb large amounts of damage without destroying the population. A dose of 1 Gy to each generation would produce an equilibrium of 14,900 genetic disorders per million live births, compared to a normal incidence of one in ten. This is an increase of only 1.5%.

The immature human oocyte is thought to be only 44% as radiosensitve for mutation induction as the male spermatocyte.[7,8] The U.N. committee has estimated that most of the genetic damage induced by low-LET radiation will be unbalanced translocations, and that a 1-Gy low-LET exposure would induce 440–17,500 unbalanced translocations per million spermatogonia but only 0–5,250 in human oocytes (Table 9-10). These estimates were based on data for spermatocytes from rhesus monkeys, marmosets, and humans. Using the direct method, 1,000–2,000 dominant mutations per million births will be expected in the first generation following paternal irradiation of 1 Gy, but only 0–900 following maternal irradiation with the same dose.

RADIATION EFFECTS *IN UTERO*

The developing embryo is extremely sensitive to ionizing radiation, and the public has shown increased awareness and concern for exposure of the fetus to low-level radiation. Human and laboratory animal data indicate that doses as low as 0.05 or 0.1 Gy may induce effects.[7,51] Thresholds are thought to exist for the induction of *in utero* responses because most occur after damage to more than one cell.[7]

Stages of Development

The gestation period can be divided into three stages of embryo development: *preimplantation*, *major organogenesis*, and *fetal*. In humans, the preimplantation stage begins with the union of sperm and egg, and continues through day 9 when the zygote becomes embedded in the intrauterine wall. During this time, the two pronuclei fuse, cleave, and form the morula and blastula.

Major organogenesis begins on day 9–11 in humans[188,189] and continues through day 45.[180,191] The organ systems undergo differentiation and development. Neural cells are the first to differentiate, starting on day 17–20.[192,193] Neural development continues throughout the major organogenesis period and into the fetal period. The fetal stage covers weeks 7–38, or term.[191]

Four general responses may occur after radiation exposure *in utero,* depending on the stage of gestation at the time of exposure. These responses range from no detectable effect to prenatal death, neonatal death, or induction of congenital anomalies.[194]

Preimplantation

The embryo is extremely radiosensitive during the preimplantation stage, and radiation can cause increased prenatal death and reabsorption of the embryonic tissue.[188,194] In humans, reabsorption does not occur, but there is an increase in prenatal death. In animals, the incidence of prenatal death decreases as development proceeds into the major organogenesis stage, and it varies with the dose and time of exposure.[7,51,188,194] During this period, the incidence of congenital anomalies is low but not absent. Surviving embryos show an all-or-none response that is essentially normal with no visible anomalies, even though radiation may have killed many cells.[188,194] During organogenesis, similar radiation doses might produce 100% incidence of a particular anomaly and probable growth retardation.[51,188,194]

Several factors, including repair capability,[188] undifferentiation, and a possible hypoxic state,[9] are thought to account for the decreased ability of radiation to induce anomalies during the preimplantation period. During the first few divisions, the cells are undifferentiated and lack predetermination for particular organ systems. If cell death were to occur following radiation exposure at this stage, the remaining cells could continue the embryonic development without gross malformation because they are still indeterminant. However, chromosomal damage at this point may be passed on to appear in later stages. When cells are no longer indeterminant, loss may lead to anomalies, growth retardation, or death. In mice, low incidences of exencephaly[195] and skeletal anomalies[196] have been observed following high-dose irradiation during preimplantation. At a critical period, 0.5 Gy may cause polydactyly.[197]

In laboratory animals, the incidence of prenatal death can vary with the dose of radiation and the time of exposure.[188,189,194] The most sensitive times of exposure in humans are at 12 hours after conception, when the two pronuclei fuse to the one-cell stage, and again at 30 and 60 hours, when the first two divisions occur.[197,198] At periods just preceding the cleavages, there would be insufficient time for repair of damage. In animals, 30% of the prenatal death at this time is because of radiation damage to the mother and a subsequent termination of pregnancy, rather than because of direct radiation damage to the embryo.[194]

Chromosomal aberrations from radiation exposure at the one-cell stage could result in the loss of a chromosome in subsequent divisions that would be uniform throughout the embryo.[7,51,199] Most chromosomal losses lead to prenatal death, although the loss of a sex chromosome in females may instead produce Turner's syndrome.[7,199] Such individuals are phenotypically female. Although this might indicate that a slightly higher proportion of phenotypic females will result from radiation exposure during this period, an altered gender ratio was not found in the children of the atomic-bomb survivors[180] or in laboratory mice irradiated during precleavage.[188] In mice, a dose of 1 Gy on day 0 (preimplantation) resulted in 50% prenatal death and produced loss of a sex chromosome in 4% of survivors. A prenatal mortality of 25% and a sex-chromosome loss in 0.5% of survivors occurred when the same dose was given 7 hours later.[199]

Major Organogenesis

Embryo malformation occurs most frequently with radiation exposure during the organogenesis stage, and the resulting incidences of abnormalities and prenatal death will peak during this time.[7-9,51,194] However, the incidence of prenatal death decreases rapidly with increasing embryo development, and becomes equal to that of the control group when three-fourths of this stage has been completed.

The produced effects depend on the stage of development in which irradiation occurs, the dose, and the dose rate.[7-9,51,194] Most anomalies have a *critical period* during which the radiation exposure will result in the highest incidence of that anomaly (Figure 9-16).[188,190,194] Critical period is sometimes misinterpreted to mean that the particular organ tissue is in its most sensitive or major developmental period. This, however, may not necessarily be the case. Increased incidence during this time may be the result of indirect effects arising from damage to the adjacent tissue or from an inducer

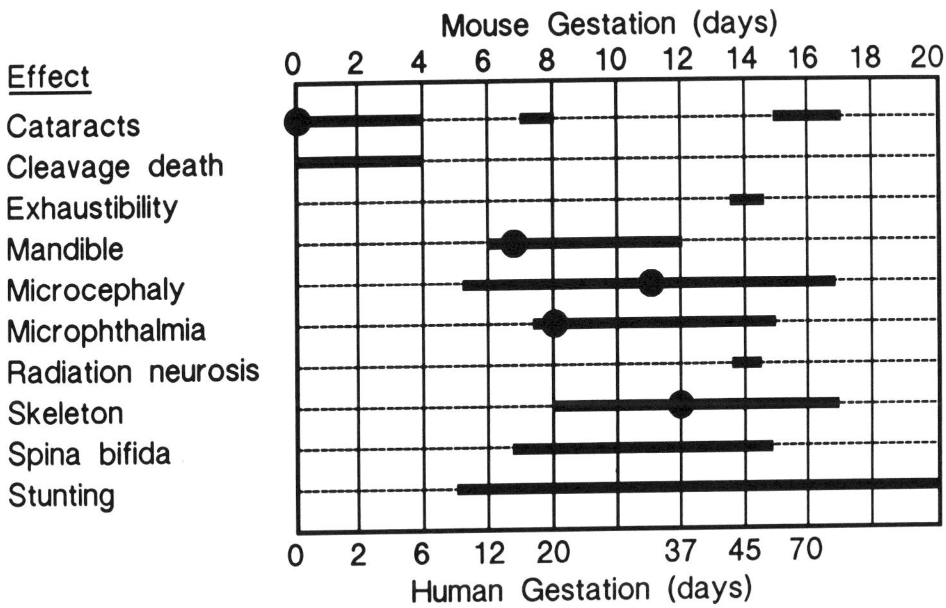

Fig. 9-16. Critical periods (solid lines) for radiation-induced birth defects in mice. Studies were performed with 1–2 Gy of acute X radiation during gestation. Corresponding days for human gestation are shown at bottom.

Source: Redrawn from reference 190

material of that organ.[51,194]

Each organ system is not at identical risk during the entire major organogenesis period because each organ is not developing at the same rate. Some organs may require the development of another organ or inducement before undergoing development themselves. Some anomalies may have more than one critical period. As a congenital anomaly in mice, cataract formation has three critical periods: 0–4 days, 8–9 days, and 14–17 days. These periods are due to the critical periods of several different systems that may in turn influence cataract formation. A slight but significant increased incidence may be observed with lower doses of radiation during the critical period.[190,194] A dose as low as 0.05 Gy may cause polydactyly,[197] skeletal malformation, decreased litter weight, and reduced tail length in mice.[200] Similar low doses have produced anomalies in the human,[201] monkey,[202] rabbit,[203] and rat.[204] *In utero* exposure to doses of less than 0.05 Gy from the Hiroshima atomic bomb resulted in an 11% increase in microcephaly.[7,204] Small continuous radiation exposures to rats from either X rays (1 cGy/day) or tritiated water (0.3–3.0 cGy/day) throughout their pregnancies produced decreases in brain weight.[7,205,206] Low doses of X radiation have also produced growth retardation[201] and behavioral defects.[207,208] Protracted low doses commonly affect the nervous system and the germ cells (ovaries and testes). The long, continuous development of the nervous system makes it sensitive to damage by even these low doses.[192,193,209-211] The range of a particular critical period may be extended by increasing the dose of radiation. Radiation does not increase the length of pregnancy in laboratory animals.[194] Fractionation of the radiation dose may produce either an increase or a decrease in the incidence of anomalies, depending on the time between exposures. If the critical period has a narrow time window, then fractionation over short periods of time may increase the damage by placing more radiation in the critical period and producing more mitotic death. Exposures at an early stage will increase the sensitivity to radiation exposure in a later critical period.

Variations in natural background radiation have not produced significant differences in the incidence of anomalies, although environmental factors may play a role in their induction.[7,51,212,213] The incidence of congenital malformations in mammals may be affected by seasonal differences, with greater sensitivity in winter.[214,215] In the human, 70% of trisomy 18 (Edward's syndrome) and trisomy 13–15 (Patau's syndrome) live births are conceived in the winter.[216] In laboratory animals, anomalies such as those for the rear appendages and eyes have a greater incidence on the right side of the body than on the left.[197,216]

Anomalies may arise in several ways. Radiation may damage the primordial tissue of a particular organ or limb by direct or indirect damage to the chromosome or gene.[194] This in turn may result either in the failure to produce a functional gene product or in the production of an altered functional product. Radiation may cause nondisjunction during mitosis, resulting in a trisomic cell and a monosomic cell. Development would be affected to the extent that either cell predominates in an organ system.

Aberrations or other damage culminating in cell death could result in a reduction in the number of stem cells available for differentiation, which affects future organ systems. Growth reduction may result in the death of differentiated cells, leaving the embryo with a cell population too small to form the proper-sized organ.[217] A reduction in the size of one organ may cause changes in the surrounding tissues, such as microcephaly and mental retardation in humans irradiated *in utero*. The development of organs requires cell cooperation, mediated by chemical messengers such as hormones, organizers, and inducers. Destruction or damage to cells that contain organizers or chemical inducers may result in prenatal death or anomalies.[209] For example, the gray crescent material is an inducer that guides formation of the dorsal lip of the blastula, and eventually (through an area called the chordamesoderm) guides the development of the nervous system itself. Loss of the gray crescent or other inducer would modify or terminate subsequent development. Alterations in tissue contacts or areas of growth also may cause abnormal organ development.

The response of each organ to the induction of malformations is unique, based on dose, gestational age, type of radiation, RBE, oxygen tension, cell types undergoing differentiation, relationships to surrounding organs, and other factors.[7,51] Neutrons and beta particles are more effective at inducing congenital anomalies than is low-LET radiation. As an internal emitter, a beta particle released from tritiated water (or an alpha particle released from plutonium-239) would cause more damage because of its high LET and because there would be no maternal reduction of the dose. The high energy levels are released within the local area of the biological target. Neutrons have an RBE of 4.5 for inducing prenatal mortality in mice.[218] Animal studies in which either the mother or the embryo was shielded indicate that the induction of malformations is due mainly to direct damage to the embryo.[219-221] It is difficult to assign an overall risk estimate to the 119 different anomalies described in the literature because, like cancers, certain malformations are more inducible than others, and accounting for the variables becomes difficult.[7,51]

The Fetal Stage

The fetal stage is the final stage of development, lasting from the end of major organogenesis until birth. In mice, this covers days 14–20 of gestation;[188,194] in humans, days 45–266.[191] Radiation-induced prenatal death and anomalies are, for the most part, negligible during this stage. Anomalies of the nervous system and sense organs are the primary types that are inducible during the fetal stage because these systems are still developing. A radiation dose of 0.2–0.4 Gy given to rats on days 16, 18, or 22 of gestation caused delayed development, irregular arrangement, and loss of neurons in the brain cortex.[222] Irradiation on day 18 resulted in a 25% loss of neurons in the outer cortex, but no decrease in brain volume because there was an associated increase in glial cells. Much of the damage present during the fetal stage may not be manifested as behavior alteration or mental retardation until later in life. The incidence of neonatal-induced death also decreases with increased development during the fetal stage. The $LD_{50/30}$ for neonatal death given on day 10 of gestation to mouse embryos is about 1.15 Gy. By day 18 of gestation, the $LD_{50/30}$ is 6 Gy and rapidly approaches that of the adult animal.[217]

Stunting (retardation of growth) that is induced during this stage is a threshold phenomenon resulting from the killing of many cells. Since differentiated tissues (such as muscles and nerves) do not divide, cell death will lead to stunting that will still be evident in the adult. This has been demonstrated in children born soon after the atomic-bomb detonation who had received radiation exposures *in utero*.[223] Stunting has not been observed in laboratory animals that received less than 0.05 Gy or in humans exposed to doses of less than 0.3 Gy,[224] except in some of the Hiroshima atomic-bomb survivors.[7,201] The sensitivity of some survivors who received lower radiation exposures may result from the contributions of neutron exposure and environmental factors.

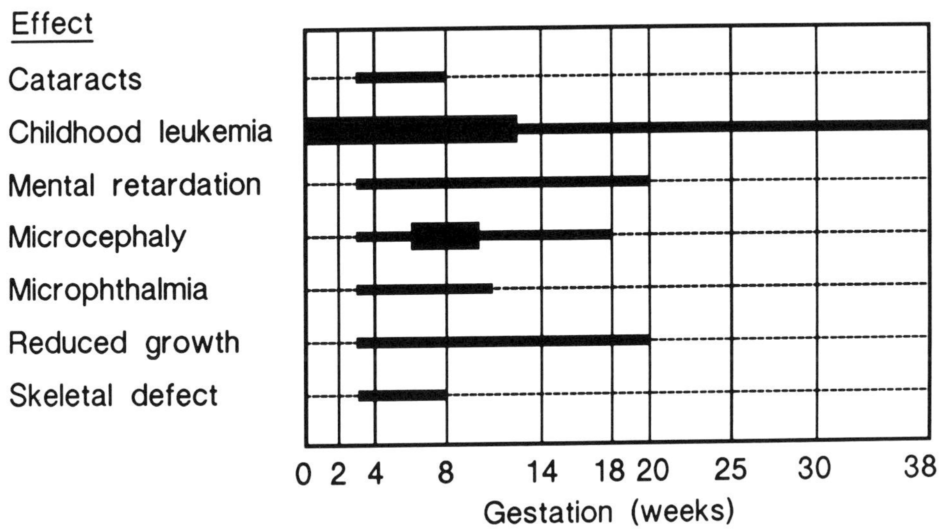

Fig. 9-17. Critical periods (solid lines) for radiation-induced birth defects in humans. Children were exposed *in utero* as a result of medical radiation treatments received by their mothers. The average dose to the midline of the pelvic region ranged from 2.5 to tens of Gy. Most children had more than one anomaly, and mental retardation was usually associated with microcephaly.

Source: Data are from reference 227

Humans Irradiated *In Utero*

Two groups of humans who have been irradiated *in utero* are children of the atomic-bomb survivors and children whose mothers received medical irradiation (therapeutic or diagnostic) during pregnancy. The predominant effects observed in humans are microcephaly, mental retardation, and growth reduction (Figure 9-17).[7,51,193,201,225-229] Eye anomalies[227,228,230] and genital and skeletal abnormalities[211] are less frequently observed.

Microcephaly observed in children exposed *in utero* to the the atomic-bomb radiation was proportional to the dose of radiation received by the mothers (Figure 9-18); even small doses carried increased incidence. Mothers with radiation sickness had higher fetal, neonatal, and infant mortalities.[231] Fetal mortality was highest in the first two trimesters, and neonatal and infant mortalities were highest in mothers who developed radiation sickness as a result of radiation exposure during the last two trimesters. In Nagasaki, four of sixteen surviving infants who *in utero* were close to the epicenter of the explosion had speech impairments. In another study of 153 of these children, 33 had a head circumference two standard deviations below average. Mental and growth retardations were also associated with the increased incidence of microcephaly,[232-234] and they remained evident in these survivors as adults.[223,234] The highest incidence of microcephaly in Hiroshima occurred with radiation exposure in weeks 6–11 of gestation.[201] No incidence of microcephaly was observed during the first week of gestation (the preimplantation period) and was negligible for exposure after the 17th week. In the Nagasaki data, microcephaly did not occur with doses below 2 Gy.

Similar observations on radiation effects *in utero* have been reported after medical irradiation.[227-229] Twenty of twenty-eight children irradiated *in utero* as a result of pelvic radium or X-ray therapy to the mother were mentally retarded, and sixteen were also micro-

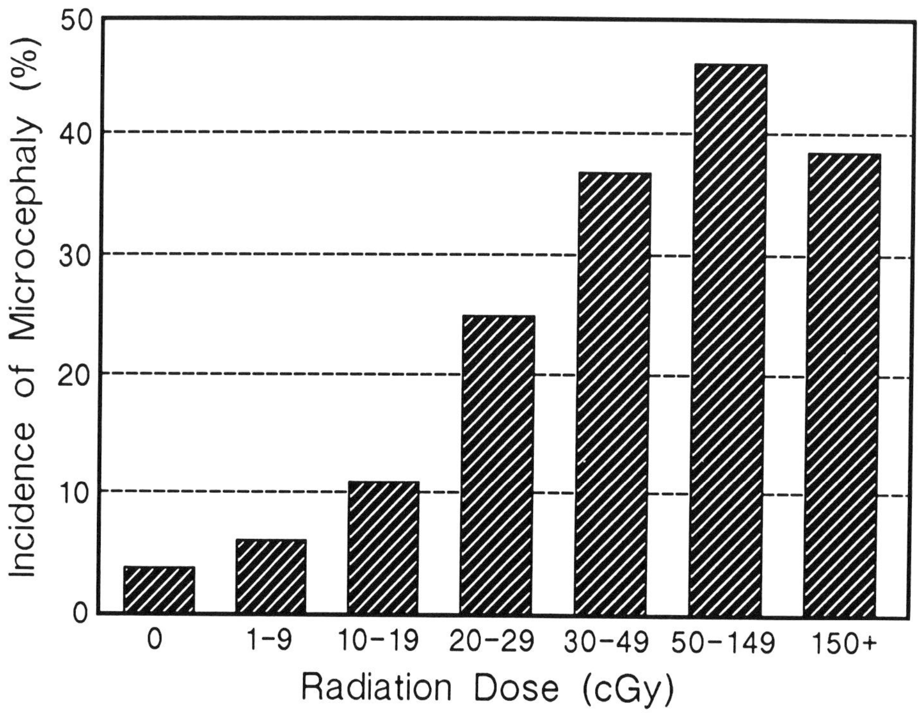

Fig. 9-18. Incidence of microcephaly in Hiroshima atomic-bomb survivors irradiated *in utero*. Data are based on T65D dose estimates.

Source: Redrawn from reference 232

cephalic.[228] Other deformities, including abnormal appendages, hydrocephaly, spina bifida, or blindness were found in eight of the children, and some also had language deficiencies. One child received a fractionated dose totaling 6.8 Gy in weeks 19, 22, and 27 of gestation and did not develop any obvious congenital anomalies or mental retardation.[235]

Increased incidence of eye anomalies has been observed following irradiation *in utero*.[227,230] In a review of twenty-six case histories, three primary eye anomalies were identified.[227] Three of twelve persons irradiated in weeks 3–8 developed cataracts; of fifteen irradiated in weeks 3–11, six had pigmentary degeneration of the retina and thirteen had microphthalmia. In the same patients, twenty-one were microcephalic; all had received radiation exposure some time in weeks 3–20, and most had been irradiated in weeks 3–11. Another study of 1,000 children exposed *in utero* showed no increase in nervous or eye anomalies but did show increased incidence of hemangioma (fifty-six versus thirty-seven in controls).[236]

Although each occurrence should be evaluated individually, the prevailing scientific opinion is that there are thresholds for the induction of congenital anomalies. Doses in the range of 0.10–0.15 Gy are thought to carry negligible risk.[7-9,51,225,226] Denmark's medical profession automatically recommends therapeutic abortion for any fetus exposed to 10 rem or more of radiation.[190] At one time, radiation was widely used to induce therapeutic abortion in cases in which surgery was deemed inadvisable. The standard treatment involved 3.6–5.1 Gy given over 2 days,[237,238] which was effective in 93% of cases.[237] Abortion usually occurred about 1 month after radiation treatment, in some cases inducing live birth.[237]

Increased Incidence of Cancer with *In Utero* Exposure

Increased incidence of leukemia and solid cancers may occur in children who received *in utero* exposure from diagnostic X-irradiation.[7,9,51,239-243] This observation was first reported in 1956 in a retrospective study of childhood cancer in Great Britain.[244] It has been confirmed by a similar study of 1.4 million children born in the northeastern United States,[243] but was not observed in the atomic-bomb survivors.[7,51] The lack of increased frequency in the bomb survivors has been attributed to the smaller sample size, where only one or two extra cases of childhood leukemia might be expected on the basis of the other studies.[9] Most of the animal studies do not demonstrate elevated rates of neoplasms following *in utero* exposure.[51] Criticisms of these studies are based on objections that as-yet-undetermined factors may have affected the results. One postulate is that the mothers of children who developed cancer may have had complicated pregnancies requiring X-ray examination, and that the cause for the examination (and not the examination itself) was associated with the increased frequency. One study pointed out that a primary reason for prenatal X-ray examinations was to confirm a diagnosis of twins.[9] The incidence of childhood cancers in twins irradiated *in utero* was higher than in twins not irradiated *in utero*.

The human data have been evaluated by several scientific bodies, including the National Academy of Sciences[7] and the United Nations.[51] These organizations have subsequently derived risk estimates for carcinogenesis that results from *in utero* irradiation. Neoplasms were three times more frequent for *in utero* exposures occurring during the first trimester than in the second or third trimesters.[7,242] The peak incidence of childhood leukemia occurred between ages 2 and 4 and was higher in males.[240] The higher risk for developing one of the leukemias continues through the 10th year of life. Children may be at increased risk for developing solid tumors for at least 14 years,[7,9] many of which will be neoplasms of the nervous system.[51] All estimates of childhood cancer induced by radiation exposure *in utero* are based on the earlier mortality data and do not reflect the advances in modern treatment. In studies performed in the late 1940s and early 1950s, leukemia was a rapid, always-fatal disease with a 3-year survival rate of 2%.[73] By the early 1970s, 3-year survival rates were 20%, and today's cure rates are 40%–60%.[73] By today's standards, the estimates are likely to overestimate the present mortality risks, because mortality is a different end point from incidence. Current estimates predict two to three leukemia deaths for each 10,000 children receiving 1 Gy of low-LET radiation *in utero*. Solid tumors will account for an additional 2.0–2.8 deaths in the same 10,000 children. The combined increased mortality from childhood cancer as a result of *in utero* exposure is 4.0–5.8 per 10,000 children per Gy. The natural total risk of mortality from malignancy through age 10 is one in 1,200. If an average chest X ray delivers 250 mGy to the fetus, the probability of that fetus developing a fatal cancer during childhood is one in a million. The NCRP recommends that fetal exposure be limited to 0.5 mSv (0.05 rem) per total gestation period or 0.05 Sv/month.[244] The increased risk for mortality in children receiving the limit of 0.05 Sv/month in a single exposure would be two to three per 100,000 children.

RELATIVE BIOLOGICAL EFFECTIVENESS OF NEUTRONS

Some doubt exists regarding the RBE of neutrons and other high-LET radiation for producing biological effects at low dose rates and doses. In general, high-LET radiation is more effective in producing biological damage. The biological effects observed in the atomic-bomb survivors are, for the most part, in agreement with human data from medical exposures. The RBE of neutrons for leukemia and breast cancer appears to be 1 in persons receiving acute or very rapid exposures.[122] As previously mentioned, the RBE of high-LET radiation increases with decreasing dose rate, because the effectiveness of low-LET gamma or X radiation decreases with decreasing dose rate. At low dose rates, the RBE for neutrons may range from 3 to 200 for tumor induction, from 10 to 45 for genetic end points, and from 25 to 200 for lens opacification.[244] These ranges are based on laboratory animal studies because no human populations have been exposed to pure neutron radiation.

REGULATORY GUIDES FOR EXPOSURE

Based on the scientific evidence, the United States government (through the Environmental Protection Agency and the Nuclear Regulatory Commission) has set regulatory guides for the occupational exposure of workers and for the general public.[123] The permissible concentrations for the occupational exposure to radiation workers (Table 9-11) are ten times higher than exposure levels for the general public. It is thought that the presumed detrimental effects on health from exposures at these limits are negligible. Scientific bodies continually reevaluate these risk estimates as additional information becomes available on radiation effects in human populations.

Modification of normal protection standards may be required in civil defense and military operations. Two limits for radiation exposure are recommended by NCRP for occupational radiation workers and for rescue personnel during radiation emergencies.[245,246] The first limit is a one-time whole-body exposure of 250 mSv, equivalent to a dose of 0.25 Gy of low-LET radiation.[246] This limit was later reduced to 100 mSv (0.1 Gy).[244] Doses of 100–250 mSv are generally asymptomatic, do not require medical treatment, and would result in three additional radiation-induced cancer mortalities over the lifetime of a battalion-sized group of 1,000 men.[7] The normal cancer incidence for this group is 250 cancers, with 200 cancer-related mortalities. It is unlikely that other somatic effects would be observed in this group. The earlier acute-exposure dose limit of 250 mSv (25 rem) is also the lower dose range estimate for inducing long-term fatigue in 10% of the individuals. Long-term fatigue occurs with doses of 250–650 mSv, with 50% incidence after a 150–mSv radiation dose received in 1 day.[10] For acute exposure in a single day, doses higher than 250 mSv may result in increased incidence of fatigue that may impair performance and alertness.

The second health limit for an acute exposure is a one-time exposure of 1 Gy of low-LET radiation in situations requiring lifesaving actions.[246] It also states that persons receiving doses greater than 1 Gy should understand the risks for somatic injury.[244] A dose of 1 Gy approaches the lower threshold limits for initiating the prodromal symptoms of nausea and vomiting and for hematological depression. At this dose level, approximately twelve extra cancer deaths would occur in a battalion-sized group of 1,000 men over their lifetimes. Minor visual opacities may occur in some of them. Both limits, 0.25 Gy (250 mSv) and 1 Gy (1 Sv), would result in temporary aspermia.[246] Lower doses of 0.01–0.02 Gy would result in 0.12–0.24 additional cancer deaths in the same battalion, assuming that no threshold for cancer exists.

The NCRP established a penalty table (Table 9-12) for making health-risk judgments in situations involving the exchange of nuclear weapons.[54] Based on the information for protracted exposures, no medical care should be required for low-LET radiation doses up to 1.5 Gy received over 1 week, or 2.0 Gy received over 1 month, or 3 Gy received over 4 months. For daily exposure of personnel over these same periods, the acceptable dose rates would be 0.21, 0.066, and 0.025 Gy/day, respectively. Animal studies have shown that the threshold dose is 0.05 Gy/day on a continuous basis, above which the stem cells are unable to compete with cell loss through maturation and depletion.[51] The immediate health concern is not cancer induction, although increased incidence will occur. Some persons exceeding these doses will require medical care,

TABLE 9-11

UNITED STATES NUCLEAR REGULATORY COMMISSION GUIDE FOR PERMISSIBLE OCCUPATIONAL EXPOSURE TO RADIATION

Body Part	Exposure (rem per calendar quarter)
Whole body	1.25
Skin of whole body	7.50
Head and trunk	1.25
Hands and forearm	18.75
Feet and ankles	18.75
Bone marrow and spleen	1.25
Lens	1.25
Gonads	1.25

Source: Data modified from reference 123

TABLE 9-12

PENALTY TABLE OF RISK ESTIMATES FOR CONTINUOUS RADIATION EXPOSURE

Persons Requiring Medical Treatment	Maximum Cancer Deaths**	Accumulated Radiation Dose* (Sv) in any period of: One Week		One Month		Four Months	
		Total	Daily	Total	Daily	Total	Daily
None	18.0	1.5	0.21	2.0	0.066	3.0	0.025
Some (5% deaths)	28.5***	2.5	0.35	3.5	0.12	5.0	0.16
Most (50% deaths)	27.0†	4.5	0.64	6.0	0.20	—	—

*RBE of neutrons increases with decreasing dose rate

**Per batallion (1,000 soldiers) over a lifetime:
16%–20% leukemia (minimal latency 3–5 years)
Remainder will be solid tumors (minimal latency 10 years)

***Based on calculations of 95% survivors using BEIR III estimates

†Based on calculations of 50% survivors using BEIR III estimates

Source: Based on NCRP Penalty Table, reference 54

and some (5% or greater) may die from the hematopoietic subsyndrome.

It is sometimes difficult for the public to place radiation risks in the proper perspective, perhaps because of their association with nuclear weapons, the documented effects from exposure, and the perception that radiation cannot be seen or controlled. Four-tenths of a minute of life are lost for each mile driven in a car due to the risk of a fatal accident, and the average smoker loses 10 minutes of life for each cigarette smoked. In comparison, an estimated average of 1.5 minutes of life are lost for each 0.0015-mSv (1.5-mrem) exposure to ionizing radiation.[245] It is expected that doubling the natural background radiation would result in an average loss of 8 days of life from the increased risk of cancer. The average coffee drinker may lose 6 days because of the increased risk of bladder cancer, and the average unmarried male may lose 9.6 years from his lifespan. For military personnel, the average loss of lifespan from a tour of duty in Vietnam was 1.1 years.[245]

The NCRP has defined a dose of 0.01 mSv per year, equivalent to 10 Gy or 1 mrad of low-LET radiation, as the negligible individual risk level.[244] This implies that almost every dose of radiation carries potential risk. In some cases, the risk is extremely small and difficult to identify, as illustrated by the comparison to smoking one cigarette. The goal is to keep exposures as low as is reasonably achievable in daily life and in emergency situations.

SUMMARY

The late effects of ionizing radiation can be divided into three major groups: somatic, genetic, and teratogenic effects. Somatic damage ranges from fibrosis and necrosis of individual organs to cataracts, epilation, and cancer.

Most somatic effects require high-threshold doses of radiation; cancer is the main health concern after exposure to low-level radiation. The three most common radiation-induced malignancies are leukemia, breast cancer, and thyroid cancer. The latency periods for the detection of cancer after radiation exposure range from 2 years for leukemia to 30–40 years for some solid tumors.

Mathematical models predicting cancer risks based on observations from high radiation exposures imply that 120–180 additional cancer deaths will occur for every million persons receiving 1 cGy of radiation. This estimate range includes the incidence of all cancers and presumes that no thresholds for induction exist. Some evidence indicates that thresholds for radiation-induced cancer do exist, ranging from 0.01 Gy for breast cancer to 0.2 Gy for leukemia.

Genetic effects are the second category of low-level or late effects of radiation. It is estimated that 5–65 additional genetic disorders will occur in the next generation for every million persons receiving 0.01 Gy of gamma or low-LET radiation. These disorders will be mainly autosomal dominant and gender-linked disorders. If each succeeding generation were to receive an additional 0.01 Gy of radiation, equilibrium would be reached in the gene pool, and an average increase of 60–1,100 genetic disorders per million persons would be observed in the population. This would result in a 1.5% increase in the overall incidence of genetic disorders. The normal incidence of genetic disorders in the population is one in ten.

The third category of late radiation damage is the teratogenic effects. The primary somatic effects seen in humans exposed *in utero* are microcephaly, mental retardation, and growth retardation. These effects have been observed with an increased incidence in the atomic-bomb survivors exposed *in utero* to doses of less than 0.10 Gy, although a neutron component may have enhanced the radiation effectiveness. In general, thresholds exist for the induction of birth defects by radiation, and effects below 0.10 Gy are negligible. The normal incidence of birth defects is one in ten live births. One concern for low-level exposure to ionizing radiation *in utero* is the increased incidence of cancer in childhood. An estimated twenty-five additional cancer deaths are predicted for every million children receiving 1 cGy of radiation *in utero*.

REFERENCES

1. Bacg, Z. M., and Alexander, P. 1966. *Fundamentals of radiobiology.* 2d ed., 45-62, 122-156. Oxford: Pergamon Press.

2. Snyder, S. L. 1977. Radiation-induced alterations in serum and splenic lysosomal hydrolases of the rat. *Radiat. Res.* 69: 306-316.

3. Donlon, M. A., and Walden, T. L., Jr. 1988. The release of biological mediators in response to acute radiation injury. *Comments on Toxicology* 2: 205-216.

4. Young, R. W. 1987. Acute radiation syndrome. In *Military Radiobiology,* edited by J. J. Conklin and R. I. Walker, 165-190. New York: Academic Press.

5. Glasstone, S. 1964. *The effects of nuclear weapons.* Rev. ed. Washington, DC: United States Atomic Energy Commission.

6. Upton, A. C. 1987. Cancer induction and non-stochastic effects. *Br. J. Radiol.* 60: 1-16.

7. Committee on the Biological Effects of Ionizing Radiation. 1980. *The effects on populations of exposure to low levels of ionizing radiation.* Washington, DC: National Academy Press.

8. United Nations Scientific Committee on the Effects of Atomic Radiation. 1982. *Ionizing radiation: Sources and biological effects.* New York: United Nations, New York.

9. Mole, R. H. 1987. Irradiation of the embryo and fetus. *Br. J. Radiol.* 60: 17-31.

10. Nuclear Regulatory Commission. 1985. *Health effects model for nuclear power plant accident consequences analysis* [U.S. Nuclear Regulatory Commission Contractor Report NUREG/CR-4214 (Sandia No. SAND85-7185)]. Washington, DC: U.S. Government Printing Office.

11. National Institutes of Health. 1985. *Report of the National Institutes of Health Ad Hoc Working Group to Develop Radioepidemiological Tables* [NIH Publication No. 85-2748]. Washington, DC: Department of Health and Human Services.

12. Upton, A. C. 1982. The biological effects of low-level ionizing radiation. *Sci. Am.* 246: 41-49.

13. Webster, E. W. 1981. On the question of cancer induction by small X-ray doses. *Am. J. Radiol.* 137: 647-666.

14. Auxier, J. A., and Dickson, H. W. 1983. Guest editorial: Concern over recent use of the ALARA philosophy. *Health Phys.* 44: 595-600.

15. National Council on Radiation Protection and Measurements. 1977. *Radiation exposure from consumer products and miscellaneous sources* [NCRP Report No. 56]. Washington, DC: National Council on Radiation Protection and Measurements.

16. Harley, J. H. 1981. Radioactive emissions and radon. *Bull. NY Acad. Med.* 57: 883-896.

17. Upton, A. C.; Christenberry, K. W.; Melville, G. S.; Furth, J.; and Hurst, G. S. 1956. The relative biological effectiveness of neutrons, X-rays, and gamma rays for the production of lens opacities: Observations on mice, rats, guinea pigs, and rabbits. *Radiology* 67: 686-696.

18. Burch, P. R., and Chesters, M. S. 1985. Natural and radiation-induced cataracts in man and mouse, and natural macular degeneration in man: Proposed mechanisms. *Phys. Med. Biol.* 30: 879-896.

19. Toda, S.; Hosokawa, Y.; Choshi, K.; Nakano, A.; and Takahashi, M. 1964. Occular changes in A-bomb survivors exposed during infancy. *Folia Ophthalmol. Jap.* 15: 96-103.

20. Hirose, K. 1956. Occular lesions development after exposure to atomic bomb in Nagasaki city. In *Research in the effects and influences of the nuclear bomb test explosions,* compiled by the Committee for Compilation of Report on Research in the Effects of Radioactivity, 1655. Ueno, Japan: Japan Society for the Promotion of Science.

21. Messerschmidt, O. 1979. *Medical procedures in a nuclear disaster: Pathogenesis and therapy for nuclear-weapons injuries,* 187-190. Munich: Verlag Karl Theimig.

22. Otake, M., and Schull, W. J. 1982. The relationship of gamma and neutron radiation to posterior lenticular opacities among atomic bomb survivors in Hiroshima and Nagasaki. *Radiat. Res.* 92: 574-595.

23. Ham, W. T., Jr. 1953. Radiation cataract. *Arch. Ophthalmol.* 50: 618-643.

24. International Commission on Radiological Protection. 1984. Non-stochastic effects of ionizing radiation. In vol. 14, *Ann. ICRP* [ICRP Publication 41]. Oxford: Pergamon Press.

25. Ash, P. 1980. The influence of radiation on fertility in man. *Br. J. Radiol.* 53: 271-278.

26. Rowley, M. J.; Leach, D. R.; Warner, G. A.; and Heller. C. G. 1974. Effect of graded doses of ionizing radiation on the human testis. *Radiat. Res.* 59: 665-678.

27. Sandeman, T. F. 1966. The effects of X-irradiation on male human fertility. *Br. J. Radiol.* 39: 901-907.

28. Clifton, D. K., and Bremmer, W. J. 1983. The effect of testicular X-irradiation on spermatogenesis in man: A comparison with the mouse. *J. Androl.* 4: 387-392.

29. Carr, B. R., and Wilson, J. D. 1983. Disorders of the ovary and female reproductive tract. In *Harrison's Principles of Internal Medicine,* 10th ed., edited by P. G. Petersdorf, R. D. Adams, E. Braunwald, K. J. Isselbacher, J. B. Martin, and J. D. Wilson, 700-720. New York: McGraw-Hill.

30. Kaplan, I. I. 1959. Genetic effects in children and grandchildren of women treated for infertility and sterility by Roentgen therapy. Report of a study of thirty-three years. *Radiology* 72: 518-521.

31. Roentgen, W. C. 1895. Uber eine neue Art von Strahlen. *Sitzunsb. d. phys.-med. Gesellsch. zu Wurzb.* : 132-141.

32. Malkinson, F. D., and Keane, J. T. 1981. Radiobiology of the skin: Review of some effects on epidermis and hair. *J. Invest. Dermatol.* 77: 133-138.

33. Marcuse, W. 1896. Nactrag zu dem Fall von Dermatitis und Alopecie nach Durchleuchtungsversuchen mit Roentgenstrahlen. *Deut. med. Wochschr.* 22: 681-686.

34. Freund, L. 1897. Ein mit Roentgen-Strahlen behandelter Fall von Naevus pigmentosus piliferus. *Wien. Med. Wochschr.* 47: 428-434.

35. Hall-Edwards, J. 1904. On chronic X-ray dermatitis. *Br. J. Med.* 2: 993-995.

36. Harris, L. H. 1906. Treatment of chronic X-ray dermatitis. *Br. J. Med.* 2: 695.

37. Drury, H. C. 1896. Dermatitis caused by Roentgen X-rays. *Br. J. Med.* 2: 1377.

38. Mutscheller, A. 1925. Physical standards of protection against Roentgen-ray dangers. *Am. J. of Roentgenol. and Radium Ther.* 13: 65-70.

39. Cronkite, E. P.; Bond, V. P.; Conard, R. A.; Durham, C. L.; Farr, R. S.; Schulman, N. R.; Sondhaus, C. A.; Cohn, S. H.; Hechter, H. H.; Sharp, R.; Alpen, E. L.; Browning, L. E.; Wood, D. A.; Rinehart, R. W.; Cong, J. K.; Robertson, J. S.; and Milne, W.L. 1956. *Some effects of ionizing radiation on human beings: A report on the Marshallese and Americans accidentally exposed to radiation fallout and a discussion of radiation injury in the human being* [U.S. Atomic Energy Commission Publication AEC-TID 5385]. Washington, DC: U.S. Government Printing Office.

40. Arlett, C., and Harcourt, S. 1980. Survey of radiosensitivity in a variety of human cell strains. *Cancer Res.* 40: 926-932.

41. Charles, M. W. 1986. Recent developments in the dosimetry of superficial tissues, I.1. *Br. J. Radiol.* (Suppl.) 19: 1-7.

42. Archambeau, J. O. 1987. Relative sensitivity of the integumentary system: Dose response of the epidermal, microvasculature, and dermal populations. *Adv. Radiat. Biol.* 12: 147-204.

43. Ernst, K., and Ehring, F. 1986. Unavoidable sequelae and accidental damage to the skin following irradiation. *Br. J. Radiol.* (Suppl.) 19: 15-18.

44. Dutreix, J. 1986. Human skin: Early and late reactions in relation to dose and its time distribution, II.1. *Br. J. Radiol.* (Suppl.) 19: 22-27.

45. Malkinson, F. D., and Wiskemann. A. 1987. Some principles of radiobiology and the effects of ionizing radiation on the skin. In *Dermatology in General Medicine.* 3d ed., 1431-1440. New York: McGraw-Hill.

46. Trott, K.-R. 1986. What can the experience of radiation therapy teach us about accidents? *Br. J. Radiol.* (Suppl.) 19: 28-30.

47. Kalz, F. 1941. Theoretical considerations and clinical use of Grenz rays in dermatology. *Arch. Dermat. Syph.* 43: 447-472.

48. Stieve, F.-E. 1986. Experiences with accidents and consequences for treatment. *Br. J. Radiol.* (Suppl.) 19: 18-21.

49. Moritz, A. R., and Henriques, F. W., Jr. 1952. Effect of beta rays on the skin as a function of the energy, intensity and duration of radiation. II. Animal experiments. *Lab. Invest.* 1: 167-185.

50. Conard, R. A. 1984. Late radiation effects in Marshall Islanders exposed to fallout 28 years ago. In *Radiation Carcinogenesis: Epidemiology and Biological Significance,* edited by J. D. Boice and J. F. Fraumeni, 57-71. New York: Raven Press.

51. United Nations Scientific Committee on the Effects of Atomic Radiation. 1977. *Sources and effects of ionizing radiation.* New York: United Nations.

52. Snyder, D. S. 1976. Effect of topical indomethacin on UVR-induced redness and PGE levels in sunburned guinea pig skin. *Prostaglandins* 11: 631-643.

53. Lushbaugh, C .C.; Fry, S. A.; Ricks, R. C.; Hubner, K. F.; and Burr, W. W. 1986. Historical update of past and recent skin damage radiation accidents. *Br. J. Radiol.* (Suppl.) 19: 7-12.

54. National Council on Radiation Protection and Measurements. 1974. *Radiological factors affecting decision-making in a nuclear attack* [NCRP Report 42]. Washington, DC: National Council on Radiation Protection and Measurements.

55. Potten, C. S. 1986. Biological dosimetry of local radiation accidents of skin: Possible cytological and biochemical methods. *Br. J. Radiol.* (Suppl.) 19: 82-85.

56. Ruben, P., and Cassaret, G. W. 1968. *Clinical radiation pathology.* Philadelphia: Saunders.

57. Daniel, J. 1896. The X-rays. *Science* 3: 562-563.

58. Brown, P. 1936. *American martyrs to science through the Roentgen rays,* 6-13, 32-42. Springfield, IL: Charles C. Thomas.

59. Upton, A. C. 1964. Cancer research 1964: Thoughts on the contributions of radiobiology. *Cancer Res.* 24: 1860-1868.

60. Grubbe, E. H. 1902. X-rays in the treatment of cancer and other malignant diseases. *Medical Record* 62: 692-695.

61. Despeignes, V. 1896. Nouvelle observation de cancer traite par les rayons de Roentgen. *Lyon Med.* 83: 550.

62. Porter, C. A., and White, C. J. 1907. Multiple carcinomata following chronic X-ray dermatitis. *Ann. Surg.* 46: 649-671.

63. Furth, J. A., and Lorenz, E. 1954. Carcinogenesis by ionizing radiations. In vol. 1, *Radiation Biology,* edited by A. Hollaender, 145-201. New York: McGraw-Hill.

64. Marie, P.; Clunet, J.; and Raoulet-Lapointe, G. 1910. Contribution a l'etude du developement des tumeurs malignes sur les ulceres de roentgen. *Bull. de l'Assoc. Franc. pour l'Etude du Cancer* 3: 404-426.

65. Weinstein, I. B.; Gattoni-Celli, S.; Kirschmeir, P.; Lambert, M.; Hsiao, W.; Backer, J.; and Jeffrey, A. 1984. Multistage carcinogenesis involves multiple genes and multiple mechanisms. *J. Cell. Physiol.* (Suppl.) 3: 127-137.

66. Chaganti, R. S. K., and Jhanwar, S. C. 1983. Oncogenes, chromosome mutation, and the development of neoplasia. In *Chromosome Mutation and Neoplasia,* 397-412. New York: Alan R. Liss, Inc.

67. Temin, H. M. 1984. Do we understand the genetic mechanisms of oncogenesis. *J. Cell. Physiol.* (Suppl.) 3: 1-11.

68. Ford, C. E., and Clarke, C. M. 1963. Cytogenetic evidence of clonal proliferation in primary reticular neoplasms. *Can. Cancer Conf.* 5: 129-146.

69. Chaganti, R. S. K. The significance of chromosome change to neoplastic development. In reference 66, 359-396.

70. Fialkow, P. J. 1977. Clonal origin and stem cell evolution of human tumors. In *Genetics of Human Cancer,* edited by J. J. Mulvihill, R. W. Miller, and J. F. Fraumeni, Jr., 439-453. New York: Raven Press.

71. Fialkow, P. J.; Gartler, S. M.; and Yoshida, A. 1967. Clonal origin of chronic myelocytic leukemia in man. *Proc. Natl. Acad. Sci. USA* 58: 1468-1471.

72. National Toxicology Program. 1985. *Fourth annual report on carcinogens. Summary 1985* [NTP 85-002]. Washington, DC: Department of Health and Human Services.

73. Doll, R., and Peto, A. 1981. Avoidable risks of cancer in the U.S. *JNCI* 66: 1196-1308.

74. Waterhouse, J.; Muir C.; Correa, P.; and Powell, J., eds. 1976. *Cancer incidence in five continents* [IARC Sci Publications #15], vol. 3, 1-584. Lyon, France: International Agency for Research on Cancer.

75. Layton, J.; Warzynski, M.; and Idiris, A. 1986. Acquired immunodeficiency syndrome in the United States: A selected review. *Crit. Care Med.* 14: 819-827.

76. Chang, E. H.; Pirollo, K. F.; Zou, Z. Q.; Cheung, H.-Y.; Lawler, E. L.; Garner, R.; White, E.; Bernstein, W. B.; Fraumeni, J. W., Jr.; and Blattner, W. A. 1987. Oncogenes in radioresistant, noncancerous skin fibroblasts from a cancer-prone family. *Science* 237: 1036-1038.

77. Croce, C. M. 1987. Role of chromosome translocations in human neoplasia. *Cell* 49: 155-156.

78. Marshall, C. J. 1987. Oncogenes and growth control: 1987. *Cell* 49: 723-725.

79. Weinberg, R. A. 1985. The action of oncogenes in the cytoplasm and nucleus. *Science* 230: 770-776.

80. Bister, K., and Jansen, H. W. 1986. Oncogenes in retroviruses and cells: Biochemistry and molecular genetics. *Advances in Cancer Res.* 47: 99-188.

81. Antoniodes, H. N.; Pantazis, P.; and Owen, A. J. 1987. Human platelet-derived factor and the sis-PDGF-2 gene. In *Oncogenes, Genes, and Growth Factors,* edited by G. Guroff, 1-40. New York: John Wiley and Sons.

82. Klein, G., and Klein, E. 1987. Myc/Ig juxtaposition by chromosomal translocations: Some new insights, puzzles, and paradoxes. In *Oncogenes and Growth Factors,* edited by R. A. Bradshaw and S. Prentis, 33-46. New York: Elsevier Science Publishers.

83. Gilman, A. G. 1984. G proteins and dual control of adenylate cyclase. *Cell* 36: 577-579.

84. Forrester, K.; Almoguera, C.; Han, K.; Grizzle, W. E.; and Perucho, M. 1987. Detection of high incidence of K-ras oncogenes during human colon tumorigenesis. *Nature* 327: 298-303.

85. Jaffe, D. R., and Bowden, G. T. 1987. Enhanced malignant progression of mouse skin tumors by ionizing radiation and activation of oncogenes in radiation induced tumors. In vol. 1, *Proceedings of 8th International Congress of Radiation Research,* edited by E. M. Fielden, J. F. Fowler, J. H. Hendry, and D. Scott, 188. London: Taylor and Francis.

86. Sawey, M. J.; Burns, F. J.; and Garte, S. J. Activation of multiple oncogenes in radiation-induced rat skin carcinomas. In reference 85, 188.

87. Guerrero, I.; Villasante, A.; Corces, V.; and Pellicer, A. 1984. Activation of a c-k-ras oncogene by somatic mutation in mouse lymphomas induced by gamma radiation. *Science* 225: 1159-1162.

88. Kudson, A. G., Jr. 1985. Hereditary cancer, oncogenes, and antioncogenes. *Cancer Res.* 45: 1437-1443.

89. Sager, A. 1986. Genetic suppression of tumor formation: A new frontier in cancer research. *Cancer Res.* 46: 1573-1580.

90. Harris, H. 1979. Some thoughts about genetics, differentiation, and malignancy. *Somatic Cell Mol. Genet.* 5: 923-930.

91. Kasid, U.; Pfeifer, A.; Weischelbaum, R. R.; Dritschilo, A.; and Mark, G. E. 1987. The raf oncogene is associated with a radiation-resistant human laryngeal cancer. *Science* 237: 1039-1041.

92. Dalla-Favera, R.; Bregni, M.; Erikson, J.; Patterson, D.; Gallo, R. C.; and Croce, C. M. 1982. Human c-myc oncogene is located on the region of chromosome 8 that is translocated in Burkitt's lymphoma cells. *Proc. Natl. Acad. Sci. USA* 79: 7824-7827.

93. Prakash, K.; McBride, O. W.; Swan, D. C.; Devare, S. G.; Tronick, S. R.; and Aaronson, S. A. 1982. Molecular cloning and chromosomal mapping of a human locus related to the transforming gene of Moloney murine sarcoma virus. *Proc. Natl. Acad. Sci. USA* 79: 5210-5214.

94. Nowell, P. C., and Hungerford, D. A. 1960. A minute chromosome in chronic granulocytic leukemia. *Science* 132: 1497.

95. de Klein, A.; Geurts van Kessel, D. A.; Grosveld, G.; Bartrum, C. R.; Hagemeirer, A.; Bootsma, D.; Spurr, N. K.; Heisterkamp, N.; Groffen, J.; and Stephenson, J. R. 1982. A cellular oncogene is translocated to the Philadelphia chromosome in chronic myelocytic leukemia. *Nature* 300: 765-767.

96. Goffen, J.; Stephenson, J. K.; Heisterkamp, N.; de Klein, A.; Bartrum, C. R.; and Grosveld, G. 1984. Philadelphia chromosomal breakpoints are clustered within a limited region, bcr, on chromosome 22. *Cell* 36: 93-99.

97. Konopka, J. B.; Watanabe, S. M.; and White, O. N. 1984. An alteration of the human c-abl protein in K562 leukemia cells unmasks associated tyrosine kinase activity. *Cell* 37: 1035-1042.

98. Bishop, J. M. 1987. The molecular genetics of cancer. *Science* 235: 305-311.

99. Cairns, J. 1975. Mutational selection and the natural history of cancer. *Nature* 255: 197-200.

100. Mossman, K. V. 1984. Ionizing radiation and cancer. *Cancer Invest.* 2(4): 301-310.

101. Upton, A. C. 1983. Environmental standards for ionizing radiation: Theoretical basis for dose-response curves. *Environ. Health Perspect.* 52: 31-39.

102. Land, C. E. 1980. Estimating cancer risks from low doses of ionizing radiation. *Science* 209: 1197-1203.

103. Jablon, S. Epidemiologic perspectives in radiation carcinogenesis. In reference 50, 1-8.

104. Robinette, C. D.; Jablon, S.; and Preston, T. L. 1985. *Mortality of nuclear weapons test participants.* Washington, DC: National Research Council.

105. Preston, D. L.; Kato, H.; Kopecky, K. J.; and Fujita, S. 1987. Studies of mortality of A-bomb survivors. 8. Cancer mortality, 1950-1982. *Radiat. Res.* 111: 151-178.

106. Neel, J. V.; Satoh, C.; Hamilton, H. B.; Otake, M.; Goriki, K.; Kageoka, T.; Fujita, M.; Neriishi, S.; and Asakawa, J. 1980. Search for mutations affecting protein structure in children of atomic bomb survivors: Preliminary report. *Proc. Natl. Acad. Sci. USA* 77: 4221-4225.

107. Auxier, J. A. 1977. *Ichiban, radiation dosimetry for the survivors of the bombings of Hiroshima and Nagasaki* [ERDA Critical Review Series, TID-27080]. Springfield, VA: National Technical Information Service.

108. U.S.-Japan Joint Reassessment of Atomic Bomb Radiation Dosimetry in Hiroshima and Nagasaki. 1987. In vol. 1, *Final report* [DS86, Dosimetry System 1986], edited by W. C. Roesch. Hiroshima: Radiation Effects Research Foundation.

109. Court Brown, W. M., and Doll, R. 1965. Mortality from cancer and other causes after radiotherapy for ankylosing spondilitis. *Br. J. Med.* 2: 1327-1332.

110. Smith, P. G. Late effects of X-ray treatment of ankylosing spondilitis. In reference 50, 107-118.

111. Smith, P. G., and Doll, R. 1982. Mortality among patients with ankylosing spondilitis after a single treatment course with X-rays. *Br. Med. J.* 284: 449-460.

112. Shore, R. E.; Albert, R. E.; and Pasternack, B. S. 1976. Follow-up study of patients treated by X-ray epilation for tinea capitis. *Arch. Environ. Health* 31: 17-28.

113. Shore, R. E.; Hemplemann, L. H.; Kowaluk, E.; Mansur, P. S.; Pasternack, B. S.; Albert, R. E.; and Haughie, G. E. 1977. Breast neoplasms in women treated with X-rays for acute postpartum mastitis. *JNCI* 59: 813-822.

114. Boice, J. D., and Monson, R. R. 1977. Breast cancer in women after repeated fluoroscopic examinations of the chest. *JNCI* 59: 823-832.

115. Boice, J. D., Jr.; Rosenstein, M.; and Trout, E. D. 1978. Estimation of breast doses and breast cancer risks associated with repeated fluoroscopic chest examinations of women with tuberculosis. *Radiat. Res.* 73: 373-390.

116. Waxweiler, R. J.; Roscoe, R. J.; Archer, V. E.; Thun, M. J.; Wagoner, J. K.; and Lundin, F. E., Jr. 1981. Mortality follow-up through 1977 of the white underground uranium miners cohort examined by the United States Public Health Service. In *Radiation Hazards in Mining,* 823-830. New York: Society of Mining Engineers.

117. Kunz, E.; Sevc, J.; Placek, V.; and Horacek, J. 1979. Lung cancer in man in relation to different time distribution of radiation exposure. *Health Phys.* 36: 699-706.

118. Ichimaru, M.; Ishimaru, I.; Belsky, J. L.; Tomiyasu, T.; Sadamori, N.; Hoshino, T.; Tomonaga, M.; Shimizu, N.; and Okada, H. 1976. *Incidence of leukemia in atomic bomb survivors, Hiroshima and Nagasaki 1950-71, by radiation dose, years after exposure, age, and type of leukemia* [Technical Report RERF 10-76]. Hiroshima: Radiation Effects Research Foundation.

119. Clark, S. S.; McLaughlin, J.; Crist, W. M.; Champion, R.; and White, O. N. 1987. Unique forms of the abl tyrosine kinase distinguish Ph1-positive CML from Ph1-positive ALL. *Science* 235: 85-88.

120. Kato, H., and Schull, W. J. 1982. Studies of the mortality of A-bomb survivors. Report 7. Mortality, 1950-1978: Part I. Cancer mortality. *Radiat. Res.* 90: 395-432.

121. Smith, P. G., and Doll, R. 1976. Late effects of X irradiation in patients treated for metropathia haemorrhagica. *Br. J. Radiol.* 49: 224-232.

122. Straume, T., and Dobson, R. L. 1981. Implications of new Hiroshima and Nagasaki dose estimates: Cancer risks and neutron RBE. *Health Phys.* 41: 666-671.

123. Nuclear Regulatory Commission. 1983. *Radiation dose standards for individuals in restricted areas* [Code of Federal Regulations. Energy. Title 10, Part 20.101], 235. Washington, DC: Office of the Federal Register.

124. Center for Disease Control. 1979. Leukemia among persons present at an atmospheric nuclear test (SMOKY). *MMWR* 28: 361-362.

125. Caldwell, G. G.; Kelley, D. B.; and Heath, C. W. 1980. Leukemia among participants in military maneuvers at a nuclear bomb test. A preliminary report. *JAMA* 244: 1575-1578.

126. Caldwell, G. G.; Kelley, D. B.; Zack, M.; Falk, H.; and Heath, C. 1983. Mortality and cancer frequency among military nuclear test (SMOKY) participants, 1957 through 1979. *JAMA* 250: 620-624 .

127. Ron, E., and Modan, B. 1980. Benign and malignant thyroid neoplasms after childhood irradiation for tinea capitis. *JNCI* 65: 7-11.

128. Hemplemann, L. H.; Hall, W. J.; Phillips, M.; Cooper, R. A.; and Ames, W. R. 1975. Neoplasms in persons treated with X-rays in infancy: Fourth survey in 20 years. *JNCI* 55: 519-530.

129. Prentice, R. L.; Kato, H.; Yoshimoto, K.; and Mason, M. 1982. Radiation exposures and thyroid cancer incidence among Hiroshima and Nagasaki residents. In *Third Symposium on Epidemiology and Cancer Registries in the Pacific Basin* [National Cancer Institute Monograph 62], 207-212. Washington, DC: Government Printing Office.

130. Wood, J. W.; Tamagaki, H.; Neriishi, S.; Sato, T.; Sheldon, W. F.; Archer, P. G.; Hamilton, H. B.; and Johnson, K. G. 1969. Thyroid carcinoma in atomic bomb survivors, Hiroshima and Nagasaki. *Am. J. Epidemiol.* 89: 4-14.

131. McTierman, M. M.; Weiss, N. S.; and Daling, J. R. 1984. Incidence of thyroid cancer in women in relation to previous exposure to radiation therapy and history of thyroid disease. *JNCI* 73: 575-581.

132. Shore, R. E.; Woodard, E.; Hildreth, N.; Dvoretsky, P.; Hemplemann, L.; and Pasternack, B. 1985. Thyroid tumors following thymus irradiation. *JNCI* 74: 1117-1184.

133. Doniach, I. 1974. Carcinogenic effect of 100, 250, and 500 rad X-rays on the rat thyroid gland. *Br. J. Cancer* 30: 487-495.

134. Conard, R. A.; Paglia, D. E.; Narsen, P. R.; Sutlow, W. W.; Dobyns, B. M.; Robins, J.; Krotsky, W. A.; Field, J. B.; Rall, J. E.; and Wolff, J. 1980. *Review of medical findings in a Marshallese population twenty-six years after accidental exposure to radioactive fallout* [Brookhaven National Laboratory Report BNL 51261]. Springfield, VA: National Technical Information Service.

135. Ron, E., and Modan, B. Thyroid and other neoplasms following childhood scalp irradiation. In reference 50, 139-151.

136. Modan, B.; Ron, E.; and Werner, A. 1977. Thyroid cancer following scalp irradiation. *Radiology* 123: 741-744.

137. National Council on Radiation Protection and Measurements. 1977. *Protection of the thyroid gland in the event of releases of radioiodine* [NCRP Report 55]. Washington, DC: National Council on Radiation Protection and Measurement.

138. Howe, G. R. Epidemiology of radiogenic breast cancer. In reference 50, 119-129.

139. Seidman, H., and Mushinski, M. H. 1983. Breast cancer: Incidence, mortality, survival, and prognosis. In *Breast Carcinoma. Current Diagnosis and Treatment,* edited by S. A. Feig and R. McLelland, 9-46. New York: Masson Publishing USA, Inc.

140. Tokunaga, M.; Land, C. E.; Yamamoto, T.; Masahide, A.; Tokuoka, S.; Ezaki, H.; Nishimori, I.; and Fujikura, T. Breast cancer among atomic bomb survivors. In reference 50, 45-55.

141. Orine, S. K.; Chambers, R. W.; and Johnson, R. H. 1967. Postirradiation carcinoma of the male breast bilaterally. *JAMA* 201: 707.

142. Boice, J. D., Jr.; Land, C. E.; Shore, R. E.; Norman, J. E.; and Tokunaga, M. 1979. Risk of breast cancer following low-dose exposure. *Radiology* 131: 589-597.

143. Tokunaga, M.; Land, C. E.; Yamamoto, T.; Asano, M.; Tokuoka, S.; Ezaki, H.; and Nishimori, I. 1982. Breast cancer in Japanese A-bomb survivors. *Lancet* 2: 924.

144. Tokunaga, M.; Norman, N. E., Jr.; Asano, M.; Tokuoka, S.; Ezaki, H.; Nishimori, I.; and Tsuju, Y. 1979. Malignant breast tumors among atomic bomb survivors, Hiroshima and Nagasaki, 1950-1974. *JNCI* 62: 13471359.

145. Hildreth, N. G.; Shore, R. E.; and Hemplemann, L. H. 1983. Risk of breast cancer among women receiving radiation treatment in infancy for thymic enlargement. *Lancet* 2: 273.

146. Land, C. E.; Boice, J. D., Jr.; Shore, R. E.; Norman, J. E.; and Tokunaga, M. 1980. Breast cancer risks from low-dose exposures to ionizing radiation: Results of parallel analysis of three exposed populations of women. *JNCI* 65: 353-376.

147. Davis, F. G.; Boice, J. D., Jr.; Kelsey, J. L.; and Monson, R. R. 1987. Cancer mortality after multiple fluoroscopic examinations of the chest. *JNCI* 78: 645-652.

148. Rowland, R. E., and Lucas, H. F. Radium-dial workers. In reference 50, 231-240.

149. Adams, E. E., and Brues, A. M. 1980. Breast canćer in female radium dial workers first employed before 1930. *J. Occup. Med.* 22: 583-587.

150. Modan, B.; Baidatz, D.; Mart, H.; Steintz, R.; and Levin, S. 1969. Radiation-induced intracranial meningiomas. *Clin. Radiol.* 20: 90-94.

151. Shore, R. E.; Albert, R. E.; and Pasternack, B. S. 1976. Followup study of patients treated by x-ray epilation for tinea capitis. Resurvey of post-treatment illness and mortality experience. *Arch. Environ. Health* 31: 17-28.

152. Asano, M.; Kato, H.; Yoshimoto, K.; Seyama, S.; Itakura, H.; Hamada, T.; and Iijima, S. 1982. Primary liver carcinoma and liver cirrhosis in atomic bomb survivors, Hiroshima and Nagasaki, 1961-75, with special reference to hepatitis B surface antigen. *JNCI* 69: 1221-1227.

153. Lewin, K., and Millis, R. R. 1973. Radiation hepatitis: A morphologic study with emphasis on the late changes. *Arch. Pathol.* 96: 21-26.

154. Prentice, R. L.; Yoshimoto, Y.; and Mason, W. W. 1983. Relationship of cigarette smoking and radiation exposure to cancer mortality in Hiroshima and Nagasaki. *JNCI* 70: 611-622.

155. Little, J. B.; Radford, E. P.; McCombs, H. L.; and Hunt, V. R. 1965. Distribution of polonium-210 in pulmonary tissues of cigarette smokers. *N. Eng. J. Med.* 273: 1343-1351.

156. Winters, T. H., and Di Franza, J. R. 1982. Radioactivity in cigarette smoke. *N. Eng. J. Med.* 306: 364-365.

157. Radford, E. P., and Hunt, V. R. 1964. Polonium-210: A volatile radioactive element in cigarettes. *Science* 143: 247-249.

158. Little, J. B.; McGandy, R. B.; and Kennedy, A. R. 1978. Interactions between polonium-210, alpha-radiation, benzo(a)pyrene, and 0.9% NaCl solution instillations in the induction of experimental lung cancer. *Cancer Res.* 38: 1929-1935.

159. Wynder, E. L., and Hoffman, D. 1979. Tobacco and health: A societal challenge. *N. Eng. J. Med.* 300: 894-903.

160. Van Dyk, J.; Keane, T. J.; Kan, S.; Rider, W. D.; and Fryer, C. J. H. 1981. Radiation pneumonitis following large single dose irradiation: A re-evaluation based on absolute dose to lung. *Int. J. Radiat. Oncol. Biol. Phys.* 7: 461-467.

161. Gross, N. J. 1977. Pulmonary effects of radiation therapy. *Ann. Intern. Med.* 86: 81-92.

162. Tokuoka, S.; Kawai, K.; Shimizu, Y.; Inai, K.; Ohe, K.; Fujikura, T.; and Kato, H. 1987. Malignant and benign ovarian neoplasms among bomb survivors, Hiroshima and Nagasaki, 1950-80. *JNCI* 79: 47-57.

163. Muller, H. J. 1927. Artificial transmutation of the gene. *Science* 66: 84-87.

164. Muller, H. J. The nature of the genetic effects produced by radiation. In reference 63, 351-474.

165. Denniston, C. 1982. Low level radiation and genetic risk estimation in man. *Annu. Rev. Genet.* 16: 329-355.

166. Russell, W. L., and Kelly, E. M. 1982. Mutational frequencies in male mice and the estimation of genetic hazards of radiation in men. *Proc. Natl. Acad. Sci. USA* 79: 542-544.

167. Selby, P. B., and Selby, P. R. 1977. Gamma-ray-induced dominant mutations that cause skeletal abnormalities in mice. *Mutat. Res.* 43: 907-975.

168. Searle, T. 1987. Radiation—the genetic risk. *Trends Genet.* 3: 152-157.

169. Abrahamson, S. 1979. Genetic effects of low level radiation. In *Proceedings of a Conference: Known Effects of Low-Level Radiation Exposure. Health Implications of the TMI Accident* [NIH Publication 80-2087], 46-60. Washington, DC: U.S. Department of Health, Education, and Welfare.

170. Popescu, H. L.; Pilat, L.; Hilt, M.; and Lancranjan, I. 1972. Evolution of biological changes noticed in three cases of accidental mild gamma irradiation. *J. Occup. Med.* 14: 317-320.

171. Dolphin, G. W.; Bolton, D.; Humphreys, D. L. O.; Speight, D. L.; and Stradling, G. N. 1970. Biological dosimetry and physical dosimetry after a radiation accident. *Nature* 227: 165.

172. Randolph, M. L., and Brewen, J. G. 1980. Estimation of whole-body doses by means of chromosome aberrations observed in survivors of the Hiroshima A-bomb. *Radiat. Res.* 82: 393-407.

173. Cohen, B. L. 1984. Perspective on genetic effects of radiation. *Health Phys.* 46: 1113-1121.

174. Strauss, B. S. 1985. Cellular aspects of DNA repair. *Adv. Cancer Res.* 45: 45-105.

175. Ward, J. F. 1975. Molecular mechanisms of radiation-induced damage to nucleic acids. *Adv. Radiat. Biol.* 5: 181-239.

176. Hook, E. B. 1981. Rates of chromosome abnormalities in different maternal ages. *Obstet. Gynecol.* 58: 282-285.

177. Freidman, J. M. 1981. Genetic disease in the offspring of older fathers. *Obstet. Gynecol.* 57: 745-749.

178. National Council on Radiation Protection and Measurements. 1979. *Tritium and other radionuclide labeled organic compounds incorporated in genetic material* [NCRP Report 63]. Washington, DC: National Council on Radiation Protection and Measurements.

179. National Council on Radiation Protection and Measurements. 1987. *Genetic effects from internally deposited radionuclides* [NCRD Report 89]. Washington, DC: National Council on Radiation Protection and Measurement.

180. Jablon, S., and Kato, H. 1971. Sex ratio in offspring survivors exposed prenatally to the atomic bombs in Hiroshima and Hagasaki. *Am. J. Epidemiol.* 93: 253-258.

181. Sigler, A. T.; Lilienfield, A. M.; Cohen, B. H.; and Westlake, J. E. 1965. Radiation exposure in parents of children with mongolism (Down's syndrome). *Bull. Hopkins Hosp.* 117: 374-399.

182. Uchida, I. A., and Curtis, E. J. 1961. A possible association between maternal irradiation and mongolism. *Lancet* 2: 845-850.

183. Uchida, I. A.; Holunga, R.; and Lawler, C. 1968. Maternal radiation and chromosomal aberrations. *Lancet* 2: 1045-1049.

184. Alberman, E.; Polani, P. E.; Roberts, J. A. F.; Spicer, C. C.; Elliot, M.; and Armstrong, E. 1972. Paternal exposure to X-irradiation and Down's syndrome. *Ann. Hum. Genet.* 36: 195-208.

185. Schull, W. J.; Otake, M.; and Neel, J. V. 1981. Genetic effects of the atomic bomb: A reappraisal. *Science* 213: 1220-1227.

186. Brewen, J. G.; Preston, R. J.; and Gengozian, N. 1975. Analysis of X-ray induced translocations in human and marmoset spermatogonial stem cells. *Nature* 253: 468-470.

187. Oftedal, P., and Searle, A. G. 1980. An overall genetic risk assessment for radiological protection purposes. *J. Med. Genet.* 17: 15-20.

188. Russell, L. B. 1950. X-ray induced development abnormalities in the mouse and their use in the analysis of embryological patterns. I. External and gross visceral changes. *J. Exp. Zool.* 114: 545-602.

189. Rugh, R. 1962. Ionizing radiations and congenital anomalies of the nervous system. *Mil. Med.* 127: 883-907.

190. Rugh, R. 1964. Why radiobiology? *Radiology* 82: 917-920.

191. Russell, L. B., and Russell, W. L. 1952. Radiation hazards to the embryo and fetus. *Radiology* 58: 369-376.

192. Rugh, R. 1971. X-ray induced teratogenesis in the mouse and its possible significance to man. *Radiology* 99: 433-443.

193. Yamazaki, J. 1966. A review of the literature on the radiation dosage required to cause manifest central nervous system disturbances from *in utero* and postnatal exposure. *Pediatrics* 37: 977-1003.

194. Russell, L. B., and Russell, W. L. 1954. An analysis of the changing radiation response of the developing mouse embryo. *J. Cell Comp. Physiol.* 43: 103-149.

195. Rugh, R., and Grupp, E. 1959. Response of the very early mouse embryo to low levels of ionizing radiations. *J. Exp. Zool.* 141: 571-587.

196. Russell, L. B. 1956. X-ray induced developmental abnormalities in the mouse, and their use in analysis of embryological patterns. II. Abnormalities of the vertebral column and thorax. *J. Exp. Zool.* 131: 329-395.

197. Ohzu, E. 1965. Effects of low dose X-irradiation on early mouse embryos. *Radiat. Res.* 26: 107-113.

198. Rugh, R. 1969. Low dose X-ray effects on the precleavage mammalian zygote. *Radiat. Res.* 37: 401-414.

199. Russell, L. B., and Montgomery, C. S. 1966. Radiation-sensitivity differences within cell-division cycles during mouse cleavage. *Int. J. Radiat. Biol.* 10: 151-164.

200. Jacobson, L. 1968. *Low-dose X-irradiation and teratogenesis: A quantitative experimental study with reference to seasonal influence on dose effects.* Copenhagen: Munksgaard.

201. Miller, R. W., and Mulvihill, J. J. 1976. Small head size after atomic irradiation. *Teratology* 14: 355-358.

202. Dobson, R. L.; Koehler, C. G.; Felton, J. S.; Kwan, T. C.; Wuebbles, B. J.; and Jones, D. C. L. 1978. Vulnerability of female germ cells in developing mice and monkeys to tritium, gamma rays, and polycyclic hydrocarbons. In *Development Toxicology of Energy-Related Pollutants. Proceedings of 17th Annual Hanford Biology Symposium* [CONF-771017], 1-14. Washington, DC: U.S. Department of Energy Symposium Series.

203. Lebedinsky, A. V.; Grigoryev, U. G.; and Demirchoglyan, G. G. 1958. The biological effects of small doses of ionizing radiation. [The cited work was done by V. V. Yokolev.] In *Proceedings of Second United Nations International Conference on the Peaceful Uses of Atomic Energy.* Vol. 22, *Biological Effects of Radiation,* 26. New York: United Nations Publications.

204. Brent, R. L. 1960. The effect of irradiation on the mammalian fetus. *Clin. Obst. Gynecol.* 3: 928-950.

205. Semagin, V .N. 1964. Higher nervous activity of adult rats irradiated daily with X-rays during the embryonic period. In *Effects of Ionizing Radiation on the Functions of Higher Nervous System of Progeny,* edited by I. A. Pintsovskoyo and translated by the U.S. Atomic Energy Commission [AEC-TR-5553], 77-103. Oak Ridge, TN: U.S. Atomic Energy Commission.

206. Cahill, D. F., and Yuile, C. L. 1970. Tritium. Some effects of continuous exposure *in utero* on mammalian development. *Radiat. Res.* 44: 727-737.

207. Bursian, S. J.; Cahill, D. F.; and Laskey, J. W. 1975. Some aspects of brain neurochemistry after intrauterine exposure to tritium. *Int. J. Radiat. Biol.* 27: 455-461.

208. Kaplan, S. 1962. Behavioral manifestations of the deleterious effects of prenatal X-irradiation. In *Effects of Ionizing Radiation on the Nervous System,* 225-243. Vienna: International Atomic Energy Agency.

209. Rugh, R., and Grupp, E. 1960. Fractionated X-irradiation of the mammalian embryo and congenital anomalies. *Am. J. Roentgenol.* 84: 125-144.

210. Russell, L. B.; Badgett, S. K.; and Saylors, C. L. 1960. Comparison of the effects of acute continuous and fractionated irradiation during embryonic development. In *Immediate and Low-Level Effects of Ionizing Radiation,* proceedings of a conference held in Venice [Special Supplement to *Int. J. Radiat. Biol.*], 343-359. London: Taylor and Francis.

211. Krigel, H., and Reihart, S. 1969. Effect of a fractionated X-irradiation of the development of the mammalian fetus. In *Radiation Biology of the Fetal and Juvenile Mammal,* edited by M. R. Sikov and D. D. Mahlum, 251-262. Washington, DC: U.S. Atomic Energy Commission, Division of Technical Information.

212. Grahn, D., and Kratchman, J. 1963. Variation in neonatal death rate and birth weight in the United States and possible relations to environmental radiation, geology and altitude. *Am. J. Hum. Genet.* 15: 329-352.

213. Hickey, R. J.; Bowers, E. J.; Spence, D. E.; Zemel, B. S.; Clelland, A. B.; and Clelland, R. C. 1981. Low level ionizing radiation and human mortality: Multi-regional studies. A preliminary report. *Health Phys.* 40: 625-641.

214. Jacobsen, L. Radiation-induced teratogenesis in relation to season and some features of reproductive biology. In reference 211, 229-242.

215. Taylor, A. I. 1968. Autosomal trisomy syndromes: A detailed study of 27 cases of Edward's Syndrome and 27 cases of Patau's Syndrome. *J. Med. Genet.* 5: 227-252.

216. Murphree, R. L., and Graves, R. B. Effect of dose rate on prenatally irradiated lambs. In reference 211, 243-250.

217. Rugh, R. Chairman's remarks. In reference 211, 381-391.

218. Friedberg, W.; Hanneman, G. D.; Faulkner, D. N.; Darden, E. B., Jr.; and Deal, R. B., Jr. 1973. Prenatal survival of mice irradiated with fission neutrons or 300 kVp X-rays during the pro-nuclear-zygote stage: Survival curves, effects of dose fractionation. *Int. J. Radiat. Biol.* 24: 549-560.

219. Brent, R. L., and Bolden, B. T. 1968. Indirect effect of X-irradiation on embryonic development: Utilization of high doses of maternal irradiation on the first day of gestation. *Radiat. Res.* 36: 563-570.

220. Brent, R. L., and Bolden, B. T. 1967. The indirect effect of irradiation on embryonic development. III. The contribution of ovarian irradiation, uterine irradiation, oviduct irradiation, and zygote irradiation to fetal mortality and growth retardation in the rat. *Radiat. Res.* 30: 759-773.

221. Brent, R. L., and McLaughlin, M. M. 1960. The indirect effect of irradiation on embryonic development. I. Irradiation of the mother while shielding the embryonic site. *Am. J. Dis. Child* 100: 94-102.

222. Hicks, S. P., and D'Amatio, C. J. 1963. Low dose radiation of the developing brain. *Science* 141: 903-905.

223. Wood, J. W.; Johnson, K. G.; and Omori, Y. 1967. *In utero* exposure to the Hiroshima atomic bomb. An evaluation of head size and mental retardation: 20 years later. *Pediatrics* 39: 385-392.

224. Brent, R. Radiation effects on the developing embryo. In reference 169, 61-75.

225. National Council on Radiation Protection and Measurement. 1977. *Medical radiation exposure of pregnant and potentially pregnant women* [NCRP Report 54]. Washington, DC: National Council on Radiation Protection and Measurement.

226. National Council on Radiation Protection and Measurement. 1977. *Review of NCRP radiation dose limit for embryo and fetus in occupationally-exposed women* [NCRP Report 53]. Washington, DC: National Council on Radiation Protection and Measurement.

227. Dekaban, A. S. 1968. Abnormalities in children exposed to X-irradiation during various stages of gestation: Tentative timetable of radiation injury to human fetus. *J. Nucl. Med.* 9: 471-477.

228. Goldstein, L., and Murphy, D. P. 1929. Etiology of ill-health in children born after postconceptional maternal irradiation. *Am. J. Roentgenol.* 22: 322-331.

229. Goldstein, L., and Murphy, D. P. 1929. Microcephalic idiocy following radium therapy for uterine cancer during pregnancy. *Amer. J. Obstet. Gynecol.* 18: 189-195, 281-283.

230. Jacobsen, L., and Mellemgaard, L. 1968. Anomalies of the eyes in descendants of women irradiated with small X-ray doses during the age of fertility. *Acta Ophthalmol.* 46: 352-354.

231. Yamazaki, J.; Wright, S.; and Wright, P. 1954. Outcome of pregnancy in women exposed to the atomic bomb in Nagasaki. *Am. J. Dis. Child* 82: 448-463.

232. Blot, W. J. 1975. Growth and development following prenatal exposure and childhood exposure to atomic radiation. *Radiat. Res.* (Suppl.) 16: 82-88.

233. Blot, W. J., and Miller, R. J. 1973. Mental retardation following *in utero* exposure to the atomic bombs of Hiroshima and Nagasaki. *Radiology* 106: 617-619.

234. Ishimaru, T.; Nakashima, E.; and Kawamoto, S. 1985. *Relationship of height, body weight, head circumference, and chest circumference at age 18, to gamma and neutron doses among in utero exposed children, Hiroshima and Nagasaki* [Technical Report RERF TR 19-84]. Hiroshima: Radiation Effects Research Foundation.

235. Kallinger, W., and Granniger, W. 1979. The effect of a high gamma dose on a human fetus. *Health Phys.* 36: 1-6.

236. Griem, M. L.; Mewissen, D. J.; Meier, P.; and Dobben, G. D. Analysis of the morbidity and mortality of children irradiated in fetal life. In reference 211, 651-659.

237. Harris, W. 1932. Therapeutic abortion produced by the roentgen ray. *Am. J. Roentgenol.* 27: 415-419.

238. Mayer, M. D.; Harris, W.; and Wimpfheimer, S. 1936. Therapeutic abortion by means of X-ray. *Am. J. Obstet. Gynecol.* 32: 945-957.

239. Stewart, A. M.; Webb, J. W.; Giles, B. D.; and Hewitt, D. 1956. Malignant disease in childhood and diagnostic irradiation *in utero*. *Lancet* 2: 447, 1956.

240. Stewart, A. M.; Webb, J. W.; and Hewitt, D. 1958. A survey of childhood malignancies. *Br. Med. J.* 1: 1495-1508.

241. Stewart, A. M., and Kneale, G. W. 1970. Radiation dose effects in relation to obstetric X-rays and childhood cancers. *Lancet* 1: 1185-1188.

242. Kneale, G. W., and Stewart, A. M. 1976. Mantel-Haenszel analysis of Oxford data. II. Independent effects of fetal irradiation subfactors. *JNCI* 57: 1009-1014.

243. Monson, R. R., and MacMahon, B. Prenatal X-ray exposure and cancer in children. In reference 50, 97-105.

244. National Council on Radiation Protection and Measurement. 1987. *Recommendations on limits for exposure to ionizing radiation* [NCRP Report 91]. Washington, DC: National Council on Radiation Protection and Measurement.

245. Cohen, B. L., and Lee, I.-S. 1979. A catalog of risks. *Health Phys.* 36: 707-722.

246. National Council on Radiation Protection and Measurement. 1971. *Basic radiation protection criteria* [NCRP Report 39]. Washington, DC: National Council on Radiation Protection and Measurement.

247. Holahan, E. V., Jr. Cellular radiation biology. In reference 4, 87-110.

Chapter 10

RADIOLOGICAL CONSIDERATIONS IN MEDICAL OPERATIONS

LARRY W. LUCKETT, C.H.P.* AND BRUCE E. VESPER, M.S.**

*Lieutenant Colonel, United States Army; Health Physicist, Office of the Director, Armed Forces Radiobiology Research Institute, Bethesda, Maryland 20814-5145
**Lieutenant Commander, United States Navy; Health Physics Advisor, Defense Nuclear Agency, Nuclear Weapons Accident Advisory Committee; Military Applications Coordinator, Armed Forces Radiobiology Research Institute, Bethesda, Maryland 20814-5145

INTRODUCTION

The success of medical support operations in a nuclear war will depend to a great extent on the adequacy of planning, training, and preparation before hostilities occur. Nuclear warfare will produce a huge disparity between the number of patients requiring treatment and the available medical resources. This problem will be further complicated by the disruption of lines of communication; the isolation of medical units; and shortages of transportation, supplies, and equipment.

Preparation problems facing medical planners and commanders can be divided into two distinct categories: *(a)* staff-level planning, including actions that must be taken before the start of a nuclear war to minimize the prompt effects of enemy nuclear attacks, and *(b)* unit preparations to minimize the immediate and delayed effects of nuclear attacks, in order to ensure continued effective medical operations in a nuclear environment.

In many instances, the experience gained during conventional wars and peacetime nuclear incidents will be applicable to the casualties of a nuclear battlefield. A rigorous training and implementation program must be instituted at all levels of medical service for professional and nonprofessional medical personnel. Emphasis must be placed on practical, problem-related training rather than on theoretical principles.

The information in this chapter on tactical operations is extracted from current NATO doctrine for medical operations in a tactical nuclear environment.[1] The information on peacetime operations is from current Department of Defense doctrine from the Defense Nuclear Agency[2] and the U.S. Army.[3]

RADIATION INTERACTION AND DETECTION

The ability to recognize the potential for radiological damage is based on a knowledge of the basic interactions of radiation particles with biological molecules, and on the ability to detect the presence of radiation or radioactive materials. The need to measure or quantify a substance that dramatically affects the human system but cannot be detected with the senses has led to the development of radiation detectors and dosimeters based on the physical principles of radiation interactions. An understanding of the nature of radiation hazards and the characteristics of various radiation types will help in the selection of a specific radiation detector for a given situation.

Interaction

Radiation arises when excited or overly energetic atomic nuclei give off excess energy as their particles convert to a more stable arrangement. The excited atoms comprise the *radioactive material*—a physical substance that, when present in sufficient quantity, can be weighed, measured, seen, or chemically separated. This radioactive material can be characterized by a *half-life*, the amount of time it takes, on average, for one-half of the excited material to convert (or decay) to stable, nonradioactive material. Depending on the material, the half-life can vary from less than seconds to many thousands of years. The shorter the half-life, the more probable it is that radiation will be emitted; the longer the half-life, the less likely are the atoms to decay. The amount of material present can be termed the *activity*, measured by the number of nuclear transformations per seconds (nts) or disintegrations per minute (dpm). The activity of a radioactive sample is a measure of its intensity. Units which measure activity are the *becquerel* (1 Bq equals one disintegration per second) and the *curie* (1 Ci equals 3.7×10^{10} disintegrations per second).

The excess energy carried away from the radioactive material comprises the radiation (Table 10-1). This energy may be carried away by particles of matter as they leave the nucleus (alpha, beta, or neutron radiation), or it may be emitted from the nucleus independently of any nuclear particles (gamma radiation). Either way, the radiation travels from the radioactive material until it interacts with the surrounding medium. The excess energy of the radiation rapidly dissipates through multiple successive interactions, until the particles recombine with the atoms in the medium. The amount of dissi-

TABLE 10-1

CHARACTERISTICS OF NUCLEAR RADIATIONS

Name	Relative Mass	Electric Charge	Emitted by	Range in Air	Tissue Penetration	Radiation stopped by
Alpha	7,300	+2	Unfissioned uranium and plutonium	5 cm	First layer of skin	Clothing Paper
Beta	1	-1	Fission products	12 m	Several layers of skin	Clothing
Gamma	0	0	Fission products	100 m	Total body	Several feet of concrete or earth
Neutron	1,830	0	Emitted only during fission	100 m	Total body	Several feet of concrete or earth

pated energy absorbed in the exposed medium is the *absorbed dose.* Units of absorbed dose are the gray (1 Gy equals 1 Joule/kg) and the rad (1 rad equals 100 ergs/g).

The interaction between radiations and any absorbing medium is *ionization.* In this process, the energy from the incoming radiation is transferred to an atom of the medium, exciting that atom and dislodging one of its orbital electrons. Each ionization event produces one ion pair, consisting of a free electron and the positively charged remainder of the atom. These free electrons, broken atomic bonds, and the resulting disrupted and distorted molecular arrangements are the basis of biological damage.

Gamma Radiation. Gamma radiation is a pure energy packet (called a *photon*), unaccompanied by any nuclear particle. Without mass or electric charge, the gamma rays have very little probability of interacting and will travel great distances through sparse media, such as air or biological tissues. This ability to penetrate and irradiate sensitive organs within the body makes gamma radiation hazardous. In order to increase the probability of interaction with and absorption of the radiation, gamma-ray shields are made of high-density concrete or lead.

Beta Radiation. Beta-particle radiation occurs when excess nuclear energy is emitted in conjunction with a high-speed nuclear electron. Because of its small mass and its one electric negative charge, the beta particle interacts more readily than does the uncharged gamma ray, traveling only several meters through air and penetrating only several layers of skin. The hazard from beta radiation is to the external skin surfaces; beta radiation cannot penetrate to internal organs unless it is inhaled or ingested. Beta-particle radiation shields may consist of lightweight materials, such as a layer of clothing.

Alpha Radiation. The heaviest particle given off in nuclear decay is the alpha particle. It is 7,300 times heavier than the beta particle, and is positively charged with twice the beta particle's electric charge. Its mass and charge make the alpha particle a highly interactive form of radiation; it will travel only 5 cm in air and can be stopped by a sheet of paper. Alpha particles will not penetrate the external layer of dead skin and thus are no direct hazard as long as they remain outside the body. Alpha-particle-emitting materials are a hazard when they can be inhaled or ingested, and are then able to irradiate sensitive organs or tissues from within.

Neutron Radiation. Neutron particle radiation is emitted only during the instant of fission by the weapon material. A neutron particle has no electric charge but does have an intermediate nuclear mass (1,830 times the mass of the beta particle but only one-fourth that of the alpha particle). Like a gamma ray, the neutron can travel great distances through sparse media and can penetrate biological tissues. Unlike other radiations that interact with orbital electrons, neutrons are more likely to interact directly with the nuclei of atoms, particularly those having low atomic numbers. Thus, effective neutron shields are composed of materials with a high hydrogen content, such as water or paraffin.

Radiation Detection

No single instrument at present has all the characteristics necessary to detect all types of radiation. Accordingly, different types of instruments must be used, depending on the nature of the radiation hazard. For any type of instrument used, the time frame over which it operates can be instantaneous or continuous. A *ratemeter* indicates the instantaneous rate at which radiation is being detected, and an *integrating meter* gives a reading of the total radiation observed since the meter was turned on or restarted (zeroed).

Radiation-detecting instruments are based on the principles of the radiation interaction being observed. A detector that merely counts the incoming radiation particles is called a *radiation counter*. An instrument designed to collect and measure the number of ion pairs produced is termed an *exposure meter;* because the unit of exposure is the roentgen (R), it is also called an *R-meter*. An instrument that measures the total energy absorbed in a detecting medium is an *absorbed dose meter;* if the detector uses a tissue-equivalent absorbing medium, the detector is called a *rem-meter*. The characteristics of some of the more commonly used detectors are summarized below.

Ionization Chambers. Ionization chambers measure dose and dose rate from gamma and X radiations. A typical ionization chamber that measures total dose is the *pocket dosimeter*, which is the size of a large fountain pen (Figure 10-1). It has a chamber containing two electrodes, one of which is a quartz fiber loop that is free to move on its mounting. Radiation entering the chamber causes ionization within the sensitive volume. The distance the fiber moves is proportional to the dose received in the chamber. Instruments of this type are sensitive to severe shock and humidity, but are small enough to be worn comfortably. The advantage of this instrument is that it can be read at any time (without the aid of a supplementary charger-reader) by simply holding it up to the light and looking into it.

Geiger-Mueller Counters. Geiger-Mueller counters are normally used for detecting single ionizing events that take place within the sensitive volume of the counter. The counters are rugged and sensitive to low levels of radiation. They are usually equipped with audible indicators of radiation detection that sound like clicks. Geiger-Mueller counters detect gamma photons or beta particles, but the detection of the former is less efficient. A discriminating shield is usually provided with Geiger-Mueller instruments; when it is opened, it admits both beta and gamma radiation. When the shield is closed, only gamma rays pass. Use of the shield may permit qualitative differentiation between the ionization caused by beta particles and that caused by gamma photons.

Proportional Counters. Proportional counters are used to detect one type of radiation in the presence of other types of radiation, or to obtain output signals greater than those obtainable with ionization chambers of equivalent size. Proportional counters may be used either to detect events or to measure absorbed energy (dose), because the output pulse is directly proportional to the energy released in the sensitive volume of the counter. Proportional counters are used for the detection of alpha particles, neutrons, and beta particles. They are often used in shielded laboratory facilities for sensitive low-level analysis.

Scintillation Counters. A scintillation counter combines a photomultiplier tube with a scintillating material, which may be a crystal or other phosphor (solid, liquid, or gas). Light pulses, produced in the scintillator by radiation, release electrons in the photomultiplier tube, and this tube then amplifies the electrons to pulses of current that can be counted. Various scintillation counters can detect alpha and beta particles, gamma rays, neutrons, protons, and electrons. The most common dosimeters for field use are alpha counters or gamma-ray detectors. Although energy dependent, scintillation counters are more efficient at detecting low-energy, low-level gamma-ray backgrounds than are Geiger-

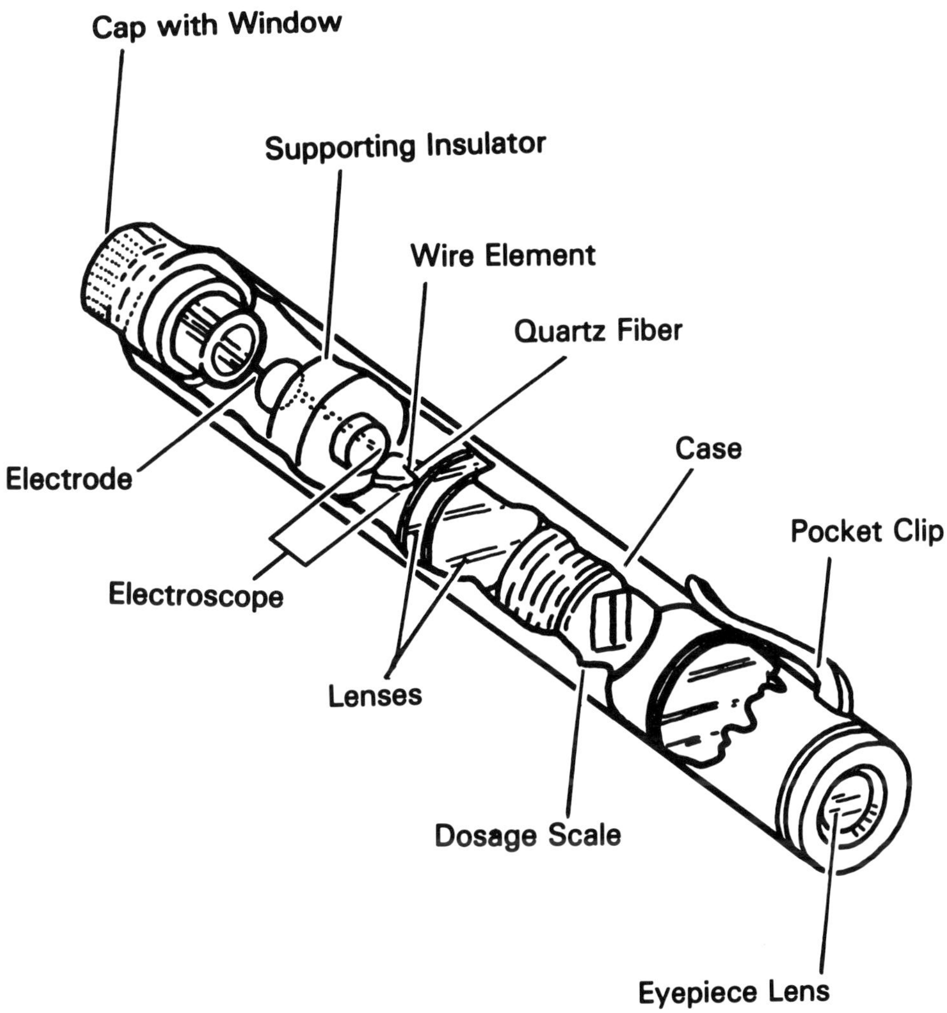

Fig. 10-1. Pocket dosimeter

Mueller counters.

Thermoluminescent Dosimeters. A thermoluminescent dosimeter (TLD) responds to ionizing radiation by trapping excited electrons in metastable states within the detector's crystalline structures. When the TLD is heated, the electrons escape these traps, releasing light as they return to their lower energy state. The amount of light is proportional to the absorbed radiation dose. The TLD is an integrating dosimeter and requires an elaborate electronic readout device to interpret the absorbed-dose data. The readout instrument will zero the TLD so that it may be used again.

Radiophotoluminescent Dosimeters. Radiophotoluminescent (RPL) glass is a dosimeter material that will luminesce following an excitation pulse of ultraviolet light if it has been exposed to ionizing radiation. This effect is caused by radiation-induced changes in the crystalline electronic structure of the glass. As with TLDs, the response is proportional to the radiation dose. The RPL dosimeter sensitivity depends on the type and manufacturer, and ranges from 0.01 to several million cGy. This type of integrating dosimeter will not be zeroed by the readout device; it gives a total cumulative dose reading that fades very slowly with time.

STAFF-LEVEL MEDICAL PLANNING

As is the case with operations planning throughout the medical support system, the staff medical officer's planning is keyed to the functions of the forces supported by the medical unit. While the problems confronted by medical units on the nuclear battlefield will be similar in some respects to those associated with conventional warfare, there are some dramatic differences. These include the vastly increased numbers of casualties requiring care, the need to operate in fallout, and the requirements to treat and decontaminate combined-injury patients.

Handling Mass Casualties

Effective techniques of evacuation, medical management, and triage become increasingly important with very large numbers of patients. The problem of handling mass casualties is not limited to hospitals. It exists throughout the chain of medical evacuation, so the basic principles of triage must be understood by all medical personnel. Flexibility in applying these principles must be an established part of medical guidance and training.

Effects of Combined Injuries. Analyses of the expected battlefield situations in a tactical nuclear environment have concluded that a high proportion of the casualties will have combined injuries, most of which will be from thermal burns and radiation exposure. Burn injuries provide portals for infection, and both burns and radiation exposure decrease the casualty's immunity to infectious microorganisms. Medical planners at all levels must anticipate *(a)* personnel with low-level exposures from nuclear weapons, who may need immediate medical attention because of combined injuries, and *(b)* personnel with otherwise recoverable conventional injuries, but whose radiation exposures make their chances for survival poor.

Effects of Psychological Stress. It is possible to estimate the number of personnel who would be injured or killed by the thermal, blast, and radiation effects of a nuclear explosion, but it is much more difficult to predict the numbers and types of psychiatric casualties. The types of acute psychological problems that would occur would probably be similar to those in other combat situations, and the treatment methods developed during past wars would be appropriate.

The most important factor in preventing stress reactions is intensive training, which will result in less fear and prompter, more effective action. Because action relieves tension, the fear response is less likely to become severe or incapacitating. Preventing or treating stress reactions in nuclear warfare may determine the continuing effectiveness of a unit's combat performance.

Public Health Concerns For centuries, the conduct and outcome of military operations have been profoundly affected by a small number of infectious diseases. Massive destruction from nuclear weapons could result in epidemics that would present serious problems for a military medical service, particularly when the effectiveness of civilian medical facilities and personnel has been diminished. In past wars, military medical forces have cared for civilian populations and have helped to rebuild nations ravaged by war. On the nuclear battlefield, the impact of classic diseases of disaster (such as dysentery, typhus, typhoid fever, cholera, and plague) may seriously affect the ability of the medical unit to treat battlefield casualties.

Logistical Support System. The success of medical support depends on the adequacy of prewar logistical preparation. Planning should provide not only for medical supplies and equipment, but also for general supplies, food, clothing, water purification apparatus, radiation-detecting and -measuring instruments, communications equipment, and modes of transportation.

The location of medical resources is crucial. Resources must be close to the area of probable greatest need, without being concentrated in areas likely to become targets for enemy attack. This means that medical planners must compromise between dispersal and the capability of the logistical system to move supplies and patients. Medical planners should take advantage of the stages of military preparedness that may precede the actual outbreak of hostilities. Because of the problems associated with long-term maintenance of medical equipment and medications in storage, extensive pre-positioning during peacetime is not practical.

Command Radiation Guidance. Line commanders at all levels will need advice from medical advisors about the effects of accumulated doses of radiation on the health of their personnel, as well as the hazards of potential exposures when operations must be conducted in areas contaminated with fallout. This advice must be practical and be based on an understanding of the requirements of the mission

TABLE 10-2

RADIATION EXPOSURE STATUS (RES) CATEGORY SYSTEM

RES	Dose (cGy)	Casualties (%)	Nuisance symptoms (%)	Risk
0	0	0	0	None
1	0–70	1.0	2.5	Negligible
2	70–150	2.5	5.0	Moderate
3	150+	5.0	—	Severe

as well as on knowledge of the diverse human responses to radiation. The effects of radiation must not be either minimized or exaggerated, and the proper place of radiation effects relative to other hazards of combat must be understood.

NATO Standardization Agreement (STANAG) 2083 has established a Radiation Exposure Status (RES) category system (Table 10-2), incorporating the most recent guidance on the operational effects of radiation exposures.[4] This system will help military commanders maintain the fighting capability of the tactical forces despite the troops' exposure to ionizing radiation. When personnel have accumulated sufficient exposure to be placed in a particular RES category, then commanders must restrict those units to activities in which additional radiation exposure is not expected, unless they are willing to accept the next higher risk to those units.

When exposures can be maintained below 150 cGy, the STANAG doctrine indicates that the overall effectiveness of combat units will not be significantly degraded. However, if the exposures become relatively large, tactical commanders must be advised of their forces' capability to continue operations. Generally, an effective military individual is one capable of carrying out assigned missions, some of which require a high degree of physical and mental effectiveness. Thus, in any attempt to relate radiation dose to this effectiveness, the complexity or physical demand of the task must be considered.

Combat-effective personnel will suffer from radiation sickness, but will be able to maintain at least 75% of their preexposure performance level. Performance-degraded personnel will be operating at 25%–75% of their preexposure performance. Combat-ineffective personnel will be capable of performing their tasks at 25% (at best) of their preexposure performance level.

Given an average dose of 400 cGy to a tactical unit required to perform a physically demanding task, the unit will become performance degraded about 2 hours after exposure and will remain so for longer than 1 month (Figure 10-2). However, if the required task is not physically demanding at that same radiation dose, performance degradation will occur at about 3 hours after exposure, and effective combat performance will recur 2 days to 2 weeks later, followed by a second performance degradation (Figure 10-3).

Of course, these predictions assume that exposure to ionizing radiation will be the combatants' only stress. The prediction of the performance capacity of irradiated persons will have to be considered with other stresses, such as conventional injury, endemic disease, continuous duty without sleep, and time in combat.

Radiological Concerns of Medical Personnel

When fallout occurs, insufficiently sheltered personnel will become contaminated. If these personnel are not wounded or sick, decontamination is not a medical responsibility; it will be done at the unit level under command supervision. If wounded personnel become contaminated, their hospitalization is more complicated. Fallout contamination can be hazardous to the patient and to attending medical personnel, although in contrast to contamination with chemical agents (in which the mere presence of the agent is life threatening), no immediate life-

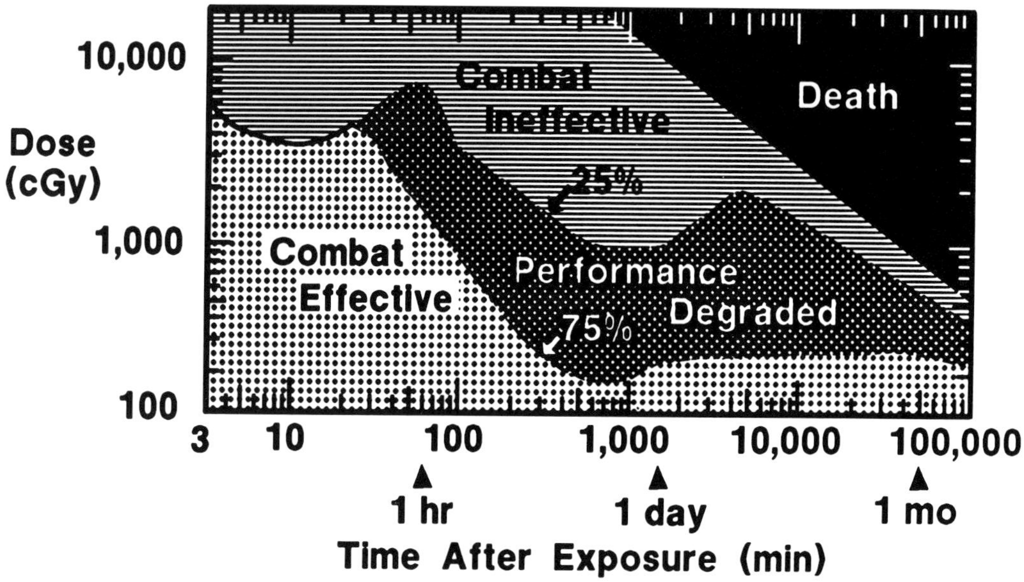

Fig 10-2. Expected response to radiation for physically demanding tasks

threatening radiation hazard exists. Thus, the decontamination of patients and contamination-control procedures within the medical facility (although important) are lower priorities than the lifesaving treatment of conventional injuries.

Radiation Hazards in Patient Treatment. Radiologically contaminated patients are those who have been contaminated with fallout, which adheres loosely to clothing and skin in the form of dust, ashes, dirt, or mud. Once these residues have been removed, the patient does not present a radiation hazard. Patient decontamination should not precede or interfere with either lifesaving procedures or surgical preparation, but rather should be an integral part of these procedures. Furthermore, care must be taken to avoid accidentally forming a real hazard by accumulating contaminated waste in the decontamination area. Effective procedures for decontamination, followed by monitoring and properly disposing of contaminated waste, must be developed and used.

Three distinct hazards are associated with radiologically contaminated patients. These are the *whole-body gamma-radiation hazard*, the *beta-contact hazard*, and the *internal hazard* from inhalation and ingestion of contaminated material.

Whole-body gamma radiation is the most important hazard because gamma radiation has a long range in air. This danger should be considerably reduced by the time the patient reaches a medical facility, however, because the loosely adhering fallout residue will drop or brush off as the patient is moved. In addition, the initial decay of residual radiation associated with a nuclear detonation is very rapid. The whole-body gamma-radiation hazard to persons handling the patient will be several orders of magnitude less than that to the patient, because of distance and elapsed time.

The beta-contact hazard is a significant problem to the patient. If fallout residue remains on the skin for an extended time (several hours to days), beta burns may occur. These resemble first- and second-degree thermal burns. Because they affect only those skin surfaces directly in contact with the radiological contamination, gently brushing or washing the dust from the skin will eliminate the hazard to the patient. Wearing rubber gloves and surgical masks, as well as practicing good hygiene, will eliminate the hazard to medical personnel.

Under conditions of nuclear war, the minute quantities of radioactive material that might be ingested, inhaled, or absorbed through wounds are a relatively minor radiation hazard. Extensive decontamination therapy is unlikely to be used because of the large number of patients and the limited time, personnel, and available logistical resources.

Patient Decontamination. Patients can easily be decontaminated without interfering with required medical care. Simply removing the patient's outer clothing and shoes before admission will remove 90%–95% of the contamination. Once removed, contaminated clothing can be placed in bags, tagged, and taken to a remote section of the medical facility. The clothing can be decontaminated or disposed of by qualified personnel, as time permits.

The second phase of decontamination consists of

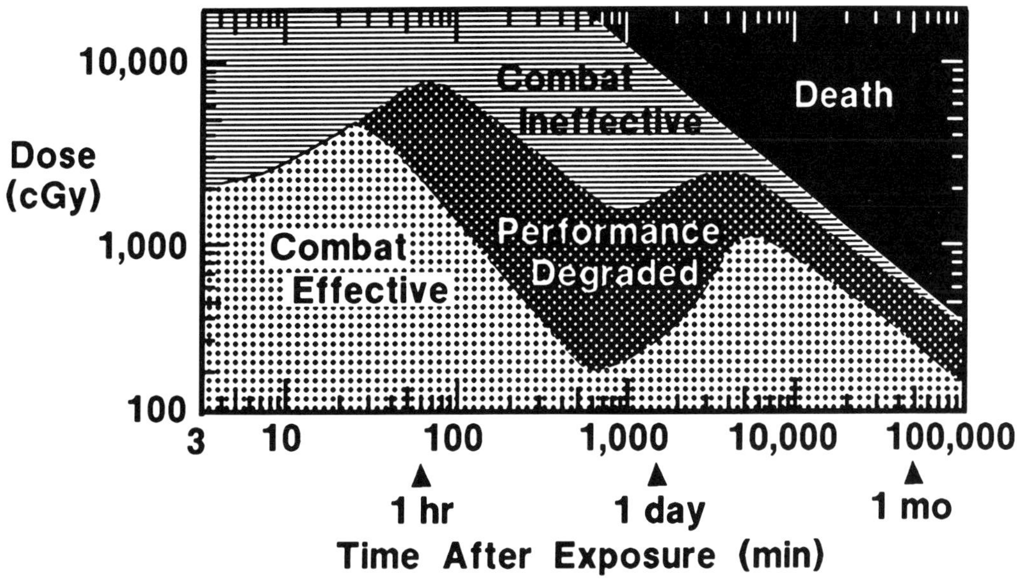

Fig. 10-3. Expected response to radiation for physically undemanding tasks

washing or wiping the patient's face, hands, and any skin surfaces not previously covered by clothing. This should leave the patient 98% decontaminated, and can be done before or after admission.

The third phase of decontamination consists of either washing or clipping the hair and washing the scalp, and is required only if the patient arrives without headgear or if monitoring indicates that the hair is contaminated.

Unit Operations in Fallout

Whenever large areas are contaminated by fallout, the operations of all units will be hampered to varying degrees, depending on the level of contamination. When a serious radiation hazard exists, the medical unit commander will be faced with the question of whether to continue operations and accept hazardous exposures to unit personnel, or to take shelter—an action that may seriously reduce the unit's ability to care for patients. To make the correct decision, the commander requires the following capabilities:

- An effective radiation-monitoring capability to correctly measure the fallout radiation hazard
- The ability to make rapid estimates of anticipated dose and dose rates
- Satisfactory lines of communication with other units and headquarters to report the fallout situation and to receive fallout warnings, information, guidance, and orders

The commander will need to know:

- Whether the unit will be in a fallout area
- The expected time of fallout arrival (or how long before most of it will be on the ground and the dose rates will begin to decline)
- The maximum dose rates expected
- The adequacy of existing facilities as fallout shelters

Decisions about operations in fallout areas should be based on actual survey data. However, because it will be not be possible or desirable to expose monitoring personnel when dose rates are very high, a reliable method of estimating fallout decay is required (Table 10-3). Note that these calculations are accurate only after all fallout is on the ground and the dose rate is beginning to decrease.

By evaluating these data along with the operational situation, the commander will be better able to make the proper decisions about moving the unit, diverting patients to other treatment units, moving into fallout shelters, or remaining in place and continuing normal operations.

Medical units that are required to remain in areas of high dose rates can survive and continue their patient-care activities if adequate shelter is available to shield against radiation. Many materials that are available on the battlefield will afford substantial shielding (Table 10-4), although some of them, such as concrete, require engineering support and prior construction. However, earth affords excellent protection and can be used with a minimum of engineering effort.

TABLE 10-3

THE 7:10 RULE FOR RESIDUAL RADIATION DECAY

Time after Detonation (in hours)	Amount of Radiation Remaining	Dose Rate Decay (cGy/hour)
1	—	1,000
7	1/10	100
49	1/100	10
343	1/1,000	1

In some cases, construction will be unnecessary; terrain and structures that will afford excellent protection from radioactive fallout (such as tunnels, caves, culverts, overpasses, ditches, ravines, and heavily constructed buildings) may be available. In existing buildings, below-ground basements give the best protection. Windows and overhead floors can be sandbagged or covered with dirt to provide additional protection with a minimum of effort.

As a matter of policy, mobile medical units should locate in or near existing shelter. When this is impossible, adequate shelter must be constructed. These shelters need not be elaborate; they have to be continuously occupied only during the period of high radiation dose rates.

Three common field-expedient fallout shelters can be constructed quickly and without extraordinary engineering support.

Dozer Trench. For this type of shelter, a trench 2.7 meters wide and 1.2 meters deep is dug with a bulldozer. It is estimated that one bulldozer can cut six 30-meter trenches in about 5 hours. About 0.6 meters of trench would be required for each person to be sheltered; thus, in 5 hours, shelters can be constructed for about 300 people. Protection and comfort can be improved later by digging the trench deeper, undercutting the walls, and erecting tents over some portions of the trench. These trenches should provide adequate shelter for most fallout situations.

Dug-In Tents of a Mobile Hospital. The tents of a mobile hospital can be dug to a depth of 1.2 meters and would be more comfortable than the dozer trench. However, dug-in tents have two drawbacks: they offer far less radiation protection than dozer trenches, and they require considerably more engineering effort.

Vehicle-Earth Shelter. A very effective shelter can be constructed combining unit vehicles and dirt. Two large tents can be joined end-to-end. A shallow trench for the vehicles can be dug around them, with the dirt piled carefully on the outside of the trench. Another 15-cm trench should be dug for the outer wheels of the vehicles. This shelter can give as much as 80% protection if fallout contamination is removed from inside the rectangle thus created. Tent liners and ponchos can be used for this purpose. This shelter requires about 2 hours to build and can be occupied or evacuated in minutes. As with other expedient shelters, it could be constructed when the medical unit occupies the position.

Regardless of the type of shelter used, a system must be developed for its efficient operation. In the case of medical units involved in the care of patients, it is usually advisable to separate the shelter management functions from those of patient care. Shelter management personnel must provide essential services, such as radiological monitoring; monitoring of water-storage facilities to prevent leaks and contamination; control of fire hazards; enforcement of health and sanitation rules; waste disposal; and provision of safe food, water, and sleeping facilities. Shelter management plans must be developed before the shelters are occupied, and the plans must be familiar to all assigned personnel.

TABLE 10-4

SHIELDING PROPERTIES OF COMMON MATERIAL FROM FALLOUT GAMMA RADIATION

Material	Half-value Layer Thickness* (cm)
Steel	2
Concrete	6
Earth	8
Water	12
Wood	22

*Thickness required to reduce the incident dose or dose rate by one half

MEDICAL RESPONSE IN PEACETIME RADIATION ACCIDENTS

A medical response to a peacetime radiation accident is similar, on a reduced scale, to the response of medical units on a tactical nuclear battlefield, although some of the radiological concerns differ. In a tactical nuclear environment (as in a large-scale nuclear reactor accident), gamma- and beta-emitting fission products become airborne fallout, exposing people to hazardous levels of external radiation. In a peacetime nuclear accident, the localized dispersal of alpha-emitting radioactive material is the governing concern. Alpha particles are not an external hazard, but when inhaled or ingested they can expose internal tissues to significant radiation doses. Due to the various levels of radiation and the different radioactive particles in tactical situations, the radiation-detecting equipment will be different from that used in peacetime.

Nuclear accidents may involve the military on short notice. Because the public will expect the response team to be knowledgeable, especially regarding medical care and public health, a review of past experiences and the current doctrine for handling nuclear accidents is essential.

Peacetime Constraints

In a peacetime nuclear accident, the medical unit is freed of some serious military concerns, such as hostile fire. Because nuclear weapons are designed so that a nuclear yield is virtually impossible without a complete sequence of deliberate actions, the major concern at a weapon-accident site is the dispersal of radioactive materials by either fire or the detonation of the conventional explosive. Thus, the consequences of a nuclear-weapon accident in peacetime are greatly reduced, and the medical response is concentrated on a few patients rather than directed toward mass casualties.

In peacetime, the concern about exposing personnel and the environment to radioactivity will have a much higher priority. Minute traces of material that would be inconsequential in wartime will assume great importance. Medical procedures must be performed to contain the contamination according to strict regulatory limits.

In managing a radiation incident, the response team will face pressure to provide details on the event. News media, public officials, and private citizens will demand information about the accident, casualties, critical aspects of the response effort, and its consequences. Medical-response personnel must be prepared to safeguard medical information in a manner that would be unnecessary during tactical operations.

Historical Perspective

The U.S. military services have experienced thirty-two accidents involving nuclear weapons through 1987.[5] The complexity of the accidents has ranged from *(a)* the simple dropping or dislocation of a weapon, resulting in physical damage but no bodily injury or dispersal of radioactive materials, to *(b)* the detonation of conventional explosives, spreading radioactive materials over hundreds of acres, contaminating private property, and requiring restoration efforts costing millions of dollars. The medical functions performed in these nuclear accidents illustrate the potential roles of military medical units that respond to future accidents.

Palomares. In January 1966, two U.S. aircraft (a KC-135 tanker and a B-52 bomber) attempted a midair refueling at 31,000 feet over the southeastern coast of Spain, but collided in the final stages of hookup. Wreckage of the two aircraft, including the four nuclear weapons aboard the B-52, rained down on the seaside farming village of Palomares, the nearby Spanish countryside, and the Mediterranean Sea. Four of the seven B-52 crew members survived the accident, but none of the four crew members of the KC-135 survived. Evacuation and treatment of the survivors were first provided by local Spanish authorities and hospitals. The first U.S. response personnel arrived at the remote site 12 hours after notification.[6]

Three of the fallen nuclear weapons came down on land; the fourth splashed down in the Mediterranean Sea and was not located for 81 days. The first weapon was found undamaged about 900 feet from the beach. The second was located the next day. It had suffered a partial high-explosive detonation, which made a crater about 20 feet wide and 6 feet deep. The third weapon was found an hour later, where it had landed within the limits of Palomares. It had also undergone high-explosive detonation, and nuclear material had spread up to 500 yards from the impact point. Luckily, no one on the ground was injured.

A contingent of American military and civilian personnel went to the Palomares area to work on recovery and the restoration of the accident site. The population rapidly increased to 747 (excluding offshore naval forces), which required establishing an on-site medical support facility to provide emergency medical treatment, supervise on-site field sanitation, and assist workers who might be exposed to radiation. As the population increased, the responsibility for obtaining routine bioassay samples from those potentially exposed was given to the camp medical facility. No cases of hazardous radiation exposure occurred. Medical cases requiring treatment beyond emergency care were evacuated.

Within days after the accident, U.S. Air Force medical officers (specialists in aviation medicine) and enlisted personnel were at the site in a field dispensary. The initial task was to identify supplies of potable water. Most medical problems involved upper respiratory infections in personnel who were exposed to high winds and cool temperatures. Members of search parties who walked in the fields and hills suffered pulled muscles, cuts, scratches, blisters, and sprains. On-site medical support ceased when the base camp was closed in April 1966, after 84 days of searching, decontaminating, and restoring the remote site.

Thule. In January 1968, a B-52 aircraft on an airborne alert mission near Thule Air Force Base, Greenland, developed a fire. The pilot was unable to extinguish it and began an emergency descent to the airbase. Shortly after the descent began, the aircraft lost all electrical power, and the order to bail out was given and executed. The aircraft struck the sea ice several miles west of the base, and disintegrated from impact, explosion, and fire. Four nuclear weapons were on board the aircraft. Of the seven crew members who ejected, six survived. The seventh person died of a head injury, probably sustained when he ejected from the aircraft.[7]

Response forces sped to the scene, and a temporary camp was erected on the sea ice. Because the accident was close to the base, medical operations were mounted from the regular base facilities. Only camp sanitation was required in addition to normal medical services. As at Palomares, the medical clinic was responsible for collecting bioassay samples throughout the recovery period.

Because of the arctic location, the next sunrise occurred 24 days later. The darkness and severe cold affected recovery operations, requiring intense cold-weather training, frequent rest breaks, and time-consuming preventive maintenance.

Time was a crucial factor because the sea ice would melt in the approaching summer season, releasing the nuclear material into the environment. The aircraft and weapons had been almost totally destroyed, but fortunately most of the radioactive material had been immobilized when it froze into the snow and ice cover. Discoloration of the snow pack from the fire was an important clue in distinguishing contaminated from uncontaminated snow.

Innovation overcame some of the difficulties. The alpha detection instruments performed poorly in the severe cold. At first, batteries lasted only 10 minutes, and the detectors were even more fragile than usual, so the operator wore the battery pack inside his parka to warm it with body heat. After site cleanup, the contaminated ice and snow were stored in old petroleum tanks and later transferred to specially modified containers for shipment to the United States.

Chernobyl. In 1986, an accident at the Chernobyl Nuclear Power Station in the Soviet Union initiated a sequence of events that mobilized civilian and military medical response forces worldwide.[8-11] Although the immediate fatalities and damage were localized, the extensive atmospheric fallout caused concern and action in health-care systems far from the accident site.

Following early reports of the accident, the U.S. European Command (EUCOM) established a Chernobyl Task Force to evaluate the accident's radiological effects on the health of American personnel in Europe. Directed by a medical corps officer, the task force was composed of representatives of public affairs and safety, and medical consultants in public health, preventive medicine, radiological hygiene, veterinary medicine/food sanitation, nuclear medicine, medical logistics, and medical operations.

The task force's initial mission was to provide medical screenings of U.S. military family members who were touring Leningrad and Kiev at the time of the reactor accident. The screening operations executed by army and air force medical units involved segregating planeloads of personnel, monitoring individuals and their baggage for external contamination, obtaining individual histories, performing thyroid counts and bioassay samples to assess internal contamination, and incorporating all analyses and interpretations into the individual's medical record.

At the request of the U.S. State Department, EUCOM deployed a radiation advisory medical team to assist the U.S. Ambassador in the USSR in defining and managing the immediate consequences of the accident. Composed of military health physicists, a physician, and a food service veterinarian, the team went to the U.S. missions in Leningrad and Moscow, evaluated the radiological environment, and advised the ambassador on potential hazards to the international community from the uncertain conditions.

Veterinary service personnel in EUCOM ensured the safety of local food supplies for consumption by American personnel. Food inspectors with radiation detectors traveled to wholesale markets, bulk issue points, and commissary distribution warehouses to monitor the supplies. Inspectors also obtained representative food and dairy-product samples for laboratory analysis. They determined that all foods met U.S. and host-nation contamination guidelines.

Although fallout data were available from State Department and host-nation authorities, the information was sometimes delayed or unavailable for some geographical areas in which Americans were stationed. The task force established an environmental monitoring program for U.S. communities, and obtained measurements of external fallout exposure rates. Samples of air, soil, rainfall, and drinking water were collected from U.S. facilities throughout the command and analyzed by medical personnel, using preventive medicine units and medical treatment facilities.

Nuclear Accident and Incident Response and Assistance Organization

The Department of Defense (DOD) has established a policy for coordinating the response to a nuclear-weapon accident which *(a)* identifies the responsibilities for command at the scene, and *(b)* clarifies the coordination among DOD and other federal agencies, such as the Department of Energy (DOE) and the Federal Emergency Management Agency (FEMA).[2,3,12]

All U.S. Army installations with custody of nuclear weapons will have a dedicated response force that is prepared to respond to any nuclear incident. Initial response and service response procedures will be included in the standard operating procedures for the installation's Nuclear Accident and Incident Response and Assistance organization.

Initial Response Force. The Initial Response Force (IRF) is the nearest military installation, regardless of size, to respond to an accident, to take immediate emergency lifesaving measures, to provide security, to reduce exposures, and to provide a federal presence and humanitarian support. IRF members will coordinate on-scene hazard containment activities with civil authorities, and will remain in charge until arrival of the Service Response Force (SRF). The IRF unit should be trained and equipped to provide 24-hour capability.[3] The IRF commander will supervise all emergency forces and direct all operations at the scene, including, but not limited to, the following:

- Securing, safeguarding, and disposing of all classified material
- Treating casualties
- Determining actual and potential hazards
- Minimizing further hazards
- Requesting required assistance
- Providing control and logistical support of on-site personnel
- Handling claims, public information, and relations with local civilian groups
- Establishing communications between the accident site and higher headquarters

Service Response Force. The capabilities of the IRF are limited. Total control of the accident response will be the responsibility of the SRF, which should arrive within 24 hours after the accident occurs. The SRF will consist of an aggregate of personnel, with a military staff as the nucleus. Members of the IRF will be integrated into the SRF and will continue to play a major role in the response. The response force will be augmented by DOE scientific and technical advisers and by specialized teams from other services, as required. The SRF commander will be a general officer, designated as the On-Scene Commander (OSC).[2] Responsibilities of the OSC include, but are not limited to, the following:

- Safeguarding national-security materials and information
- Coordinating with federal, state, and local authorities (a liaison officer should be provided to local, state, or host-nation authorities and to the senior FEMA official by the OSC as soon as possible)[2]
- Ensuring that a public-health hazard assessment is made
- Notifying civil authorities of the precautions and other measures required for protecting public health and safety
- Establishing the priorities for response, recovery, and restoration efforts
- Coordinating, reviewing, and approving public information and news releases
- Communicating all required information and situation reports to the National Military Command Center and service operations center
- Coordinating with the senior FEMA official (in the continental United States) and state or host-nation authorities to restore the accident site

- Coordinating with the accident investigation board
- Obtaining assets required to support response operations

Guidelines for Medical Advisors

The Installation Medical Authority (for the IRF) and the Medical Staff Advisor (for the SRF) are responsible for planning the medical support required for their respective portions of the nuclear-accident response. They should maintain up-to-date plans and be prepared to train and supervise other medical personnel. Procedural guides should be prepared and distributed to any medical facility that may become involved in the support of such a response.

These medical advisors must be prepared to deal with the question of how much long-term radiation hazard exists for the local population in the contaminated area. Another concern is the development of definitive treatment regimens for individual radiation casualties and combined-injury casualties. Several army, DOD, and DOE advisory teams will assist the medical advisors in determining appropriate medical guidance. Although these teams will respond to the accident site or treatment facility on request, prior coordination between the IRF and SRF medical advisors and the special teams is recommended.

Radiological Advisory Medical Team. The army has established the Radiological Advisory Medical Team (RAMT), which is staffed with health physicists, physicians, and technicians trained to evaluate radiological health hazards and manage radiation casualties.[13] At the accident scene and at the medical facility, the RAMT will assist with the following:

- Potential health hazards from radioactive contamination
- Medical treatment and decontamination of casualties
- Decontamination procedures for personnel, facilities, and equipment
- Control methods for radiation exposure during on-site recovery and restoration operations
- Medical surveillance or bioassay procedures during site-restoring operations

Medical Radiobiology Advisory Team. The Defense Nuclear Agency has established a Medical Radiobiology Advisory Team (MRAT) located at the Armed Forces Radiobiology Research Institute in Bethesda, Maryland.[2] This team is trained in the biomedical consequences of radiation exposure. It will help medical authorities to make definitive treatment decisions for individual casualties. The MRAT maintains treatment protocols that are relevant to the handling of radiation-accident injuries, based on state-of-the-art radiobiology research and human radiobiology data from previous accident victims.

Department of Energy Assistance. Major DOE installations have medical support capabilities that can be called on for assistance, if needed. Also, DOE facilities that routinely handle radioactive material are equipped to give medical treatment to radiological casualties. The Radiation Emergency Assistance Center Training Site (REAC/TS) in Oak Ridge, Tennessee, is prepared to deal with all types of radiation exposure and can provide expert advice and assistance.[2]

Rescue and Evacuation of Injured Persons at a Nuclear Accident Site

An accident involving a nuclear weapon will probably result in casualties. The injuries may be severe and numerous, like those from a serious multi-vehicle accident. Emergency personnel sent to an accident site must be well trained in trauma first aid. By the time medical personnel arrive at the scene, initial rescue may have been effected and some first aid given. The medical personnel should assist in further rescue operations and begin evacuating casualties to the closest medical facility as soon as possible. They should notify the receiving facility of the nature of the accident and the number and type of patients involved.

The weapons materials give off short-range alpha radiation, which is not a hazard to attending personnel unless the actual radioactive material itself is inhaled. Standard military protective masks provide excellent protection. They should be worn by personnel inside ambulances until the patients are brought to the medical facility. Hospital personnel can safely wear a standard surgical mask.

After the patients have been brought to the hospital, the ambulance personnel and their vehicles should be decontaminated as soon as possible, even if monitoring facilities are not available. They must not be released until monitoring indicates that they are no longer contaminated. This requires special alpha-sensitive radiation equipment, which is generally not available at hospitals, and will have to be obtained from teams at the accident site.

The place for decontaminating ambulance personnel can be the same place used by other hospital personnel (such as the emergency room staff), preferably away from the emergency room. The place should have two entrances and a shower. A number of laundry bags should be set up and tagged. The personnel should strip off all clothing and put it into appropriate bags. If necessary, large tags should be attached to the clothing. Personal items, such as watches and jewelry, should be put into plastic bags. Protective masks should also be put into a special bag. A complete set of clean clothing should be available to personnel. If this is not possible, clean scrub suits should be provided until fresh clothing can be obtained. Complete monitoring is essential after showering.

Initial Care, Resuscitation, and Admission of Contaminated Patients

Every medical facility must have a plan for handling contaminated patients, while still restricting any changes in basic operations to those that are absolutely essential. The most important objective is to give injured patients proper, efficient, and rapid care without spreading the contamination. Traffic should be restricted, and a diagram of traffic changes should be posted in the emergency room area. If possible, contaminated patients should be treated in a room into which they can be brought without crossing main corridors in the building.

If the hospital has been warned of possible contamination, the route over which the patients are to be brought may be covered with paper. After the patients enter the treatment room, this paper should be carefully rolled up by personnel wearing caps, gowns, masks, and gloves. The paper then should be put into tagged bags. The process can be repeated as often as necessary. If patients are brought in over uncovered floors, the floors should be immediately covered with paper. The paper must be left in place until personnel with the proper monitoring equipment arrive to help evaluate the hazard. Traffic over the paper must be limited to that which is absolutely essential.

Several laundry hampers should be available in the treatment rooms and adjacent hallways. They should be tagged so that all linens and clothing can be properly identified for later decontamination.

A treatment team should be organized to function like an operating-room team, and will require a moderate amount of prior training so that it will function smoothly and effectively. All members should wear caps, gowns, masks, and gloves. The physician and an assistant (if required) should be restricted to the area immediately around the patient. Circulating personnel in the room should bring supplies to the physician but should not touch the patient or the equipment. These personnel should not leave the room. There should be other circulating personnel who would bring supplies to the room but who should not enter the room.

The treatment priorities for a contaminated patient will vary with the seriousness and nature of the basic injuries. As lifesaving resuscitative measures are progressing, certain decontamination procedures can be performed without compromising the care of the patient. The patient's clothing should be removed carefully and put into a tagged bag for later decontamination or disposal. Valuables should be put into a tagged bag (preferably plastic) and held in a designated place for monitoring and decontamination; they should not be mixed with the valuables of other patients. The patients should be thoroughly washed, especially their exposed surfaces. The rinse water must be collected. Later disposal must be in accordance with the limitations of the laws of the nation in which the accident occurred. Consultation with expert personnel from among those at the accident site will be necessary to assure that this is done properly. Normal surgical management of wounds will be more than adequate for removal of radioactive contamination. Special debridement procedures are not required. Again, the rinse water or sponges should not be disposed of until expert advice has been obtained. Material objects from the wounds must be saved. If they can be separated from the rest of the waste, they should be put into marked bags. These fragments will be studied by experts and then disposed of through special procedures.

Patients should be admitted to designated wards or rooms and kept in semi-isolation to limit the spread of the contamination. All personnel should put on gowns, gloves, caps, masks, and shoe covers before entering the room and should remove them after each visit. All waste materials and linens must be marked and monitored. Frequent monitoring by trained health-physics personnel will be required to determine when it is proper to discontinue isolation techniques.

The patient's urine should be saved to be analyzed for radiological contamination. Normal urinalyses can be done safely on portions of the sample, but the laboratory should be notified that there is a potential hazard of contamination with radioactive material. The laboratory must keep a record of the volumes of urine so that later calculations can be made of estimated body burdens of radioactive materials by appropriate laboratories. Fecal samples should also be taken and retained, in addition to nose blows and swabs, when directed.

Operating-Room Care of Contaminated Patients

Some of the patients from a nuclear accident may be injured severely enough to require extensive surgical care. These patients may be contaminated with any of a variety of radioactive and nonradioactive materials. Most of the materials will not be a significant hazard to operating-room personnel if simple precautions are taken. The basic organization and routine of the operating room should not be changed.

Since the hazard from any contaminating material will be respiratory, all personnel in the operating room should wear surgical masks at all times. Personnel with monitoring equipment will be able to advise the operating-room staff when it is safe to unmask.

Once an operating room has been used for the surgical care of nuclear-accident patients, decontamination and monitoring will be necessary before the room can be used for normal surgical cases. The surgical service must be prepared to lose the use of the room for the time needed for these procedures. In some cases, it may be practical for a hospital to set up a temporary operating room close to but not in the regular operating-room area. Alternative surgical areas may be used, such as a plastic surgery clinic or an outpatient surgical facility.

The actual surgery can be managed according to standard operating procedures for handling persons contaminated with infectious hazards, with the following additions or exceptions:

- All waste material must be saved in appropriate containers. Large plastic bags are the most suitable because they do not leak, if properly handled. The containers must be tagged so that they can be identified later and examined by qualified personnel.
- Used surgical gowns, caps, and gloves must also be considered contaminated. They must be removed carefully, and persons assisting in their removal must be wearing caps, gowns, and gloves. The masks should be put in a marked container.
- All personnel should shower completely after working on such cases and must not be released from the area until after they are monitored. This monitoring must be done by qualified technical-team personnel with special equipment.

SUMMARY

A nuclear event exposes people to a blast wave, thermal pulse, and ionizing radiation. If medical units are near the target area, injury and damage may disrupt their ability to perform. Thorough prior planning to adjust medical operations to the nuclear environment is essential. Intensive mission-oriented training that addresses the concerns of medical personnel can reduce their stress and lead to more prompt, effective action. The experience gained through medical operations in peacetime radiation incidents provides skills that are directly transferable to the medical support of the tactical nuclear battlefield. Unless medical personnel recognize and plan for the radiological effect on unit operations, the health-care delivery system may become a casualty of the nuclear event.

NUCLEAR WEAPONS ACCIDENT CHECKLISTS

Predeployment

Publications. Establish necessary publications, including the *Nuclear Weapons Accident Response Procedures Manual* (Defense Nuclear Agency Manual 5100.1) and pertinent service and local directives.

Medical Matériel. Establish necessary medical gear that can be immediately transferred to the accident site, ensuring that all shelf-life items are still effective. The gear will be based on the expected number of casualties and the amount of medical matériel that can be carried by the initial response team(s).

Directory. Establish a directory of local radiological resources, including their locations and telephone numbers. This should include military and civilian health-physics personnel and equipment, as well as the nearest whole-body counters and persons trained to use them. Also include the telephone numbers for REAC/TS as well as for local and state or regional coroners. Ensure that the lists include Autovon, FTS, and commercial numbers, as appropriate.

Training Plans. Establish regular and routine training for medical personnel in the handling of radiological hazards from a nuclear accident. This may be a part of nuclear/biological/chemical training, but it should be emphasized that the hazards from a nuclear weapons accident differ from the hazards from most other radiation accidents. Ensure that medical team members from other units are also trained and aware of their roles.

Organization and Communications. Review the local organization chart for persons and groups to be notified in case of a nuclear weapons accident, and ensure that the lines of communication and the duties of medical organization are clear and thoroughly understood. Review the communications assets to be used in the field, and ensure that personnel are aware of proper operational procedures.

Transportation. Review the transportation assets to ensure that equipment and personnel can be quickly transported. Establish a priority list for personnel and equipment in case the accident site is difficult to reach. Establish contingency plans for movement by four-wheel-drive vehicles and by helicopter.

Field Deployment

Casualty Treatment and Triage. The first medical personnel to arrive on the scene should begin immediately to treat casualties. If casualties have already been treated, contact the treatment facilities (in conjunction with radiological controls personnel) to follow up on patient treatment and to perform radiological surveys of the facilities, as needed. Treatment should always be given in priority of medical condition. Radiation injury or contamination should not upset the normal triage pattern.

Mortuary Affairs. Make arrangements with local coroners or civil officials for the removal of fatalities from the accident site, if necessary. This should be coordinated with the legal and public affairs staffs.

REFERENCES

1. Department of the Army. 1973. *NATO handbook on the medical aspects of NBC defensive operations* [AMedP-6; FM 8-9]. Washington, DC: Department of the Army (revision in press).

2. Defense Nuclear Agency. 1984. *Nuclear weapons accident response procedures (NARP) manual* [DNA Manual 5100.1]. Washington, DC: Defense Nuclear Agency.

3. Department of the Army. 1988. *Nuclear accident and incident response and assistance* (NAIRA) [TC 3-15]. Washington, DC: Department of the Army.

4. North Atlantic Treaty Organization. 1981. *Commander's guide on nuclear radiation exposure of groups* [STANAG 2083]. Brussels: North Atlantic Treaty Organization.

5. Reese, H. L. 1986. *DOD nuclear mishaps* [Special Report SP86-2]. Bethesda, MD: Armed Forces Radiobiology Research Institute.

6. Lewis, F. 1987. *One of our H-bombs is missing.* New York: Bantam Books.

7. Project Crested Ice. *USAF nuclear safety* [special ed., March 1970] 65(2).

8. Gus'kovaya, A. K., ed. 1987. *Early acute effects among the victims of the accident at the Chernobyl Nuclear Power Plant* [USSR Ministry of Health Order Number 4851], translated by U.S. Defense Intelligence Agency [LN 818-87]. Moscow: USSR Ministry of Health.

9. Linneman, R. E. 1987. Soviet medical response to the Chernobyl nuclear accident. *JAMA* 258(5): 637-643.

10. Parker, J. S. 1986. 7th MEDCOM Task Force monitors contamination. *MEDCOM Examiner* 17(6): 1.

11. Dickey, C. 1986. Chernobyl danger slight in EUCOM. *The Stars and Stripes* 45(63): 1.

12. Department of the Army. *Nuclear surety* [AR 50-5]. 1986. Washington, DC: Department of the Army.

13. Department of the Army. 1985. *Medical support—nuclear/chemical accidents and incidents* [AR 40-13]. Washington, DC: Department of the Army.

RECOMMENDED READING

American Medical Association. 1984. *A guide to the hospital management of injuries arising from exposure to or involving ionizing radiation.* Chicago: American Medical Association.

Conklin, J. J., and Walker, R. I., eds. 1987. *Military radiobiology.* Orlando, FL: Academic Press.

Halperin, J. A.; Shleien, B.; Kahana, S. E.; and Bilstad, J. M. 1981. *Background material for the development of the FDA recommendations on thyroid-blocking with potassium iodide* [HHS Pub FDA81-8158]. Washington, DC: Department of Health and Human Services.

Nishiyama, H.; Lukes, S. J.; and Saenger, E. L. 1984. Low-level internal radionuclide contamination: Use of gamma camera for detection. *Radiology* 150(1): 235-240.

Department of the Army. 1969. *Nuclear Handbook for Medical Service Personnel* [TM 8-215]. Washington, DC: Department of the Army.

Shleien, B. 1983. *Preparedness and Response in Radiation Accidents* [HHS Pub FDA83-8211]. Washington, DC: Department of Health and Human Services.

Shleien, B.; Schmidt, G. D.; and Chiacchierini, R. P. 1982. *Background for protective action recommendations: accidental radioactive contamination of food and animal feeds* [HHS Pub. FDA82-8196]. Washington, DC: Department of Health and Human Services.

Chapter 11

PROSPECTS FOR RADIOPROTECTION

LEO I. GIAMBARRESI, Ph.D.* AND RICHARD I. WALKER, Ph.D.**

*Lieutenant, United States Navy; Armed Forces Radiobiology Research Institute, Bethesda, Maryland 20814-5145
**Captain, United States Navy; Director, Enteric Disease Program, Naval Medical Research Institute, Bethesda, Maryland 20814-5055 and Armed Forces Radiobiology Research Institute, Bethesda, Maryland 20814-5145

INTRODUCTION

One of the longest-sought and most elusive goals in radiobiology has been the development of a pharmacological agent that can mitigate the early damage produced in cells and tissues by ionizing radiation. The search for such an agent began in 1949 with the simultaneous demonstration by two different laboratories of survival in rodents exposed to a lethal dose of radiation and treated with the sulfur-containing compounds cysteine or glutathione.[1,2] Since that time, many diverse compounds have been shown to have protective activity (Table 11-1).

With new advances in immunology, biochemistry, radiobiology, and pharmacology, the achievement of that goal may be at hand. Over the longer term, newer concepts and techniques in molecular biology, arising from the so-called biotechnology revolution, are providing exciting approaches for developing specific and effective means to mitigate radiation injury.

The primary objective is to develop an agent or combination of agents that will substantially increase survival and enhance the postattack effectiveness of military personnel on a nuclear battlefield. This radioprotective agent differs from the medical interventions discussed in previous chapters in that it must be easily self-administered shortly before or after radiation exposure to reduce early molecular, cellular, and tissue damage. This chapter briefly reviews the relevant radiobiological concepts, presents the strategies and mechanisms for mitigating radiation injury, and discusses some of the more promising agents being investigated.

RADIATION INJURY

To understand the various strategies being used to mitigate ionizing radiation injury, it is first necessary to define ionizing radiation and to consider the events that occur in the development of ARS.

Ionizing Radiation

Ionizing radiation can be defined as any type of electromagnetic radiation (such as X or gamma rays) or particulate radiation (such as neutrons or alpha particles) that has sufficient energy to ionize atoms or molecules; that is, to eject electrons from their outer orbits.

In considering the effects of radiation on biological systems, it is important to distinguish the different types of ionizing radiation according to their LET. This term describes the amount of energy deposited by a particular type of radiation per unit of path length. Low-LET radiation (X and gamma rays) is sparsely ionizing because it causes few ionizations per micron of path length, whereas high-LET radiation (neutrons and alpha particles) is densely ionizing because it produces many ionizations per micron of path length. Generally, high-LET radiation is much more efficient in producing biological damage than low-LET radiation.[3,4]

Biological Damage

Death from radiation injury is the result of a sequence of events that occurs over a period of less than a billionth of a second to several weeks (Figure 11-1).[28,29] The first step in this sequence is the transfer of radiation energy from the photon or particle to atoms and molecules in its path. This results in the production of the first discrete lesion in the sequence: a chemical alteration in macromolecules that are critical for biological function. Although the importance of membrane damage is still being evaluated, much of the evidence suggests that damage to DNA may be the most important factor in cell death.[28,30] This initial chemical injury can occur in one of two ways. If a critical biological molecule is in the radiation path, it becomes chemically altered by direct interaction with radiation energy. If that molecule is not in the radiation path, it can still become chemically altered indirectly, via reactions with free radicals and reactive oxygen species produced primarily from the radiolysis of water.

These free radicals and oxygen species are important in the overall scheme of radiation injury because their lifetime in solution is sufficiently long to allow them to diffuse and extend the damage be-

TABLE 11-1

RADIOPROTECTIVE COMPOUNDS

Compounds	Protective Effectiveness*	Probable Mechanism of Action	References
Aminothiols		Free-radical scavenging, hydrogen donation	
Cysteine	(+++)		3–6
WR-2721	(+++)		3,6,7
MPG	(++)		3,8,9
Other Sulfur Compounds		Free-radical scavenging	
Dimethylsulfoxide**	(++)		4,10,11
Thiourea	(+)		10,12
Cyanide derivatives***		Hypoxia	
Cyanide	(++)		12–14
Hydroxyacetonitrile	(+++)		10,12, 14
Chelating Agent		Uncertain	
EDTA	(+)		10,12
Metabolites		Free-radical scavenging	
Glucose†	(+)		12
Fructose†	(+)		12
Hypoxia inducers		Hypoxia	
Paraminopropiophenone	(+++)	Hemoglobin changes	6,12,14
Carbon monoxide	(++)		14
Ethanol†	(++)	Respiratory-center depression	14
Morphine	(++)		14
Serotonin	(+++)	Hemodynamic alterations	14
Immunomodulators		Hematopoietic system regeneration	
Glucan	(++)		3,15
Trehalose dimycolate	(++)		16,17
Endotoxin	(++)		3,18–20
Cytokines		Hematopoietic system regeneration	
Interleukin-1	(++)		21
Tumor necrosis factor	(+)		21
Antioxidants		Free-radical scavenging	
Vitamin E	(+)		22,23
Vitamin A (beta-carotene)	(+)		24
Superoxide dismutase	(+++)	Oxygen detoxification	25
Selenium	(+)		22
Eicosanoids		Uncertain	
DiPGE$_2$	(++)		26,27

*Data taken from studies using mice exposed to X or gamma radiation. Grading is according to following scale: (+) slight protection (DRF < 1.2); (++) moderate protection (DRF < 1.5); (+++) good protection (DRF > 5).

**Provides protection when administered topically

***Highly toxic: Protective dose is very close to toxic dose

†Provides protection only at extremely high dose (glucose and fructose, 13,500 mg/kg; ethanol 6–7.5 ml/kg)

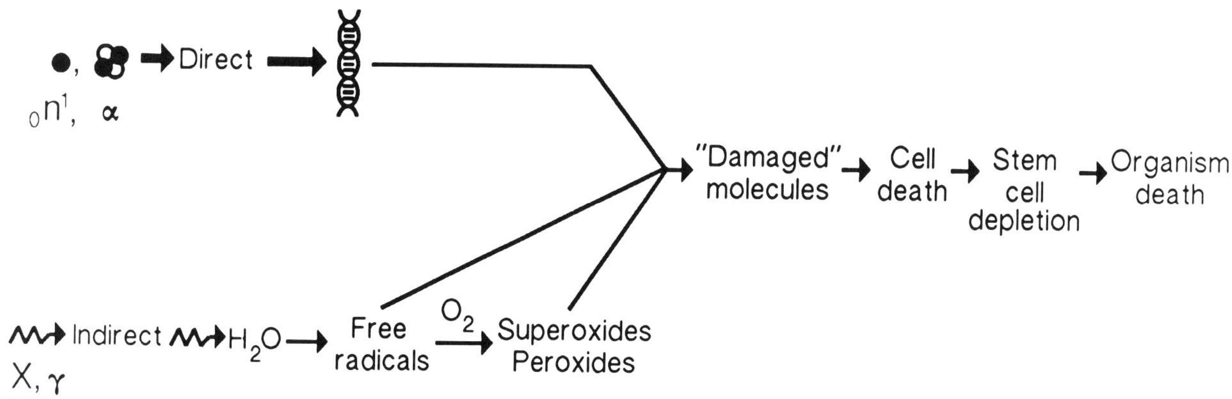

Fig. 11-1. Direct and indirect radiation effects on key biological molecules, which can lead to death of critical cells. Without those cells, the organism cannot survive.

yond the primary path of radiation. In this way, the effects of ionizing radiation within the cell are greatly amplified. Most radiation injury from low-LET radiation is the result of this indirect damage, while that from high-LET radiation is from direct damage.[31] The net effect of direct and indirect damage is the disruption of molecular structure and function, leading to altered cell metabolism. When DNA is damaged, this is followed by altered cell division, cell death, depletion of stem-cell pools, organ system dysfunction, and, if the radiation dose is high enough, death of the organism.

There are several strategies for reducing radiation injury and mortality. Pharmacological agents can *protect* against indirect damage, *repair* damage once it occurs, or stimulate the *regeneration* of depleted cell populations (Figure 11-2). Spanning these strategies are new genetic approaches that are just beginning to be used in the development of advanced pharmacological agents. Combinations of agents that exploit the operative mechanisms in at least two of these strategies may substantially improve drug effectiveness.

PROTECTION AGAINST RADIATION INJURY

As indicated in Figure 11-2, almost nothing can be done pharmacologically to protect against the initial transfer of radiation energy to either water or critical biological molecules. The transfer occurs too rapidly (within 10^{-14} seconds after irradiation) and is a purely physical process.[28]

The failure of radioprotective agents to protect against direct damage to critical molecules indicates an inherent upper limit to the degree of protection that can be achieved pharmacologically. Because injury from high-LET radiation is due primarily to direct damage, and because the relative yields of water radiolytic products and reactive oxygen species decrease with increasing LET, protection against high-LET radiation injury is more difficult to achieve.[3] Protective agents would be most effective against a low-LET radiation hazard.

The earliest point at which a protective effect from pharmacological agents can be detected is around 10^{-12} seconds after irradiation.[29] At that time, the pharmacological agents can begin to repair chemical damage produced in the critical biological molecules and also react with the chemical intermediates that indirectly damage these molecules. Protection depends on the ability of chemical agents to reduce the intracellular concentration of free radicals and reactive oxygen species that are produced within the first millisecond after irradiation.

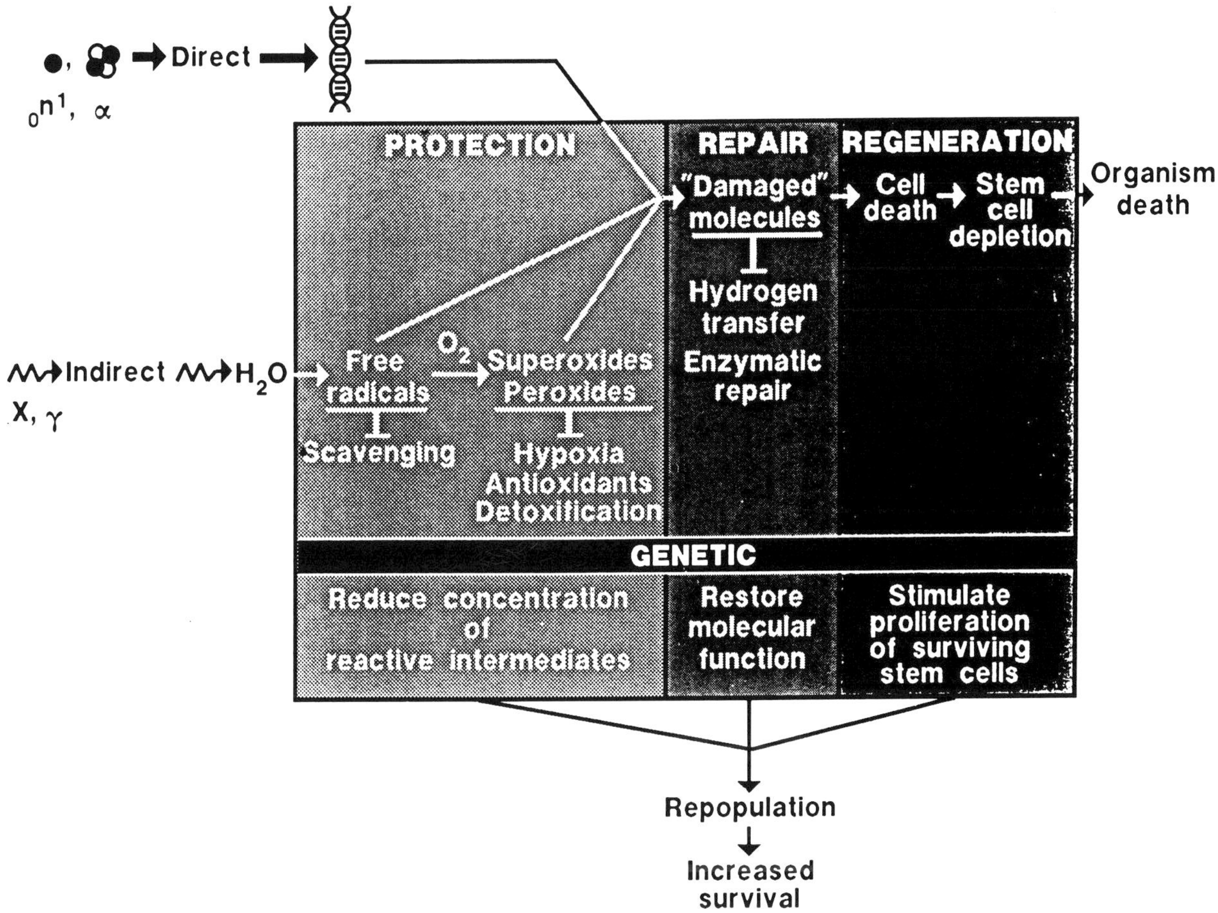

Fig. 11-2. Strategies of protection, repair, and regeneration may prevent cell and organism death after radiation exposure

Mechanisms

The damage induced by the products of radiation interactions with water can be reduced either by inhibiting the formation of these reactive radical intermediates, or by eliminating them from the cellular environment. This can be accomplished by using agents that induce hypoxia or that scavenge toxic products.

Hypoxia. The formation of reactive oxygen species can be inhibited by the induction of hypoxia. The extent of radiation damage in a tissue is directly related to the degree of oxygenation of that tissue; agents capable of reducing oxygenation will mitigate the injury.[3,32] Many of these chemical agents are known to induce transient systemic or localized hypoxia.[3-5] Systemic hypoxia can be achieved in several ways: induction of hemodynamic cardiovascular alterations, interference with hemoglobin function, increased tissue oxygen utilization, and depressed respiratory-center function. At the cellular and molecular levels, localized hypoxia can be achieved by agents that take part in the chemical and biochemical reactions that use oxygen.

Induction of hypoxia is a widespread protective mechanism that accounts, at least in part, for the protective action of many different chemicals, drugs, and physiological mediators (Table 11-1). In spite of that, the usefulness of this mechanism must be considered with caution because of the potential effects of hypoxia on normal physiological function. This caution may apply more to agents that induce a systemic hypoxic state than to those that create localized hypoxia.

Scavenging. Free-radical scavenging and enzymatic detoxification refer to the ability of chemicals and endogenous enzymes to remove products of water radiolysis and highly reactive oxygen species before they can damage molecules of biological importance.[2,33] In essence, these are competitive reactions between protective agents and biological molecules. In aqueous solutions, protective agents and enzymes react with free radicals and oxygen species to form relatively stable, nontoxic end products, thereby reducing the concentration of these reactive species and sparing the biological target. Many protectants are very efficient scavengers of water-derived free radicals.

Candidate Agents

Agents currently available as candidates for protection against indirect damage fall into three main groups: *aminothiols, naturally occurring antioxidants,* and *eicosanoids* (Tables 11-2 and 11-3). Research is also being conducted using various *genetic approaches.*

Aminothiols. The vast majority of agents that have been developed and tested in laboratory models for their ability to increase survival after irradiation are the aminothiols.[34] These compounds are chemical analogues of the sulfur-containing amino acid, cysteine. Like cysteine, they have a sulfhydryl group separated by two or three carbon atoms from a strongly basic nitrogen group (Figure 11-3).

As a group, the aminothiols are very effective protectants, and they must be present in the system during irradiation. Optimal protection in laboratory animals is generally obtained by intravenous injection 15–30 minutes before irradiation. The aminothiols function primarily through free-radical scavenging[5] and hydrogen transfer.[3,33] Hypoxia induction may also play a part in their functioning.[4,6]

One of the most significant events in the development of radioprotective agents was the 1969 synthesis of an aminothiol derivative known as WR-2721 (ethiofos).[35] This drug was developed through a program sponsored by the Walter Reed Army Institute of Research, and is the most thoroughly studied of over 4,000 compounds developed and tested to date. WR-2721 has been reported to reduce the effect of a radiation dose by a factor of 2.7 in mice given this drug intraperitoneally 30 minutes before exposure to gamma radiation.[36,37] This is the highest dose reduction factor (DRF) against mouse lethality at 30 days reliably reported for a single injection of a conventional radioprotectant. Increased 30-day survival is commonly interpreted as protection against death due to hematopoietic-system failure.

WR-2721 also exerts differing protective effects for normal tissue and at least some types of solid tumors.[37] In addition, the drug significantly reduces the toxicity of the tumor chemotherapeutic agents, cyclophosphamide and cisplatin,[38,39] without altering their chemotherapeutic effectiveness. For these reasons, WR-2721 is undergoing clinical trials as an adjunct to tumor radiation and chemotherapy. Two other potentially beneficial clinical side effects of this drug are that WR-2721 is a hypocalcemic agent and inhibits parathyroid hormone secretion.[40]

WR-2721 is still not available as a field-useable radioprotective agent because it induces nausea and vomiting.[41,42] Although no cumulative or irreversible toxicity has ever been observed in humans or experimental animals that received this drug (even at relatively high doses), the animals did show significant performance degradation after its parenteral administration.[43,44] Another problem that must be overcome is the drug's poor oral bioavailability, due primarily to first-pass metabolism by the intestinal mucosa during absorption.[45] In addition, the drug is hydrolyzed in the acidic environment of the stomach, a factor that is aggravated by its ability to slow gastric emptying.[46]

Research is in progress to overcome these bioavailability problems by using different formulations and by developing prodrugs that are not susceptible to first-pass metabolism. Researchers are also seeking to control or minimize the side effects by combining WR-2721 with antiemetics, or by using subtoxic amounts of the drug in combination with other agents that act synergistically or additively. A DRF of about 1.2 has been obtained with WR-2721 administered intraperitoneally to mice at a dose that produced no observable side effects or performance degradation.[44]

The side effects of WR-2721 and the pharmacological problems associated with its administration are serious obstacles that must be overcome before it can be fielded as a military radioprotective agent. However, a number of other compounds have been developed through the army's program that may more readily satisfy the requirements of a militarily useful agent (Table 11-4).

To compare these compounds for their potential military usefulness, it is necessary to consider a variety of characteristics in addition to the DRF. These include the route of administration, effective drug dose, and *therapeutic index*.[47] The therapeutic index, as used here, refers to the ratio between the toxic LD_{50} and the protective dose used to produce a specific DRF. Although it would also be advantageous to compare information on acute side effects pro-

TABLE 11-2

SUMMARY OF PROTECTIVE SCAVENGING AGENTS

Mechanism and Agent	Level of Protection	Side Effects and Therapeutic Index*	Deliverability	Advantages	Disadvantages
WR-2721	DRF > 2.0 Duration of effect > 3 hr	Nausea, vomiting, hypotension, hypocalcemia, behavioral changes TI = 1.4 (DRF = 2.7) TI = 3.5 (DRF = 1.2)	Dose** = 400 mg/kg Route:*** i.v. or i.p. Time: 30 minutes before irradiation	Very high DRFs possible; DRF = 1.2 at behaviorly non-toxic dose in human clinical trials	Large doses (> 200 mg/kg); ineffective p.o.; high DRFs only at doses that produce serious side effects
WR-159243	DRF = 1.3	Unknown side effects TI = 7.5	Dose = 40 mg/kg Route: p.o. Time: 30 minutes before irradiation	Effective p.o.; fairly low dose (< 50 mg/kg); large TI (>5.0)	Unknown
WR-76841	DRF = 1.19	Unknown side effects TI = 5.1	Dose = 175 mg/kg Route: p.o. Time: 30 minutes before irradiation	Effective p.o.; large TI (> 50.0)	Fairly large doses (> 100 mg/kg); DRF < 1.2
WR-1551	DRF = 1.3	Unknown side effects TI = 3.0	Dose = 100 mg/kg Route: p.o. Time: 30 minutes before irradiation	Effective p.o.	Unknown
WR-3302	DRF = 1.39	Unknown side effects TI = 6.0	Dose = 5 mg/kg Route: i.p. Time: 30 minutes before irradiation	Low doses (≤ 20 mg/kg); large TI (> 5.0)	Oral effectiveness not established
WR-2926	DRF = 1.7	Unknown side effects TI = 2.5	Dose = 50 mg/kg Route: i.p. Time: 30 minutes before irradiation	DRF > 1.5	Oral effectiveness not established; TI < 3.0
WR-1607	DRF = 1.4	Nausea, vomiting TI = 3.4	Dose = 5 mg/kg Route: i.p. Time: 30 minutes before irradiation	Low doses (> 20 mg/kg); mitigates performance decrement	Oral effectiveness not established
Mercapto-propionyl glycine (MPG)	DRF = 1.4	Unknown side effects TI = 100.0	Dose = 20 mg/kg Route: i.p. or i.v. Time: 30 minutes before irradiation	Low doses (≤ 20 mg/kg); extremely high TI in clinical use (Japan); effective after irradiation	Oral effectivess not established; protection at 20 mg/kg is difficult to reproduce
Vitamin E	DRF = 1.1	Unknown side effects	Dose = 3 x dietary requirement Route: p.o. Feeding Regimen: 1 week before irradiation 4 weeks after irradiation	Effective p.o.; naturally occurring dietary component	Dietary regimen may be impractical for field use; single dose effectivess not established; DRF < 1.2; conflicting reports in literature on effectiveness
Vitamin A	DRF = 1.26	Unknown side effects	Dose = 28 x dietary requirement Route: p.o. Feeding Regimen: 1 week before irradiation (3 x dietary requirement) 4 weeks after irradiation (28 x dietary requirement)	Effective p.o.; naturally occurring dietary component	Dietary regimen may be impractical for field use; single dose effectivess not established; large vitamin dose required

*Therapeutic index (TI): ratio of toxic LD_{50} to the drug dose required to produce the DRF specified in the table
**Dose: dosage of drug required to produce the DRF indicated under "Level of Protection"
***Routes of administration: i.v. (intravenous), i.p. (intraperitoneal), p.o. (oral), s.c. (subcutaneous)

TABLE 11-3

SUMMARY OF DETOXIFICATION AGENTS, REGENERATION AGENTS, AND OTHER AGENTS OF UNDEFINED ACTION

Mechanism and Agent	Level of Protection	Side Effects and Therapeutic Index*	Deliverability	Advantages	Disadvantages
DETOXIFICATION AGENTS					
Selenium	DRF ≤ 1.1	Unknown	Dose** = 4 ppm in drinking water Route:*** p.o. Regimen: 2 months before irradiation Dose =1.6 mg/kg Route: i.p. Time: 24 hours before irradiation	Effective p.o.; naturally occurring dietary component	Oral regimen may be impractical for field use; single p.o. dose effectiveness not established; DRF < 1.2
Superoxide dismutase	DRF = 1.56	Unknown side effects	Dose and Time = 200 mg/kg (1 hour before irradiation) and 35 mg/kg (1 hour after irradiation) Route: i.v.	DRF > 1.5; effective as single doses given 1 hour before irradiation	Oral effectivess not established; large molecular size
REGENERATION AGENTS					
Glucan F	DRF ≤ 1.2	Unknown side effects	Dose = 250 mg/kg Doses > 250 mg/kg provide no increased protection Route: i.v. Time: 24 hours before irradiation	Effective after irradiation	Oral effectiveness not established; DRF < 1.2; optimum protection at 20 hours after irradiation is impractical for field use
Trehalose dimycolate (TDM)	70% survival at LD_{100}	Unknown side effects	Dose ≅ 1.7mg/kg Route: i.p. Time: 2 hours after irradiation delivered as a squalene emulsion	Effective after irradiation; low dose (≤ 20 mg/kg)	Oral effectiveness not established; DRF unknown
Interleukin-1 (IL-1)	DRF = 1.25	Unknown side effects	Dose = 0.004 mg/kg Route: i.p. Time: 20 hours before irradiation	Extremely low doses (≤ 0.01 mg/kg)	Oral effectiveness not established; optimum protection at 20 hours after irradiation is impractical for field use; effectiveness is strain dependent
Tumor-necrosis factor (TNF)	DRF = 1.16	Unknown side effects	Dose ≅ 0.2 mg/kg Route: i.p. Time: 20 hours before irradiation	Very low doses (< 0.5 mg/kg); effectiveness is not strain dependent	Oral effectiveness not established; optimum protection at 20 hours before irradiation is impractical for field use
AGENTS OF UNDEFINED ACTION					
16,16-Dimethyl prostaglandin E_2 ($DiPGE_2$)	DRF = 1.72	Diarrhea; decreased ambulation	Dose = 1.6 mg/kg Route: s.c. Time: 5–15 minutes before irradiation	Low doses (< 20 mg/kg); DRF > 1.5	Oral effectiveness not established; severe diarrhea at protective doses
Leukotriene C_4 (LTC_4)	DRF = 1.9	Unknown side effects	Dose = 0.4 mg/kg Route: s.c. Time: 5 minutes before irradiation	Very low doses (< 0.5 mg/kg); DRF > 1.5	Oral effectiveness not established
Platelet-activating factor (PAF)	DRF = 1.9	Unknown side effects	Dose = 0.3 mg/kg Route: s.c. Time: 5–10 minutes before irradiation	Low doses (< 20 mg/kg); DRF > 1.5	Oral effectiveness not established

*Therapeutic index (TI): ratio of toxic LD_{50} to the drug dose required to produce the DRF specified in the table
**Dose: dosage of drug required to produce the DRF indicated under "Level of Protection"
***Routes of administration: i.v. (intravenous), i.p. (intraperitoneal), p.o. (oral), s.c. (subcutaneous)

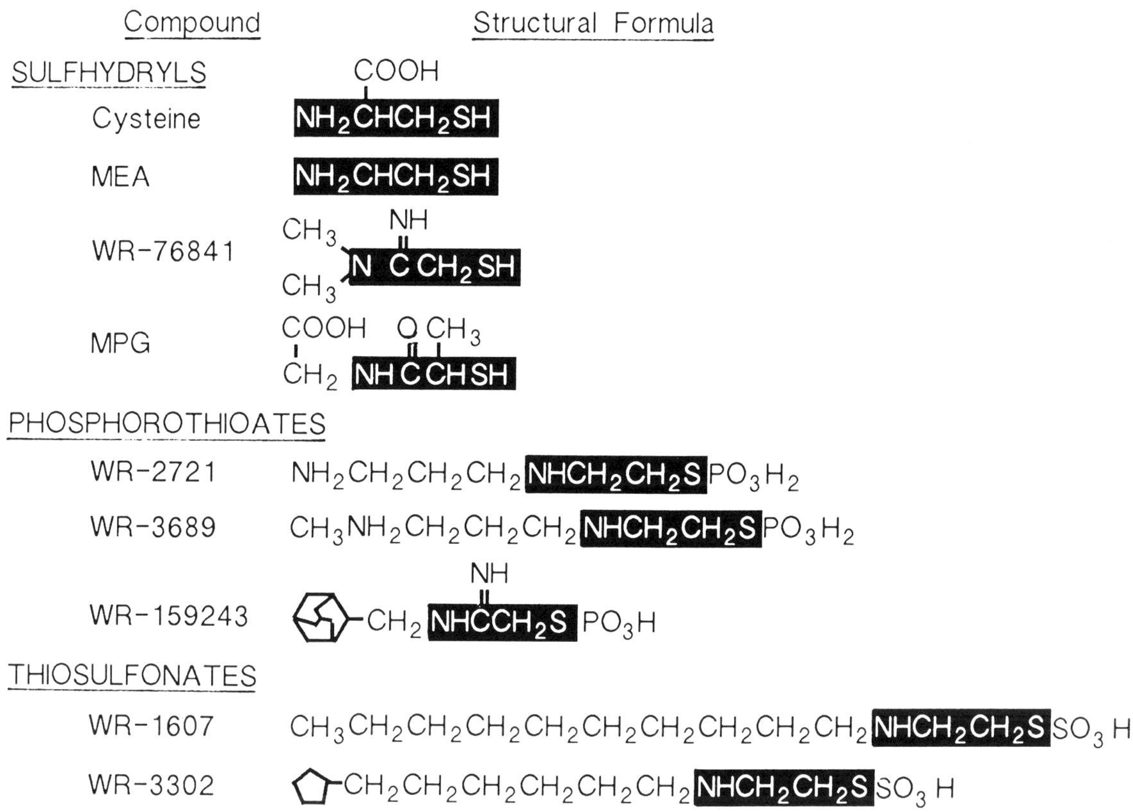

Fig. 11-3. Structural formulas for selected sulfur-containing radioprotectants. All compounds are chemical analogues of cysteine and MEA.

duced by these agents at protective doses, the data are so limited that these factors cannot be included at this time.

The compound that stands out as the most promising candidate is the phosphorothioate WR-159243. Although its DRF is only 1.3, it is effective in mice when given orally, the protective dose is less than 50 mg/kg, and it has the highest safety margin or therapeutic index (7.5) of all the compounds listed. Other compounds with therapeutic indices greater than 2.5 that are being considered include *(a)* the sulfhydryl WR-76841, because of its oral effectiveness and relatively high therapeutic index (5.1); and *(b)* the thiosulfonates WR-1551, because of its oral effectiveness; WR-3302, because of its very low effective dose (5 mg/kg) and high therapeutic index (6.0); and WR-2926, because of its relatively low effective dose (50 mg/kg) and relatively high DRF (1.7). The thiosulfonate WR-1607 is particularly interesting because *(a)* it has a very low effective dose (5 mg/kg) in protecting against radiation-induced lethality, and *(b)* it is one of the few compounds available that not only enhance survival but also ameliorate ETI.[48,49] This latter effect may be related to the drug's ability to minimize postirradiation hypotension.[48]

WR-2721 has a therapeutic index of only 1.4 at the dose required to produce a DRF of 2.7. However, the therapeutic index increases dramatically to 7.0 at a dose that produces minimal side effects (200 mg/kg). The DRF obtained at this dose is 1.2.

WR-3689 is identical in structure to WR-2721, except that WR-3689 possesses a terminal methyl group (Figure 11-3). When given intraperitoneally at a dose of 450 mg/kg, it provides a DRF of 1.7 with a therapeutic index of 2.5. When given orally at a similar dose (500 mg/kg), WR-3689 is still capable of providing significant protection (DRF: 1.2). With this regimen, the therapeutic index for WR-3689 increases to greater than 3.5 because the lethally toxic

TABLE 11-4

CANDIDATE SULFUR COMPOUNDS STUDIED AT WRAIR*

Walter Reed Number	Type**	Administration Route***	Protective Dose † (mg/kg)	Toxic LD_{50} Dose (mg/kg)	DRF	Therapeutic Index††
WR 2721	Phosphorothioate	i.p.	500	704	2.72	1.4
WR 2926	Thiosulfonate	i.p.	50	125	1.70	2.5
WR 3689	Phosphorothioate	i.p.	450	1,120	2.22	2.5
WR 176240	Phosphorothioate	p.o.	200	580	1.20	2.9
WR 1551	Thiosulfonate	p.o.	100	300	1.30	3.0
WR 2347	Sulfhydryl	i.p.	600	1,800	1.53	3.0
WR 3562	Thiosulfonate	i.p.	100	300	1.55	3.0
WR 2754	Thiosulfonate	i.p.	100	300	1.80	3.0
WR 2824	Phosphorothioate	i.p.	200	675	1.33	3.4
WR 1607	Thiosulfonate	i.p.	5	17	1.40	3.4
WR 3689	Phosphorothioate	p.o.	500	>1,750	1.22	3.5
WR 76841	Sulfhydryl	p.o.	175	900	1.19	5.1
WR 3302	Thiosulfonate	i.p.	5	30	1.39	6.0
WR 2721	Phosphorothioate	i.p.	100	704	1.20	7.0
WR 159243	Phosphorothioate	p.o.	40	300	1.30	7.5

*Data derived from studies using mice exposed to whole-body X or gamma radiation

**Compounds are listed in order of increasing therapeutic index

***Route of administration: i.p. (intraperitoneal), p.o. (oral)

†Dose: Dosage of drug used to obtain the DRF listed

††TI is the ratio between toxic LD_{50} and protective dose

Source: Data taken from a report presented to NATO NBC Panel VII, AC 225/GEC, October 1987. Colonel David E. Davidson, Jr., Veterinary Corps, United States Army, compiled these data from the archives of the Division of Experimental Therapeutics, Walter Reed Army Institute of Research (WRAIR), Washington, D.C. 20307-5100.

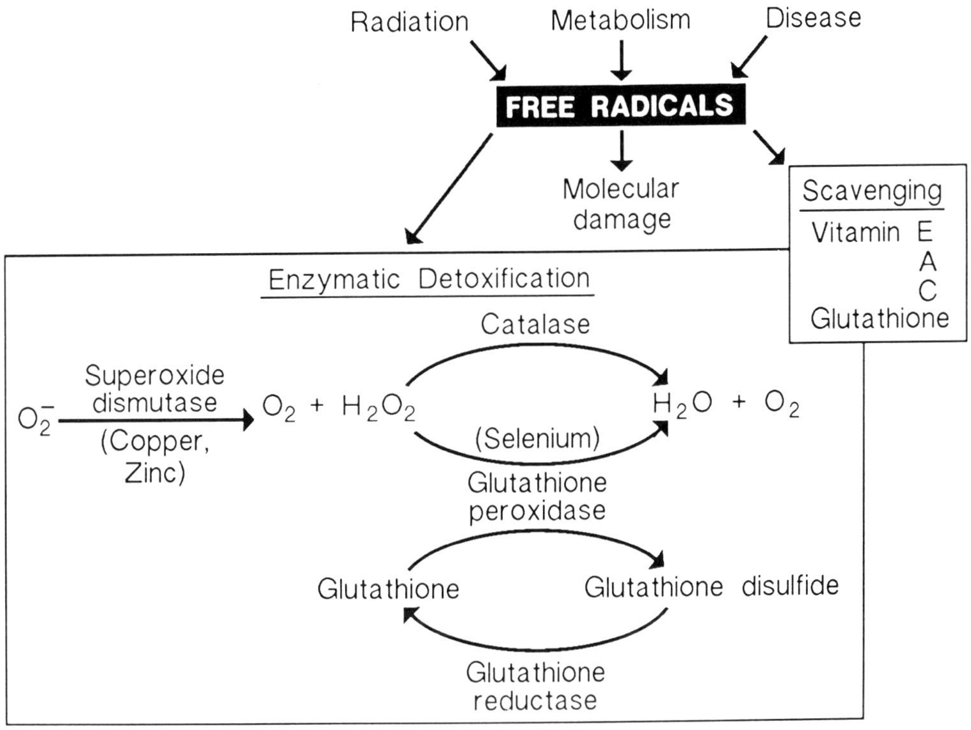

Fig. 11-4. Natural biochemical defense system of the cell, which scavenges free radicals and detoxifies reactive oxygen species

oral dose is much higher than that for the intraperitoneal dose.

Another potentially promising aminothiol compound is mercaptopropionylglycine (MPG). Under the trade name Thiola, this drug has been available in Japan since the 1970s. It has been used as a detoxifying agent for heavy-metal poisoning, among other clinical applications.[50] Evidence suggests that MPG is also radioprotective. In the most promising studies, it has provided a DRF of up to 1.4 when injected intraperitoneally at a dose (20 mg/kg) that is about 100-fold lower than its toxic dose (2,100 mg/kg).[51,52]

Naturally Occurring Antioxidants. Naturally occurring compounds that function as antioxidants, such as certain vitamins, minerals, and enzymes, are also being evaluated. These are part of a natural biochemical defense system that has evolved to protect cells against free radicals and reactive oxygen species arising from normal metabolic processes. This defense can be divided into two components: compounds of low molecular weight that scavenge free radicals, and enzymes that detoxify reactive oxygen species (Figure 11-4).[53]

The low-molecular-weight compounds that function as free-radical scavengers in this defense system include vitamins A and E, which are lipophilic, and vitamin C, which is hydrophilic. The enzymatic arm of this system includes superoxide dismutase, which catalyzes the conversion of superoxide anions to hydrogen peroxide and molecular oxygen. The hydrogen peroxide produced by this reaction is removed from the system by two other enzymes: catalase and glutathione peroxidase. Selenium contributes to this scheme in that it is a cofactor for glutathione peroxidase.

Vitamin E has been shown to increase survival after irradiation.[22] Groups of mice were fed either a basal control diet or a diet supplemented with three times the normal daily mouse requirement of vitamin E (dl-alpha-tocopherol) for 1 week before an 8.5-Gy dose of cobalt-60 gamma radiation and for 30 days after exposure. All of the control animals succumbed by day 30, whereas 60% of the vitamin E-fed animals survived. At 7.5 Gy, 10% of the controls survived, while 100% of the vitamin E-fed animals survived. DRFs for vitamin E have not been determined experimentally.

Vitamin A is also able to increase postirradiation survival when fed to mice as a dietary supplement.[23] In these experiments, mice were maintained on a basal control diet containing three times the daily mouse requirement of vitamin A for 1 week before irradiation from a cesium-137 source. Immediately following irradiation, they were maintained for the remainder of the experiment on *(a)* the basal diet, *(b)* a diet supplemented with about twenty-eight times the normal requirement of vitamin A, or *(c)* a diet supplemented with an amount of beta-carotene equivalent to about ten times the normal requirement of vitamin A. The vitamin A diet was able to produce DRFs of 1.12–1.25. The beta-carotene diet produced a DRF of 1.26. Significant mitigation of radiation lethality was also provided by vitamin A when diet supplementation was delayed for up to 2 days after irradiation, although delaying the supplementation for 6 days resulted in no increase in survival over the basal-diet-fed animals. Vitamin A fed to mice for 3 days before partial-body irradiation can substantially reduce the effects of localized (hind limb) X irradiation.[54]

In addition to its radioprotective ability, vitamin A or beta-carotene may also be able to promote recovery from burn injury by reversing postburn immunosuppression.[55] This point is significant because burns are expected to be the most common type of injury on the nuclear battlefield.

Selenium is protective when administered either orally or parenterally. When given orally as sodium selenite in drinking water (4 ppm)[21] or injected (1.6 mg/kg) 24 hours before exposure to 900 Gy of cobalt-60 radiation,[56] selenium was able to provide slight but significant increases in survival. The real potential for using selenium as a radioprotective agent lies in its ability to act synergistically with other agents. Selenium can also reduce the toxicity of the sulfur-containing radioprotective compound WR-2721.[56]

Vitamins A and E and selenium are being considered as potential radioprotectant candidates because they are normal dietary components, and considerable data on their toxicity, metabolism, and pharmacological action in the human are available. They are also effective when given orally.

The parenteral administration of superoxide dismutase has increased survival in mice exposed to ionizing radiation.[25] Intravenous injection of this enzyme to mice at a dose of 200 mg/kg given 1 hour before irradiation with X rays resulted in a DRF of 1.38. A single injection of only 35 mg/kg given 1 hour before irradiation with X rays was also able to increase survival (DRF: 1.12). The highest DRF reported for this enzyme is 1.56, achieved in mice given two intravenous injections: one at a dose of 200 mg/kg given 1 hour before irradiation with X rays, and the other at a dose of 35 mg/kg given 1 hour after irradiation.[25]

Eicosanoids. The eicosanoids are a large group of potent inflammatory mediators derived from the 20-carbon fatty-acid precursor, arachidonic acid. The compounds in this family that are being examined for their ability to increase the survival of irradiated animals include 16,16-dimethyl prostaglandin E_2 ($DiPGE_2$, a synthetic analogue of the naturally occurring prostaglandin GE_2), leukotriene C_4 (LTC_4), and platelet-activating factor (PAF). In one study, $DiPGE_2$ was given subcutaneously to mice at a dose of 1.6 mg/kg and was able to elicit a DRF of 1.72, although severe diarrhea occurred at protective doses.[27] The optimal time for injection is 5–15 minutes before cobalt-60 gamma irradiation, but protection can still be achieved when the compound is given 1 hour before irradiation. LTC_4 has just recently been shown to be effective in increasing the survival of hematopoietic stem cells of mice exposed to cobalt-60 gamma radiation.[57] A DRF of 1.9, using 30-day lethality as the end point, has been achieved with LTC_4 in mice exposed to cobalt-60 gamma radiation.[58] Similarly, PAF is capable of producing fairly high DRFs (about 1.7).[59]

Genetic Approaches. Work is also under way, using molecular biology techniques, to define sequences in the DNA molecule that may be particularly sensitive to radiation. By precisely defining the mechanisms and sites of damage, it may be possible to develop protective agents that can be targeted to specific sensitive sites on the DNA molecule. Additionally, because enzymes are part of the body's natural defense against reactive chemical intermediates, it should be possible to identify the factors involved in regulating their synthesis and to define the encoding gene sequences. This may provide a means by which the synthesis can be activated to increase radioresistance.

REPAIR OF RADIATION INJURY

The aim of this strategy is to restore the chemical structure and normal function of damaged biological molecules so that the injury or death of critical cells is avoided.

As with protection, the effectiveness of the repair varies with the LET. High-LET radiation is densely ionizing and produces very intensive local chemical damage. As the density of damage increases, the ability of chemicals and enzymes to repair this damage becomes overwhelmed. Therefore, repair strategies are more effective for low-LET radiation. Repair can be achieved either chemically (by hydrogen transfer) or enzymatically.

Chemical Repair by Hydrogen Transfer

Radiation damage to a critical biological molecule results in the transformation of that molecule into an organic free radical. In this form, the molecule can then react with oxygen or other free radicals and become permanently altered chemically. However, if a suitable hydrogen donor is in the vicinity of the damaged molecule, it can compensate for the damage by donating or transferring a hydrogen atom.[3,33] Hydrogen atom transfer can be thought of as an instantaneous repair process, in which the original molecular structure is restored before the damaged critical molecule becomes permanently altered by further chemical reaction. Many of the agents that function as free-radical scavengers also have the ability to donate a hydrogen atom.

No radioprotective agents that function primarily or exclusively by chemical repair are available. However, the aminothiols, which act as free-radical scavengers, are all capable of hydrogen transfer and therefore can function in the repair strategy.[3]

Genetic Repair

Similar chemical alterations may also be induced by natural biological processes and disease states that generate free radicals. In the case of DNA, mammalian cells have evolved an elaborate and remarkably efficient system of enzymes that continually repair lesions in that critically important molecule. This system is complex, involving a number of different enzymes and a variety of regulatory molecules that control their synthesis and activity. One of the potentially useful features of this system is that it is inducible; that is, the synthesis of the repair enzymes and regulatory factors is activated when the need arises.

Strains of prokaryotic organisms exist that are capable of surviving very high doses of radiation. One that has received attention is *Deinococcus radiodurans*, which is an extremely radioresistant strain of bacteria.[60] Although study of these relatively simple prokaryotic systems may provide some insight into the genetic mechanisms involved in radiation sensitivity, their lack of complexity compared to mammalian cells is a limitation.

About 25 years ago, a radiosensitive mammalian cell line was isolated in tissue culture from a relatively radioresistant mouse lymphoma cell line.[61] With the advent of new biotechnology techniques, this extensively characterized strain is just beginning to be exploited to its full potential in uncovering genetic mechanisms in radiosensitivity.[62] Recent evidence indicates that the radiosensitivity of this cell line is due to a lower rate of DNA repair.[63] The genomes of the resistant parental line can be compared with the sensitive daughter line by DNA hybridization techniques, making it possible *(a)* to determine if genes are induced by radiation to activate the repair process, *(b)* to identify the genes that are so induced, and *(c)* to determine the proteins that are encoded.

It may be possible (as a long-term goal) to develop agents that will function exclusively in genetic repair. By increasing molecular repair capabilities, these agents may prevent the effects of cellular damage from overwhelming the organism.

REGENERATION AFTER RADIATION INJURY

The aim of this strategy is to increase survival by stimulating the function and regeneration of stem-cell populations that have decreased in number due to radiation-induced cell death. Conceptually, this strategy can be applied to any organ system (such as the hematopoietic system and the gastrointestinal

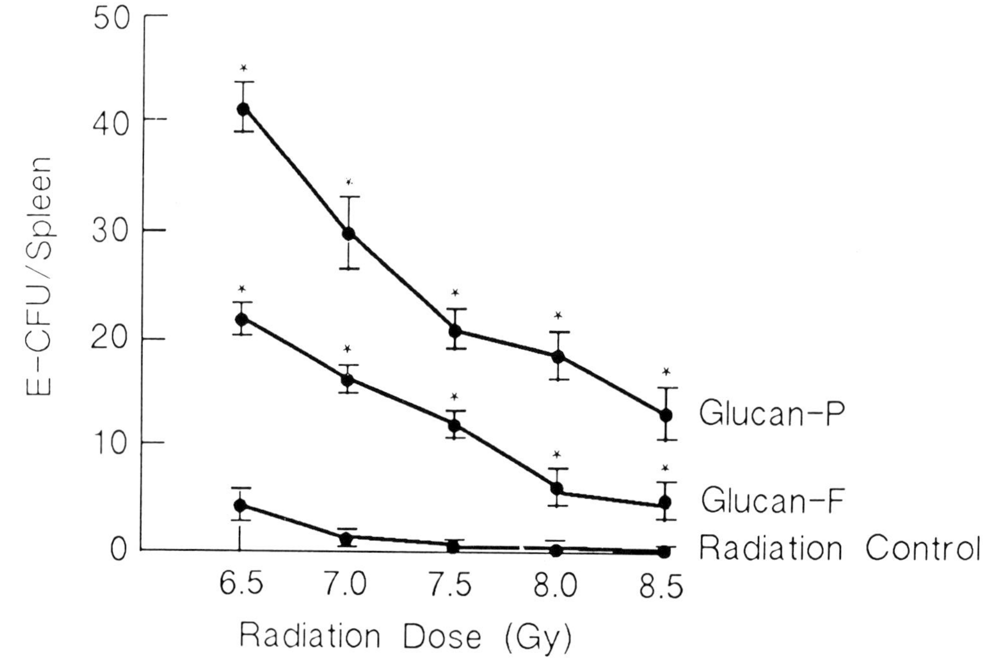

Fig. 11-5. Hematopoietic stem-cell survival as a function of radiation dose treated or not treated with glucan, an agent useful in promoting regeneration of stem cells. Glucan effectiveness decreases as increased numbers of stem cells are killed by higher doses of radiation.

system) that relies on stem-cell proliferation to provide mature differentiated cells for proper functioning. However, because hematopoietic stem cells are the most radiosensitive, only regeneration of the hematopoietic system is discussed here.

Regeneration is a feasible strategy for mitigating radiation injury at radiation doses below the threshold dose that would result in 100% death of hematopoietic stem cells. Figure 11-5 examines hematopoietic stem-cell survival as measured by the number of colony-forming units found in the spleens (E-CFU/spleen) of irradiated mice. Some of the mice were treated with the regenerating agent glucan. In the radiation control animals, which were not given glucan, the number of E-CFU/spleen decreased with increasing radiation dose. Similarly, the effectiveness of glucan in increasing the survival of these cells also decreased with increasing dose. This indicates that the effectiveness of these agents depends on the number of surviving stem cells. Above the threshold radiation dose that results in 100% stem-cell death (greater than 8.5 Gy in Figure 11-5), regeneration becomes ineffective.

The utility of this strategy depends on the threshold point, a factor that can be influenced greatly by partial shielding or by agents that operate in the protection or repair strategies. Because hematopoietic stem cells are among the most radiosensitive in the body, this threshold occurs at a fairly low radiation dose. For uniform whole-body radiation exposure, the threshold dose is approximately equal to the $LD_{100/30}$ radiation dose. However, in battlefield or accident situations, it is likely that the apparent threshold will be substantially higher. Because the inherent radiosensitivity of the hematopoietic stem cells would not change, other factors related to the nature of radiation exposure contribute to this apparent increase. In battlefield or accident situations, some element of shielding, either deliberate or coincidental, is likely to be present. This will provide inhomogeneous exposures, so that high levels of radiation reaching one part of the body may not reach

TABLE 11-5

PRIMATE SURVIVAL FOLLOWING 8 Gy OF COBALT-60 IRRADIATION

Category	No Supportive Therapy	Supportive Therapy Only	Supportive Therapy (allogeneic bone-marrow transplant)*	Partial Shielding**
Survivors	0	0	5	4
Total primates	4	4	5	4
Mean survival time in days	12.5	16.3	>30.0	>30.0

*Antibiotics, fluids, platelets
**Less than 1% surviving stem cells

others, thereby permitting increased stem-cell survival. In these situations, it may also be possible to increase stem-cell survival by minimizing the time spent in high-radiation fields and maintaining some distance from radiation sources. The contribution of these protective measures was evident in the Chernobyl accident victims, in whom bone-marrow grafts apparently failed. These failures were due, at least in part, to host-versus-graft reactions initiated by surviving stem cells, even in patients who were exposed to doses of radiation much greater than those expected to completely deplete stem cells.

The effectiveness of minimal local shielding in protecting even small numbers of stem cells is demonstrated in experiments done with monkeys (Table 11-5).[64] Supportive therapy (fluid, platelets, and antibiotics) significantly increased the $LD_{50/30}$ of irradiated animals. In monkeys exposed to a lethal dose (8 Gy) of whole-body cobalt-60 radiation, supportive therapy extended survival for a few days but had no effect on 30-day survival rates because the radiation dose completely depleted the stem-cell population. However, when the tibias of these animals were shielded so that less than 1% of their bone-marrow stem cells survived, regeneration occurred and many of the animals survived.

Mechanisms

The regeneration of depleted stem-cell populations is brought about by agents that stimulate the proliferation and function of hematopoietic and immunopoietic stem cells. The precise biochemical mechanisms by which this stimulation occurs are complex and are as yet incompletely understood.

Exactly which cell type becomes stimulated depends on the type of agent involved (Figure 11-6). Nonspecific immunomodulators are exogenous agents that can bind to and stimulate a variety of different cell types, particularly macrophages. These agents are thought to induce the stimulated cells to release a variety of peptides (cytokines) that act specifically on immunopoietic and hematopoietic progenitor and stem cells to stimulate their growth and differentiation into mature, functional cells.[65]

Candidate Agents

Agents that mitigate radiation injury via regeneration can be grouped into two broad categories: *immunomodulators* and *cytokines*. Immunomodulators can be thought of as inducer molecules, and cytokines as effector molecules.

Figure 11-7 traces the development of early immunomodulators to cytokines. Original immunomodulators were generally crude whole-cell microbial preparations (such as *Bacillus Calmette-Guerin* [BCG] and *Corynebacterium parvum*) that were used because they could nonspecifically stimulate host immune responses. Later, the active components of these cells (such as endotoxin and zymosan) were identified and isolated from their cell walls. Further

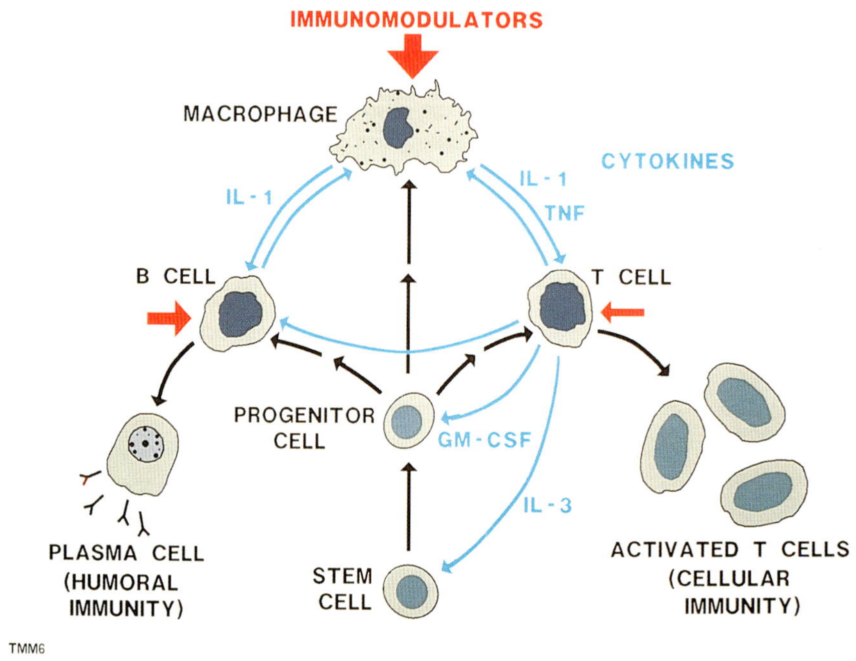

Fig. 11-6. Relationship of immunomodulators with host-produced mediators (cytokines), which regulate immunological and hematological functions

work led to the purification, identification, and synthesis of the specific portions of the cell fragments that were actually responsible for stimulating immune responses (such as lipid A from endotoxin and glucan from zymosan). Stimulation of cells by immunomodulators results in the release of cytokines, which act as specific stimulators of host immune responses. Recent advances have seen the development of biologically defined molecules and recombinantly produced cytokines (such as interleukin-1 [IL-1] and granulocyte-macrophage colony-stimulating factor [rGM-CSF]), which are relatively nontoxic but allow specific manipulation of various components of the immune and hematological systems.

Immunomodulators. Immunomodulators are generally nonspecific immunostimulants that function as external stimuli for a broad range of cell types in the hematopoietic system. To reduce radiation injury, the most effective compounds appear to be those that act primarily on the macrophage. Glucan and trehalose dimycolate (TDM) are two immunomodulators that are currently being evaluated as potential mitigating agents for radiation injury.

Glucan is a beta-1,3-linked polysaccharide isolated from the cell wall of the yeast *Saccharomyces cerevisiae*. This agent is a potent immune modulator that is capable of enhancing a variety of immunopoietic and hematopoietic responses.[15,66]

The effect of glucan on preventing infection and enhancing the regeneration of bone-marrow cells after irradiation is shown in Figure 11-8. In this experiment, mice were injected with either saline or glucan 24 hours before exposure to 9 Gy of cobalt-60 gamma radiation.[15] The number of saline-treated mice showing evidence of infection increased substantially at 7–15 days following irradiation, and no detectable marrow regeneration was evident. However, glucan was able to reduce infection signifi-

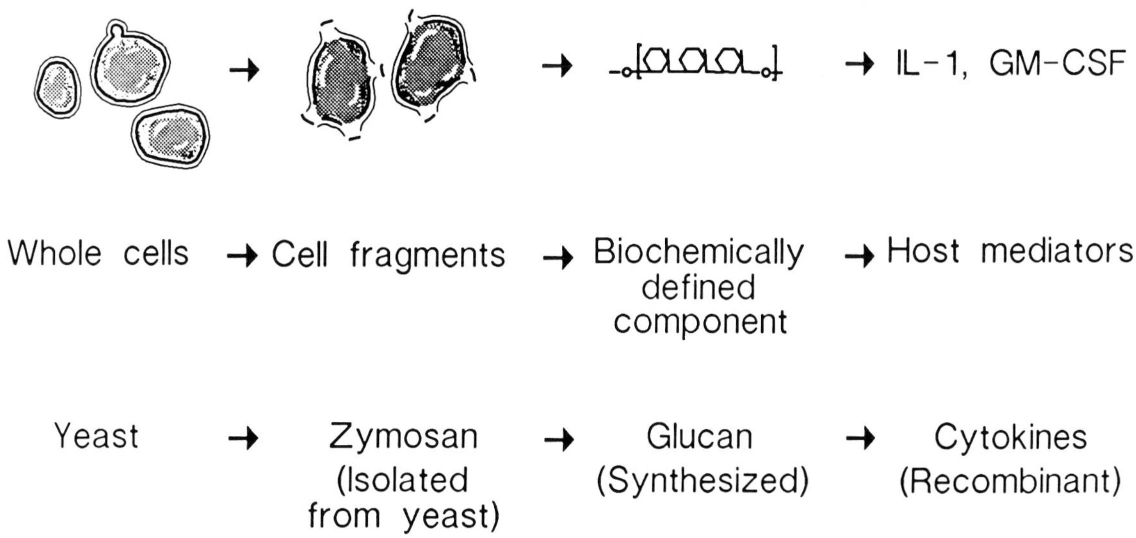

Fig. 11-7. Evolution of immunomodulators from crude cell preparations to biochemically defined molecules and host factors produced by recombinant DNA technology

cantly and to produce a substantial increase in marrow regeneration. A temporal relationship was seen between the two effects: the ability of glucan to control infection occurred well before its demonstrable effect on marrow regeneration. This suggests a dual role for glucan in enhancing postirradiation survival: *(a)* this compound can stimulate the remaining mature, relatively radioresistant macrophages to control infection, and *(b)* it can also induce the stimulation of stem and progenitor cells to proliferate and repopulate the marrow.

These data correlate with the ability of this compound to increase the survival of irradiated animals. Administered intravenously to mice 24 hours before 9 Gy of cobalt-60 gamma radiation, glucan increased the 30-day survival from 0% in the saline-injected control mice to 63% in the glucan-treated mice (DRF: 1.2).[67] In addition, glucan is capable of slightly enhancing survival (DRF: 1.08) in mice when it is administered 1 hour after an exposure to 9 Gy of cobalt-60 gamma radiation.[68]

Trehalose dimycolate (TDM), also known as cord factor, is a glycolipid consisting of 6,6'-diesters of the sugar D-trehalose. It is isolated from the cell walls of *Mycobacteria*, *Nocardia*, and *Corynebacteria*, and is an active component of Freund's complete adjuvant. Like glucan, TDM is a potent immunostimulant that is capable of increasing host defense mechanisms against a variety of organisms and of increasing survival after irradiation.[16,17]

Cytokines. Cytokines are hormone-like peptides that function as molecular signals between cells. They are synthesized and released primarily by macrophages and lymphocytes that have been stimulated by inflammatory agents or immunomodulators. Included in this class of compounds are the interleukins-1 through -6, tumor necrosis factor (TNF), a variety of hematopoietic growth factors (such as granulocyte-macrophage colony-stimulating factor, granulocyte colony-stimulating factor, and erythropoietin), and the alpha-, beta-, and gamma-interferons. All of these act in a variety of ways to stimulate proliferation, differentiation, or function of cells in the hematopoietic system. Several have been examined for their ability to mitigate radiation injury, and of these, IL-1 and TNF have been found to be the most effective.

IL-1 is released by activated macrophages. It has a number of local immune effects, including the activation of resting T cells and the stimulation of cytokine synthesis and release.[69]

Although a significant increase in survival (43% for treated versus 0% for control mice) is seen when IL-1 is given 4 hours before irradiation, optimum survival (greater than 80% versus 0% in controls) is obtained when IL-1 is administered intraperitoneally 20 hours before exposure to 9.5 Gy of cobalt-60 gamma radiation.[70] Using that regimen, DRFs of up

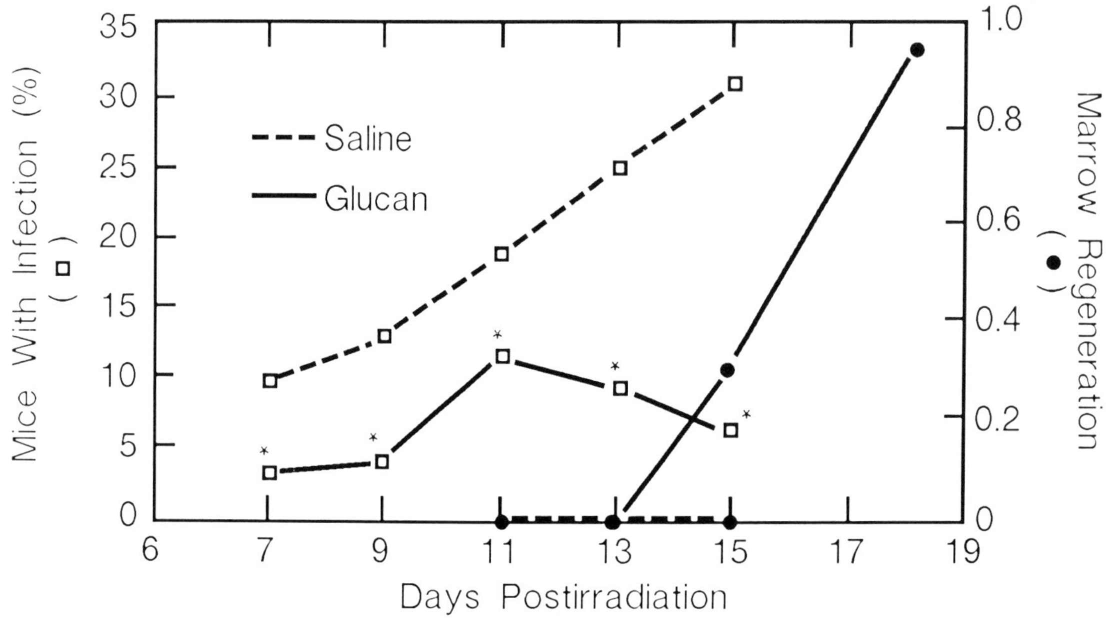

Fig. 11-8. Effect of glucan on enhancement of nonspecific resistance to infection and marrow hematopoiesis in mice exposed to 9 Gy of radiation

to 1.25 have been achieved with IL-1 in C57BL/6 mice. IL-1 is particularly attractive as a pharmacological means of mitigating radiation injury because only very small doses are required. The DRF of 1.25 was achieved with a dose of only 0.1 µg of IL-1 per mouse (approximately 0.004 mg/kg). The effectiveness of IL-1 in mice is strain dependent. While all strains of mice examined showed different degrees of increased survival, optimum survival was obtained with the C57BL/6 strain.[71]

TNF is also released by activated macrophages. It was named for its ability to act as a direct cytotoxin for some tumor cells. Like IL-1, it has several local immune effects, including the stimulation of cytokine synthesis and release.[69] Unlike IL-1, however, its effectiveness does not depend on the mouse strain. In most strains, TNF is less effective than is IL-1, and in others it is more effective due to the variability in effectiveness of IL-1. TNF is optimally effective (with DRFs of 1.08–1.16) when given intraperitoneally 20 hours before irradiation at a dose of 5–10 g per mouse (approximately 0.2 mg/kg).[72]

Two other cytokines may be potentially useful agents: GM-CSF and interleukin-3 (IL-3). Several growth factors that are specific for different hematological cell populations have been discovered and can be produced by recombinant DNA methodologies. One of these, a specific human recombinant GM-CSF (rGM-CSF), accelerates marrow repair or engraftment and may contribute to increased nonspecific resistance. It functions by increasing the number of circulating granulocytes and platelets in normal animals and accelerating the recovery of these cells after irradiation. This factor was used in treating some victims of the radiation exposure accident in Brazil.

The effectiveness of this factor in ameliorating radiation-induced cytopenia can be seen from data obtained in the minimal-shielding experiment.[64] In that experiment, the survival of partially shielded monkeys that were given supportive therapy was enhanced. Unshielded animals rapidly became neutropenic and died within 15 days. In the shielded animals that survived beyond 30 days, peripheral granulocytes began to recover slowly between days 20 and 40. In contrast, shielded animals treated with a growth factor showed evidence of granulocyte recovery well before day 20, and granulocyte levels quickly reached supranormal levels. Therefore, it appears that this factor is a useful adjunct to radiation-injury therapy. However, its effectiveness as a regeneration agent in radioprotective regimens is much lower than that for IL-1 and TNF when it is given alone in the protocols described above for those cytokines.[70] In spite of that, evidence suggests that it may act synergistically when combined with other cytokines.[72]

IL-3 has not yet been evaluated for its ability to increase survival after irradiation. Unlike the described action of the cytokines (whose major target cells are primarily the more mature functional cells in the system), IL-3 is reported to act specifically in stimulating the growth of pluripotent stem cells.[69] Because hematopoietic stem cells are among the most radiosensitive in the body, this cytokine may be particularly effective as a regenerating agent.

COMBINATION AGENTS

Rationale

Agents that function in the three strategies (protection, repair, and regeneration) contribute in different ways to the mitigation of radiation injury. Each of the three strategies also has its limitations. Neither chemical nor enzymatic means of protection are able to minimize direct damage. In addition, it is almost impossible for any protective or repair agent either to completely eliminate all of the reactive intermediates formed or to repair all of the damaged molecules. Regardless of the efficiency of scavengers and repair agents and their concentration within the cell at the time of irradiation, some molecular damage and cell death will occur. The effectiveness of agents that function in the regeneration strategy is limited because the agents require a pool of surviving functional cells on which to work. That pool of highly radiosensitive hematopoietic stem cells becomes depleted after fairly low radiation doses.

It is reasonable to expect that optimal survival would be provided by an agent or combination of agents that would operate within two or more of these strategies. Such a formulation would maximize the effectiveness of each strategy and minimize its limitations. Protective and repair agents reduce the concentration of reactive species that are produced from the radiolysis of water and also repair the damage to critical target molecules. In so doing, the agents increase the surviving fraction of stem cells, progenitor cells, and mature cells of the hematopoietic system after irradiation. By allowing stem cells to survive higher radiation doses, the net effect is to increase the threshold radiation dose that limits the effectiveness of regeneration agents. Regeneration agents further enhance the organism's survival by capitalizing on the advantages provided by protective and repair agents; that is, they maximize the proliferation and function of the extra cells provided.

It would be difficult to produce one drug that would be able to mitigate radiation injury by all three strategies. Two or more agents might be used either together or at intervals, but this is not desirable. The simplest dosing regimen (single dose) is the most desirable for military personnel under battlefield conditions. Therefore, the goal is a single treatment consisting of a combination of two or more agents that function in *(a)* either the protection or repair strategy, and *(b)* the regeneration strategy.

Examples of Combination Agents

The concept of using combinations of agents that function by different mechanisms to achieve protection was developed and studied in the 1950s and 1960s.[3] In many of the combinations examined, synergistic effects were seen. These results are particularly significant because increased protection with the combinations was often achieved using substantially lower doses of individual drugs than those required for protection when each agent was given alone. For example, one study examined various combinations of five different radioprotective agents: cysteine, beta-mercaptoethylamine (MEA), aminoethylisothiouronium (AET), glutathione, and serotonin.[73] AET, MEA, or serotonin used alone provided similar protection (DRF: 1.7), cysteine was less effective (DRF: 1.12), and glutathione was marginally protective (DRF: 1.05). The most effective regimen was a combination of all five agents, which produced a DRF of 2.8. In this combination, the doses were two-thirds that of the AET and one-half that of the MEA used when the drugs were given individually.

More recently, additive and synergistic effects were demonstrated with various combinations of aminothiols, antioxidant vitamins and minerals, immunomodulators, and cytokines. It is likely that a first-generation agent will be a combination of subtoxic doses of two or more of these agents. The effectiveness of several combinations is shown in Table 11-6.

TABLE 11-6

EFFECTIVENESS OF PHARMACOLOGICAL AGENT COMBINATIONS*

Agents and Agent Combinations			Dose Reduction Factor (DRF)**					
A	B	C	A	B	C	A+B	A+B+C	References
IL-1***	TNF***	—	1.19	1.12	—	1.38	—	64
Glucan P†	WR 2721†	Selenium†	1.22	1.33	1.01	1.51	1.64	67
Glucan F††	WR 2721††	—	1.07	1.32	—	1.53	—	68
Selenium‡	WR 2721‡	—	1.10	2.20	—	2.50	—	54
DiPGE$_2$¥	WR 2721¥	—	1.40	1.90	—	2.20	—	70

*Data obtained using mice exposed to gamma radiation from a cobalt-60 source

**DRF calculated as a ratio between radiation-treated group ($LD_{50/30}$) and radiation control group ($LD_{50/30}$)

***IL-1 (150 ng/mouse) and TNF (5 µg/mouse) injected i.p., 20 hours after irradiation

†Glucan P (particulate) injected i.v., 75 mg/kg, 20 hours before irradiation
WR-2721 (200 mg/kg) injected i.p., 30 minutes before irradiation
Selenium (0.8 mg/kg) injected i.p., 20 hours before irradiation

††Glucan F (soluble) injected i.v., 250 mg/kg, 1 hour after irradiation
WR-2721 (200 mg/kg) injected i.p., 30 minutes before irradiation

‡Selenium (1.6 mg/kg) injected i.p., 24 hours before irradiation
WR-2721 (400 mg/kg) injected i.p., 30 minutes before irradiation

¥DiPGE$_2$ (0.4 mg/kg) injected s.c., 15 minutes before irradiation
WR-2721 (200 mg/kg) injected i.p., 15 minutes before irradiation

Mitigation of Performance Decrement

Because a single, self-administrable agent is sought as a radioprotectant, it might also be necessary to include moderators of performance decrements in any regimen that is developed. While measures to enhance resistance to the lethal effects of radiation have been extensively studied, relatively little attention has been given to the application of pharmacological interventions to mitigate performance and behavioral deficiencies, even though these are of immediate military concern. Although it is possible for radioprotective agents to prevent some performance decrements, drugs that increase survival generally have not enhanced performance. In fact, except for a few notable exceptions, they usually exacerbate radiation-induced performance decrements.[43,44] Groups of drugs are being developed that will, perhaps, stabilize performance by modulating cellular permeability, altering regional blood flow, and interrupting the release or action of various mediators. Drugs are being identified that can modulate postirradiation emesis, ETI, and other performance decrements.

Radioprotectants and Supportive Therapy

Radioprotectants will be most effective in personnel exposed to radiation doses within the ranges re-

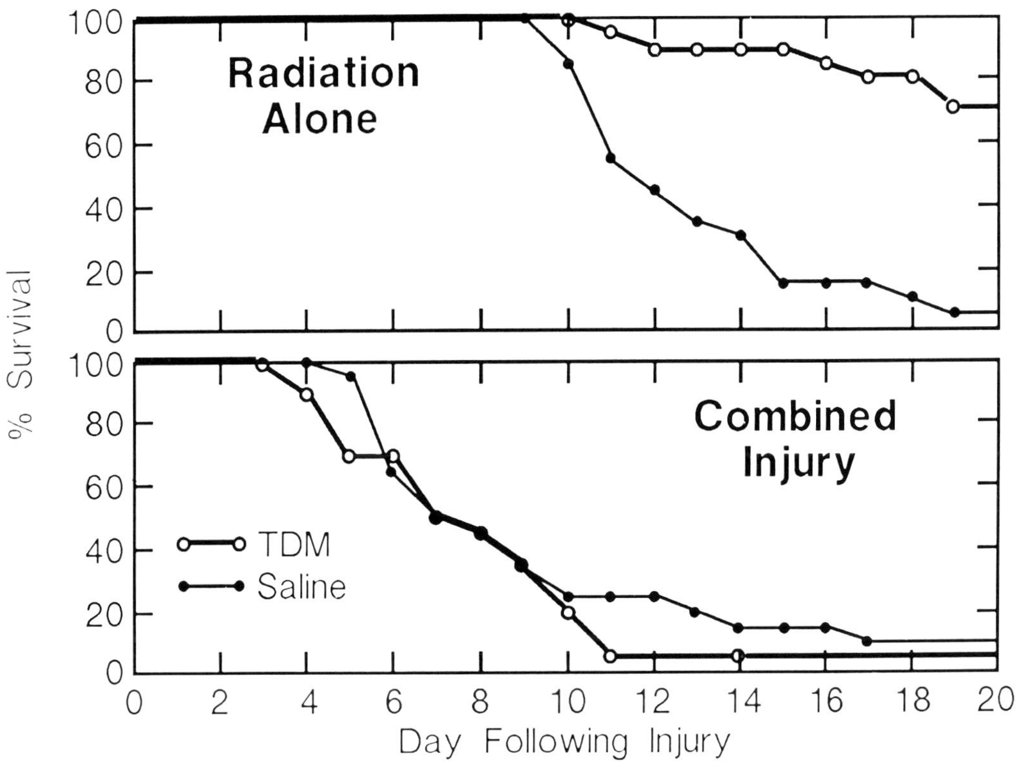

Fig. 11-9. Comparative effects of trehalose dimycolate (TDM) on enhancement of survival in mice receiving either radiation alone or radiation and a 30% body-surface-area wound (combined injury)

quired to produce the hematopoietic subsyndrome (approximately 2.0–8.0 Gy) and mild gastrointestinal subsyndrome (approximately 8.0–10.0 Gy), and in whom no associated injuries are present. In the event of more severe radiation injury, or if radiation injury is combined with traumatic or burn injuries (a likely occurrence on the battlefield), then radioprotective measures alone will be insufficient, and additional supportive therapy will be required. Although the effectiveness of radioprotectants may be reduced in the face of more severe radiation injury or combined injury, their use at the time of irradiation will likely increase the effectiveness of supportive therapies provided days later.

Traumatic injury can reduce the ability of pharmacological agents to increase survival (Figure 11-9).[16] Mice that were given TDM dissolved in squalene within 2 hours after exposure to 10.25 Gy of cobalt-60 gamma radiation were protected against the infectious consequences of this exposure (70% survival versus 5% in vehicle-injected control animals). However, this protection was not seen in animals given a 1.0-by-1.5 inch skin wound and irradiated with only 8.5 Gy. In the irradiated and wounded mice, death began to occur about 1 week earlier than in the irradiated-only animals, and all mice died at the same rate regardless of treatment with TDM.

This difference in protective response between irradiated-only and combined-injury animals may be due to a more profound immunosuppression (Figure 11-10) and/or physiological perturbations. To avoid infection, the natural and artificial defenses must be in balance so that host resistance is sufficient to control the number of microorganisms. Therefore, as normal defenses are compromised (suppression), artificial interventions (enhancement) are required to maintain the resistance above the threshold for infection.

The potential synergy between therapeutic agents, such as antibiotics, and substances that may be used as radioprotectants is indicated by recent

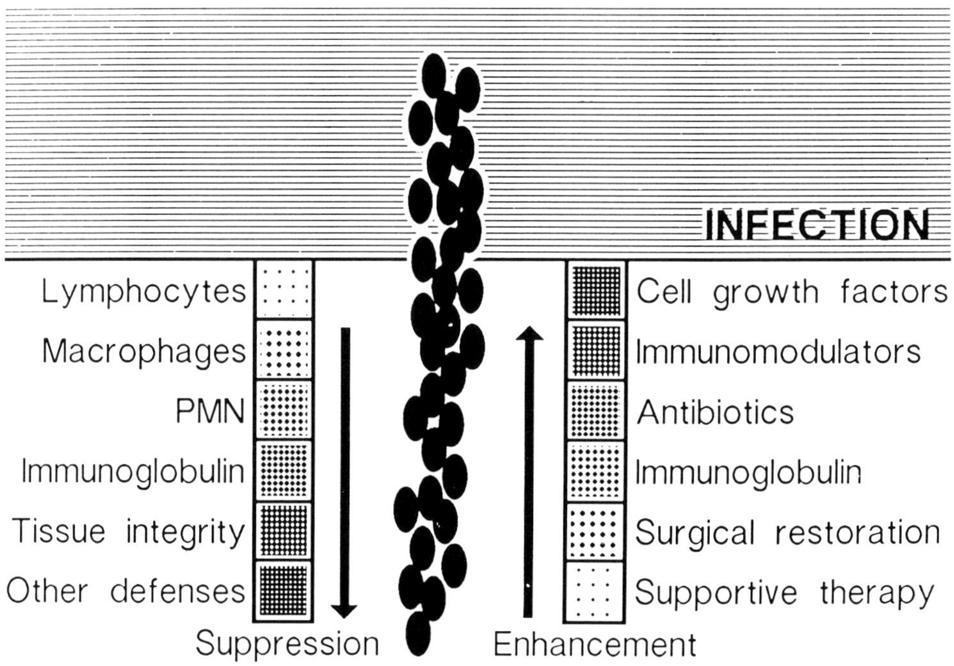

Fig. 11-10. Suppression of resistance to infection when normal defenses are lost. Various interventions to enhance resistance may be used in combination to prevent infection in severely injured subjects.

data on the use of glucan and the antibiotic pefloxacin in the management of postirradiation mortality.[74] In this experiment, only 30% of mice given 7.9 Gy of whole-body cobalt-60 gamma radiation survived. Treatment with glucan alone at 1 hour after irradiation, or incorporation of pefloxacin in the animal's drinking water for 24 days after exposure, had little or no effect on survival. However, if the two treatments were combined, survival was greater than 90%.

DEVELOPMENT OF A RADIOPROTECTIVE REGIMEN

A variety of factors must be considered in evaluating and developing candidate radioprotectant drugs for military use, and a compromise must be reached between the ideal and the achievable (Table 11-7).

Level of Protection

The problem of defining a suitable minimum level of effectiveness in promoting survival is still not fully resolved. For many years, the goal was that pharmacological agents should have a DRF of at least 2 against exposure to gamma radiation. This goal may have caused promising drugs with lower DRFs to be overlooked. Protection at a DRF greater than 2 is achievable in the laboratory, but the required doses produce side effects that are unacceptable in type and severity for military use.

Although it may not be possible to field a first-generation drug with a DRF of 2, it is likely that one can be developed with a DRF of less than 2. A reasonably achievable lower limit would be a DRF of about 1.4. Although this level of mitigation is generally considered to be low to moderate, it is far from trivial. First, because the animals used in research are immunologically naive, a laboratory-derived DRF of 1.4 is likely to underestimate the degree of protection actually realized in the field by normal, healthy persons. Second, as discussed previously, it is likely that many cases of accidental exposure will be accompanied by some degree of partial shielding. In light of evidence that even small amounts of partial shielding are beneficial, shielding should augment the effectiveness of pharmacological agents. Third, the difference between a dose of radiation that is lethal to 95% of a population (LD_{95}) and a dose lethal to 5% (LD_5) is commonly less than 1.0–2.0 Gy. Therefore, the use of an agent with a DRF of 1.4 for most species (including humans) can result in a reduction of the LD_{95} to a value near the LD_5. For persons exposed to doses greater than those resulting in LD_{95}, the use of an agent with a DRF of 1.4 may mean the difference between life and death, especially if even minimal postirradiation therapy is available. Over a large population, the net effect is a substantial increase in survival. It is possible that this level of protection might be achieved with minimal side effects.

Toxicity

Side effects are a major obstacle to the fielding of agents to mitigate radiation injury. Acute side effects (such as nausea, vomiting, and hypotension) are common, especially with the sulfur compounds. For a fieldable drug, any acute side effects will have to be reduced in severity so that military performance is not impaired. If that is not possible, these effects should be at least controllable by other conveniently applied therapies.

In addition, these agents must not significantly increase the user's vulnerability to chemical or biological agents or antidotes, exacerbate other battlefield injuries, negatively affect behavior, or interfere significantly with wound healing. The agent should have a wide safety margin (therapeutic index) to compensate for the "if one is good, then two must be better" philosophy.

Deliverability

A prime requirement for an agent that will be used by many people under battlefield conditions is that it be easily self-administered. The route of administration, drug dose, and simplicity of schedule are important. Oral administration is the most desirable route, but this may be difficult to achieve, at least for a first-generation agent. Transdermal administration (for example, via a dermal patch) is also acceptable, but is limited by the fact that only microgram or smaller quantities of the drug can be delivered. Most of the agents under study are effective in milligram to gram quantities. The major exceptions are the cytokines, which are effective in very small dosages, and may be administrable by the transdermal route. The transdermal route may have greater applicability for second- and third-generation agents

TABLE 11-7

PHARMACOLOGICAL REQUIREMENTS

Administration
Repeated administration
Easily self-administered
Order of preference:
Oral > transdermal >sublingual > intramuscular
Biological Action of Drug
Adequate duration of effect
Compatible with other drugs
Chemical Characteristics
High chemical stability (long shelf-life)
Dose
DRF > 1.4 (30-day lethality, gamma radiation)
Single-dose regimen
Manageable dose quantities (weight or volume)
Pharmacological Side Effects
No chronic toxicity
Minimal behavioral toxicity
Minimal or controllable acute side effects
Minimal increased vulnerability to chemical or biological agents
Minimal effect on wound healing
Wide safety margin

developed via the genetic approaches described above. The next most acceptable route of administration is sublingual. The least acceptable practical method is intramuscular injection. Intravenous and subcutaneous injection and suppository administration are unacceptable routes for a self-administered field-deployed drug.

For oral, sublingual, or intramuscular administration, the drug dose must be small enough to be dispensed as a reasonably sized tablet or capsule, or in a manageable volume. If taken as a liquid, either orally or parenterally, the agent must also be soluble and stable in a vehicle that is appropriate for administration. Finally, for simplicity of use in the field, the agent should be designed as a single treatment, rather than a regimen of two or more different and sequentially spaced medications.

Other Factors

Ease of administration, simplicity of dose schedule, minimal side effects, and a wide safety margin are particularly important because it may be necessary to take a radioprotective drug repeatedly for several days. The agent should be compatible with the other drugs and antidotes available to the soldier in the field, and it should have optimum effectiveness for an adequate duration (up to 6 hours following a single administration). Two hours of effectiveness should be considered the minimum. Finally, the agent should be formulated and packaged so that it has a shelf life of at least 5 years, to allow stockpiling. It should retain its potency under a wide variety of adverse conditions and, for an injectable, should not deteriorate in solution.

SUMMARY

Historically, the development of radioprotective agents has been dominated by the study of sulfhydryl compounds, particularly the aminothiols. These compounds function by a variety of mechanisms, almost all of which increase survival in the irradiated organism by minimizing the radiation-induced damage to critical biological molecules. The ability of aminothiols to provide high levels of protection has been demonstrated repeatedly. However, as a group, these compounds suffer from one major drawback: high levels of protection have been achieved only at doses that are accompanied by unacceptable side effects. Therefore, it has been necessary to look at less-toxic compounds in the search for a radioprotective agent.

Among the candidates being evaluated are naturally occurring dietary components (selenium and vitamins E and A) and drugs of low toxicity that are being used clinically (such as MPG). The drawback to these latter agents is that, generally, the protection achieved is relatively low.

The net effect of protective compounds, such as the aminothiols and dietary components, is an increase in the number of stem cells and progenitor cells that survive the initial radiation insult. To exploit this early benefit, agents that stimulate the proliferation and differentiation of those cells would help effect optimum repopulation of the organ systems that were depleted by radiation-induced cell death. The use of such regeneration agents (such as immunomodulators and cytokines) alone has been shown to enhance survival after irradiation, although the effect is relatively low. But when these agents are administered along with a protective agent, additive and synergistic effects are seen. Most important, these effects are often achieved using subtoxic doses of the individual agents.

Combining those agents that function in the protection or repair strategy with those that function in the regeneration strategy offers the advantages of *(a)* circumventing the side effects of aminothiols, *(b)* enhancing the effectiveness of relatively nontoxic agents that provide only mild protection when given alone, and *(c)* maximizing the therapeutic benefit provided by each agent.

The use of pharmacological agents to increase survival after irradiation will be most effective for personnel exposed to low or intermediate doses of radiation who have minimal associated traumatic or burn injuries. Indeed, in a mass-casualty situation, these agents may be the only type of medical intervention that is available. On the other hand, with smaller numbers of casualties, especially those with combined injuries, it is likely that additional supportive therapies will be available. When considered in this context, radioprotection should be thought of as part of the holistic management of radiation injury (Figure 11-11) Here, in the face of increasing injuries, various dose-reducing events occur to minimize the effect of the injury. The early application of radioprotector agents will minimize the need for subsequent interventions and will enhance the effectiveness of the interventions that are provided.

Many factors must be considered in defining the desired properties of a potentially fieldable first-generation agent. Since the development of WR-2721,

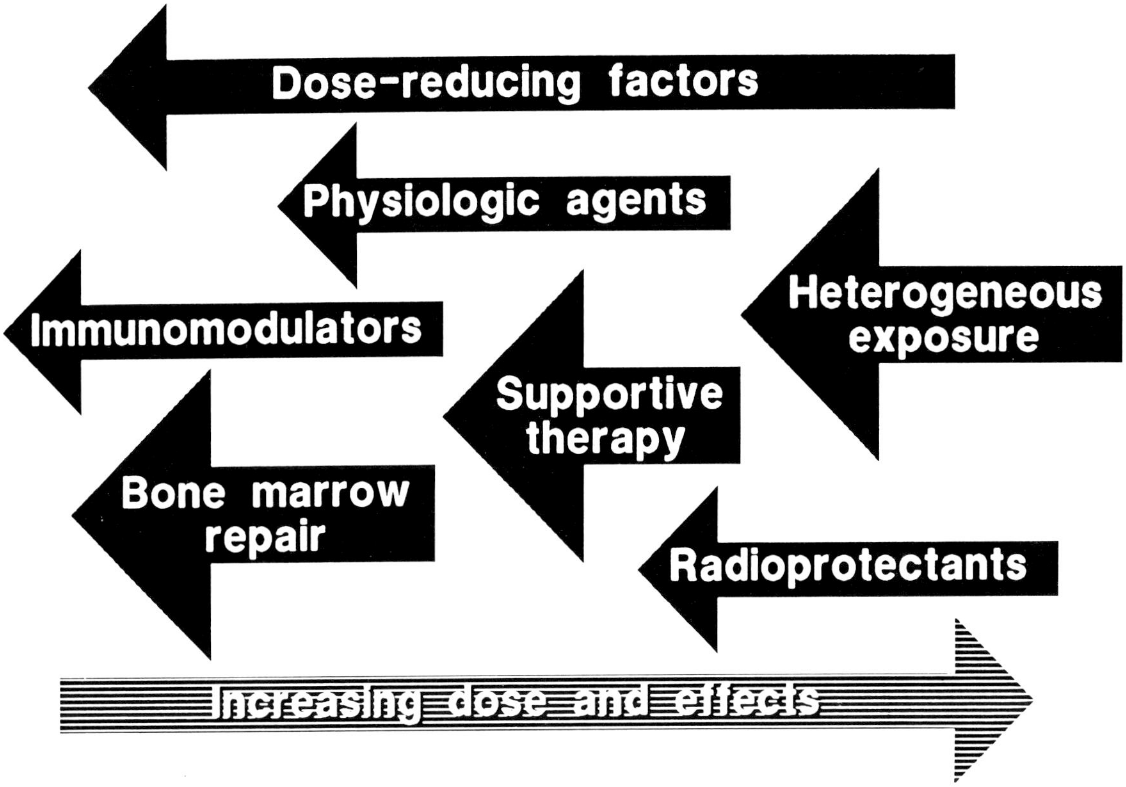

Fig. 11-11. A variety of factors can act together to reduce lethality of increasing radiation doses

emphasis has been placed on studying agents that produce DRFs greater than 2. This emphasis may actually have hampered efforts to field a suitable agent. Some agents with lower DRFs can provide significant protection and may be more appropriate for field use. Thus, the DRF used in evaluating a radioprotective drug need not be the maximum obtainable. Rather, the DRF should be that obtainable at doses resulting in minimal acute side effects and behavioral toxicity. The agent should also have a high therapeutic index, because it will most likely be self-administered. Whether or not the agent can be taken orally is an important consideration.

Based on the strategies and candidate agents now available, it should soon be possible to recommend several protective agents that sufficiently meet the requirements. After an agent has been recommended, it will be evaluated as a first-generation field-usable radioprotective drug (or drug combination) in humans. The agent should have a DRF greater than or equal to 1.4 and be effective when given as a single oral or intramuscular dose. The agent will probably be a combination of at least two of the candidate agents described above. Regardless of the number of candidates in this combination, it is likely that at least one will be a protective agent and one will be a regeneration agent.

Fielding a first-generation agent that satisfies most of the requirements discussed above is an achievable near-term goal that will satisfy, at least in part, a critical immediate need of the armed forces. Success will depend on making intelligent choices from the many available agents.

However, it is critical to note that fielding this first-generation agent is only an initial step. Much work needs to be done to develop an agent that is effective against high-LET radiation. This need will become increasingly urgent as the human presence in space expands. Second- and third-generation agents will be developed only through intense studies that are aimed at defining the mechanisms of radiation injury on the molecular and cellular levels and determining how organisms can be stimulated to protect themselves against this injury.

REFERENCES

1. Patt, H. M.; Tyree, E. B.; Straube, R. L.; and Smith, D. E. 1949. Cysteine protection against X-irradiation. *Science* 110: 213-214.

2. Chapman, W. H.; Cipte, C. R.: Elizholtz, D. C.; Cronkite, E. P.; and Chambers, F. W., Jr. 1949. *Sulfhydryl-containing agents and the effects of ionizing radiations. I. Beneficial effect of glutathione injection on X-ray induced mortality rate and weight loss in mice* [Naval Medical Research Institute Project NM006012.08.25]. Bethesda, MD: Naval Medical Research Institute.

3. Giambarresi, L., and Jacobs, A. A. 1987. Radioprotectants. In *Military Radiobiology,* edited by J. J. Conklin and R. I. Walker, 265-301. Orlando, FL: Academic Press, Inc.

4. Alper, T. 1979. *Cellular radiobiology.* London and New York: Cambridge University Press.

5. Fabrikant, J. I. 1972. *Radiobiology.* Chicago: Year Book Medical Publications, Inc.

6. Carr, C. J.; Huff, J. E.; Fisher, K. D.; and Huber, T. E. 1970. Protective agents modifying biological effects of radiation. *Arch. Environ. Health* 21: 88-98.

7. Yuhas, J. M.; Proctor, J. O.; and Smith, L. H. 1973. Some pharmacologic effects of WR-2721: Their role in toxicity and radioprotection. *Radiat. Res.* 54: 222-233.

8. Sugahara, T. 1974. 2-Mercaptopropionylglycine (MPG) and the recent development of chemical radioprotection. In *Proceedings of the Second International Symposium on Thiola,* 17-22. Osaka: Santen Pharmaceutical Co., Ltd.

9. Ayene, S. I., and Srivastava, P. N. 1985. Radioprotective effect of 2- mercaptopropionylglycine on radiation-induced microsomal lipid peroxidation. *Int. J. Radiat. Biol.* 48: 197-205.

10. Foye, W. O. 1969. Radiation-protective agents in mammals. *J. Pharm. Sci.* 58: 283-300.

11. Kim, S. E., and Moos, W. S. 1967. Radiation protection by topical DMSO application. *Health Phys.* 13: 601-606.

12. Bacq, Z. M. 1965. *Chemical protection against ionizing radiation.* Springfield, IL: Charles C. Thomas.

13. van der Meer, C.; Brocades Zaalberg, O.; Vos, O.; Vergroesen, A. J.; and van Bekkum, D. W. 1961. On the mechanism of the radioprotective action of cyanide. *Int. J. Rad. Biol.* 4: 311-319.

14. Thomson, J. F. 1962. *Radiation protection in mammals.* New York: Reinhold Publishing Corporation.

15. Patchen, M. L.; D'Alesandro, M. M.; Brook, I.; Blakely, W. F.; and MacVittie, T. J. 1987. Glucan: Mechanisms involved in its radioprotective effect. *J. Leukocyte Biol.* 42: 95-105.

16. Madonna, G. S.; Ledney, G. D.; Elliott, T. B.; Brook, I.; Ulrich, J. T.; Myers, K. R.; Patchen, M. L.; and Walker, R. I. Trehalose dimycolate enhances resistance to infection in neutropenic animals. *Infect. Imm.,* in press.

17. Madonna, G. S.; Ledney, G. D.; Funckes, D. C.; and Ribi, E. E. 1988. Monophosphoryl lipid A and trehalose dimycolate therapy enhances survival in sublethally irradiated mice challenged with *Klebsiella pneumoniae.* In *Immunomodulators and Nonspecific Host Defence Mechanisms against Microbial Infections,* edited by K. N. Masihi and W. Lange, 351-356. Oxford: Pergamon Press.

18. Ainsworth, E. J.; Larsen, R. M.; Mitchell, F. A.; and Taylor, J. F. 1970. Survival-promoting effects of endotoxin in mice, dogs, and sheep. In *Radiation Protection and Sensitization,* edited by H. L. Moroson and M. Quintiliani, 381-388. London: Taylor and Francis.

19. Bertok, L. 1980. Radio-detoxified endotoxin as a potent stimulator of nonspecific resistance. *Perspect. Biol. Med.* 24: 61-66.

20. Snyder, S. L.; Walker, R. I.; MacVittie, T. J.; and Sheil, J. M. 1978. Biologic properties of bacterial lipopolysaccharides treated with chromium chloride. *Can. J. Microbiol.* 24: 495-501.

21. Neta, R. 1988. Role of cytokines in radioprotection. *Pharmacol. Ther.* 39: 261-266.

22. Jacobs, A. J.; Rankin, W. A.; Srinivasan, V.; and Weiss, J. F. 1983. Effects of vitamin E and selenium on glutathione peroxidase activity and survival of irradiated mice. In *Proceedings of the 7th International Congress of Radiation Research,* edited by J. J. Broerse, G. W. Barendsen, H. B. Kal and A. J. van der Kogel, D5-D15. Amsterdam: Martinus Nijhoff Publishers.

23. Srinivasan, V.; Jacobs, A. J.; Simpson, S. A.; and Weiss, J. F. 1983. Radioprotection by vitamin E: Effects on hepatic enzymes, delayed type hypersensitivity, and postirradiation survival of mice. In *Modulation and Mediation of Cancer by Vitamins,* 119-131. Basel: Karger.

24. Seifter, E.; Rettura, G.; Padawar, J.; Stratford, F.; Weinzweig J.; Demetriou, A. A.; and Levenson, S. M. 1984. Morbidity and mortality reduction by supplemental vitamin A or beta-carotene in CBA mice given total-body-radiation. *JNCI* 73: 1167-1177.

25. Petkau, A. 1978. Radiation protection by superoxide dismutase. *Photochem. Photobiol.* 28: 765-774.

26. Walden, T. L., Jr. 1987. Enhanced radiation survival in mice receiving a combined pretreatment of 16,16 dimethyl prostaglandin E_2 and WR-2721. *Abstracts of Papers for 35th Annual Meeting of Radiation Research Society,* 120. Atlanta: Radiation Research Society.

27. Walden, T. L., Jr.; Patchen, M.; and Snyder, S. L. 1987. 16,16-Dimethyl prostaglandin E_2 increases survival in mice following irradiation. *Radiat. Res.* 109: 440-448.

28. Chapman, J. D., and Reuvers, A. P. 1977. The time-scale of radioprotection in mammalian cells. *Experientia* (Suppl.) 27: 9-18.

29. Singh, A., and Singh, H. 1982. Time-scale and nature of radiation-biological damage: Approaches to radiation protection and post-irradiation therapy. *Prog. Biophys. Mol. Biol.* 39: 69-107.

30. Holahan, E. V. Cellular radiobiology. In reference 3, 87-110.

31. Greenstock, C. L. 1981. Redox processes in radiation biology and cancer. *Radiat. Res.* 86: 196-211.

32. Pizzarello, D. J., and Colombetti, L. G., eds. 1982. *Radiation biology.* Boca Raton, FL: CRC Press.

33. Copeland, E. S. 1978. Mechanisms of radioprotection—a review. *Photochem. Photobiol.* 28: 839-844.

34. Davidson, D. E.; Grenan, M. M.; and Sweeney, T. R. 1980. Biological characteristics of some improved radioprotectors. In *Radiation Sensitizers: Their Use in the Clinical Management of Cancer,* edited by L. W. Brady, 309-320. New York: Masson.

35. Piper, J. R.; Stringfellow, C. R., Jr.; Elliot, R. D.; and Johnston, T. P. 1969. S-2-(omega-aminoalkylamino)ethyl dihydrogen phosphorothioates and related compounds as potential antiradiation agents. *J. Med. Chem.* 12: 236-243.

36. Yuhas, J. M. 1970. Biological factors affecting the radioprotective efficiency of S-2-(3-aminopropylamino)ethylphosphorothioic acid (WR-2721): $LD_{50(30)}$ doses. *Radiat. Res.* 44: 621-628.

37. Yuhas, J. M., and Storer, J. B. 1969. Differential chemoprotection of normal and malignant tissues. *JNCI* 42: 331-335.

38. Glover, D. J.; Glick, J. H.; Weiler, C.; Hurowitz, S.; and Kligerman, M. 1986. WR-2721 protects against the hematologic toxicity of cyclophosphamide: A controlled phase II trial. *J. Clin. Oncol.* 4: 584-588.

39. Glover, D. J.; Glick, J. H.; Weiler, C.; Fox, K.; and DuPont, G. 1987. WR-2721 and high dose cisplatin: An active combination in the treatment of metastatic melanoma. *J. Clin. Oncol.* 5: 574-578.

40. Glover, D.; Riley, L.; Carmichael, K.; Spar, B.; Glick, J.; Kligerman, M. M.; Agus, Z. S.; Slatopolsky, E.; Attie, M.; and Goldfarb, S. 1983. Hypocalcemia and inhibition of parathyroid hormone secretion after administration of WR-2721 (a radioprotective and chemoprotective agent). *N. Eng. J. Med.* 309: 1137-1141.

41. Phillips, T. L. Rationale for initial clinical trials and future development of radioprotectors. In reference 33, 321-329.

42. Turrisi, A. T.; Glover, D. J.; Hurwitz, S.; Glick, J.; Norfleet, A. L.; Weiler, C.; Yuhas, J. M.; and Kligerman, M. M. 1986. Final report of the Phase I trial of single-dose WR-2721 [S-2-(3-aminopropylamino)ethylphosphorothioic acid]. *Cancer Treat. Rep.* 70: 1389-1393.

43. Bogo, V.; Jacobs, A. J.; and Weiss, J. F. 1985. Behavioral toxicity and efficacy of WR-2721 as a radioprotectant. *Radiat. Res.* 104: 182-190.

44. Landauer, M. R.; Hirsch, D. D.; Dominitz, J. A.; and Weiss, J. F. 1987. Dose and time relationships of the radioprotector WR-2721 on locomotor activity in mice. *Pharmacol. Biochem. Behav.* 27: 573-576.

45. Fleckenstein, L.; Swynnerton, N.; Ludden, T. M.; and Mangold, D. Bioavailability and newer methods of delivery of phosphorothioate radioprotectors. *Pharmacol. Ther.,* in press.

46. Dubois, A.; Gueta, O.; LaPorte, J. L.; and Conklin, J. J. 1986. Relation between gastric emptying and gastric motility in primates. *Gastroenterology* 91: 1051A.

47. Katzung, B. G. 1984. *Basic and clinical pharmacology.* 2nd ed. Los Altos, CA: Lange Medical Publications.

48. Turbyfill, C. L.; Roudon, R. M.; Young, R. W.; and Kieffer, V. A. 1972. *Alteration of radiation effects by 2-(n-decylamino) ethanethiosulfuric acid (WR1607) in the monkey* [Scientific Report SR72-3]. Bethesda, MD: Armed Forces Radiobiology Research Institute.

49. Sharp, J. C.; Kelly, D. D.; and Brady, J. V. 1968. The radio-attenuating effects of n-decylaminoethanethiosulfuric acid in the rhesus monkey. In *Use of Nonhuman Primates in Drug Evaluation,* edited by H. Vagtborg, 338-346. Austin and London: University of Texas Press.

50. Santen Pharmaceutical Co., Ltd. 1974. *Proceedings of the Second International Symposium on Thiola.* Osaka: Santen Pharmaceutical Co., Ltd.

51. Sztanyik, L. B., and Santha, A. 1976. Synergistic effect of radioprotective substances having different mechanisms of action. In *Modification of Radiosensitivity of Biological Systems, Proceedings of Advisory Group,* 47-59. Vienna: International Atomic Energy Agency.

52. Sugahara, T., and Srivastava, P. N. MPG (2-mercaptopropionylglycine): A review on its protective action against ionizing radiations. In reference 50, 77-87.

53. Freeman, B. A., and Crapo, J. D. 1982. Biology of disease: Free radicals and tissue injury. *Lab. Invest.* 47: 412-426.

54. Seifter, E.; Mendecki, J.; Holtzman, S.; Kanofsky, J. D.; Friedenthal, E.; Davis, L.; and Weinzweig, J. 1988. Role of Vitamin A and beta-carotene in radiation protection: Relation to antioxidant properties. *Pharmacol. Ther.* 39: 357-365.

55. Fusi, S.; Kupper, T. S.; Green, D. G.; and Ariyan, S. 1984. Reversal of postburn immunosuppression by the administration of vitamin A. *Surgery* 96: 330-335.

56. Weiss, J. F.; Hoover, R. L.; and Kumar, K. S. 1987. Selenium pretreatment enhances the radioprotective effect and reduces the lethal toxicity of WR-2721. *Free Rad. Res. Comms.* 3: 33-38.

57. Walden, T. L., Jr.; Patchen, M. L.; and MacVittie, T. J. 1988. Leukotriene-induced radioprotection of hematopoietic stem cells in mice. *Radiat. Res.* 113: 388-395.

58. Walden, T. L., Jr. Personal communication.

59. Hughes, H. Personal communication.

60. Serianni, R. W., and Bruce, A. K. 1968. Role of sulphur in radioprotective extracts of *Micrococcus radiodurans*. *Nature* 218: 485-487.

61. Alexander, P. 1961. Mouse lymphoma cells with different radiosensitivities. *Nature* 192: 572-573.

62. Beer, J. Z.; Budzicka, E.; Niepokojczycka, E.; Rosiek, O.; Szumiel, I.; and Walicka, M. 1983. Loss of tumorigenicity with simultaneous changes in radiosensitivity and photosensitivity during *in vitro* growth of L5178Y murine lymphoma cells. *Cancer Res.* 43: 4736-4742.

63. Wlodek, D., and Hittelman, W. N. 1987. The repair of double-strand breaks correlates with radiosensitivity of L5178Y-S and L5178Y-R cells. *Radiat. Res.* 112: 146-155.

64. Monroy, R. L.; Skelley, R. R.; Taylor, P.; Dubois, A.; Donahue, R. E.; and MacVittie, T. J. 1988. Recovery from severe hematopoietic suppression using recombinant human granulocyte macrophage colony stimulating factor. *Expt. Hematology* 16: 344-348.

65. Cohen, S.; Pick, E.; and Oppenheim, J. J., eds. 1979. *Biology of the lymphokines.* New York: Academic Press.

66. Patchen M. L. 1983. Immunomodulators and hemopoiesis. *Surv. Immunol. Res.* 2: 237-242.

67. Patchen, M. L.; D'Alesandro, M. M.; Chirigos, M. J.; and Weiss, J. F. 1988. Radioprotection by biological response modifiers alone and in combination with WR-2721. *Pharmac. Ther.* 39: 247-254.

68. Patchen, M. L.; MacVittie, T. J.; and Jackson, W. E. 1989. Postirradiation glucan administration enhances the radioprotective effects of WR-2721. *Radiat. Res.* 117: 59-69

69. Dinarello, C. A., and Mier, J. W. 1987. Lymphokines. *N. Engl. J. Med.* 317: 940-945.

70. Neta, R.; Vogel, S. N.; Oppenheim, J. J.; and Douches, S. D. 1986. Cytokines in radioprotection. Comparison of the radioprotective effects of IL-1 to IL-2, GM-CSF and IFN. *Lymphokine Res.* (Suppl.) 5: S105-S110.

71. Neta, R.; Oppenheim, J. J.; Douches, S. D.; Giclas, P. C.; Imbra, R. J.; and Karin, M. 1986. Radioprotection with Interleukin-1: Comparison with other cytokines. *Progress in Immunology* 6: 900-908.

72. Neta, R.; Oppenheim, J. J.; and Douches, S. D. 1988. Interdependence of IL-1, TNF, and CSFs in radioprotection. *J. Immunol.* 140: 108-111.

73. Maisin, J. R.; Mattelin, G.; Fridman-Manduzio, A.; and van der Parren, J. 1968. Reduction of short- and long-term radiation lethality by mixtures of chemical protectors. *Radiat. Res.* 35: 26-44.

74. Brook, I. Personal communication.

ADDRESSES

AFRRI
Armed Forces Radiobiology Research Institute
Office of the Director
Bethesda, MD 20814-5145
301-295-1210

DNA
Defense Nuclear Agency
6801 Telegraph Road
Alexandria, VA 22310-3398
701-325-7060

FEMA
Federal Emergency Management Agency
500 C Street, SW
Washington, DC 20472
Emergency Information Center: 202-646-2400

IAEA
International Atomic Energy Agency
Wagramerstrasse 5
PO Box 100
A1400 Vienna, Austria
For publications only:
UNIPUB
4611-F Assembly Drive
Lanham, MD 20706-4391
800-274-4888

ICRP
International Commission on Radiological Protection
Scientific Secretary
PO Box 35
Didcot, Oxfordshire, OX11-0RJ United Kingdom

MRAT
Medical Radiobiology Advisory Team
Armed Forces Radiobiology Research Institute
Office of the Director
Bethesda, MD 20814-5145
24-hour emergency number: 301-295-3909
Administrative offices: 301-295-0316

NTIS
National Technical Information Service
5285 Port Royal Road
Springfield, VA 22161
703-487-4600

OCLC
Online Computer Library Center
6565 Frantz Road
Dublin, OH 43017
800-848-5800

REAC/TS
Radiation Emergency Assistance Center/Training Site, Oak Ridge Associated Universities
PO Box 117
Oak Ridge, TN 37831-0117
615-576-2210

RAMT
Radiological Advisory Medical Team
Walter Reed Army Medical Center
Attention: HSHL-QHP/RAMT
Washington, DC 20307
(AV) 291-5107
202-576-5107

EUCOM
U.S. European Command Headquarters
Attention: ECMD
APO New York 09128-4209
(AV) 430-7166
Seventh Medical Command, Heidelberg
APO New York 09102-3304
(AV) 370-8816 and
(AV) 370-552-826
49-6211-572-55

WRAIR
Walter Reed Army Institute of Research
Office of the Director
14th and Dahlia Streets, NW
Building 40, Room 1062
Washington, DC 20307-5100
202-576-3551
Library: 202-576-3314

INDEX

☆U.S. GOVERNMENT PRINTING OFFICE: 1989-223-543
PIN 902241-000